Appleton & Lange's

Outline Review for the Physician Assistant Examination

Albert F. Simon, MEd, PA-C
Chairman, Department of Physician Assistant Sciences
Saint Francis College
Loretto, Pennsylvania

Anthony A. Miller, MEd, PA-C
Associate Dean, School of Allied Health
Assistant Professor, Department of Physician Assistant Studies
Medical College of Ohio
Toledo, Ohio

Appleton & Lange Reviews/McGraw-Hill
Medical Publishing Division

New York   St. Louis   San Francisco   Auckland   Bogotá   Caracas   Lisbon   London
Madrid   Mexico City   Milan   Montreal   New Delhi   San Juan
Singapore   Sydney   Tokyo   Toronto

McGraw-Hill

A Division of The McGraw·Hill Companies

Appleton & Lange's Outline Review for the Physician Assistant Examination

Copyright © 2000 by The **McGraw-Hill Companies,** Inc. All rights reserved. Printed in the United States of America. Except as permitted under the United States Copyright Act of 1976, no part of this publication may be reproduced or distributed in any form or by any means, or stored in a data base or retrieval system, without the prior written permission of the publisher.

1 2 3 4 5 6 7 8 9 0   PBT/PBT   0 9 8 7 6 5 4 3 2 1 0

ISBN 0-8385-0373-X

This book was set in New Baskerville by Rainbow Graphics, LLC.
The editor was Sally J. Barhydt.
The production supervisor was Minal Bopaiah.
The production service was Rainbow Graphics, LLC.
The cover designer was Aimee Nordin.
The index was prepared by Rainbow Graphics, LLC.

Phoenix Book Technology was the printer and binder.

This book is printed on acid-free paper.

Contributors

Salah Ayachi, PhD, PA-C
Associate Professor
Department of Physician Assisted Studies
School of Allied Health Science
University of Texas Medical Branch
Galveston, Texas

Tonya Babbitt, PA-C
General Surgery/Surgical Endoscopy
Walter Ruf MD, Inc.
Akron, Ohio

J. Dennis Blessing, PhD, PA-C
Associate Professor
Department of Physician Assistant Studies
Clinical Associate Professor
Department of Family Medicine
University of Texas Medical Branch
Galveston, Texas

Kathryn Boyer, MS, PA-C
Leukemia Department
University of Texas
M.D. Anderson Cancer Center
Houston, Texas

Patricia A. Francis, MS, PA-C
Assistant Professor and Chair
Department of Physician Assistant Studies
Medical College of Ohio
Toledo, Ohio

Anita Duhl Glicken, MSW
Associate Professor, Pediatrics
University of Colorado Health Sciences Center
Denver, Colorado

Roderick S. Hooker, PhD, PA-C
Department of Physician Assistant Studies
University of Texas Southwestern Medical Center
Dallas, Texas

Brenda L. Jasper, PA-C
Renal-Endocrine Associates, P.C.
Forbes Regional Hospital
Monroeville, Pennsylvania

P. Eugene Jones, PhD, PA-C
Physician Assistant Program
Allied Health Science School
University of Texas Southwestern Medical Center
Dallas, Texas

Ricky E. Kortyna, MMS, PA-C
Instructor, Department of Physician Assistant
Duquesne University
Pittsburgh, Pennsylvania

Rebecca Luebke, MSBS, PA-C
Fallen Timbers Family Physicians, Inc.
Maumee, Ohio

Dana S. Martin, PA-C
Clinical Coordinator
Physician Assistant Program
Baylor College of Medicine
Houston, Texas

Dawn Morton-Rias, RPA-C
Assistant Professor and Chairperson
Physician Assistant Program
Associate Dean for Primary Care
College of Health Related Professions
State University of New York
Health Science Center of Brooklyn
Brooklyn, New York

Maura Polansky, MS, PA-C
Medical Oncology Outpatient Clinic
The University of Texas
M.D. Anderson Cancer Center
Houston, Texas

John W. Rafalko, MS, PA-C
Assistant Professor
Physician Assistant Program
Nova Southeastern University
Fort Lauderdale, Florida

Richard R. Rahr, EdD, PA-C
Professor and Chair
Department of Physician Assistant Studies
School of Allied Health Science
University of Texas Medical Branch
Galveston, Texas

Allan M. Rubin, MD, PhD, FACS
Professor and Chairman
Department of Otolaryngology—Head and Neck
    Surgery
Medical College of Ohio
Toledo, Ohio

Douglas R. Southard, PhD, MPH, PA-C
President, Health Management Consultants of
    Virginia, Inc.
Floyd, Virginia

Stephen M. Thomas, BHS, PA-C
Department of Physician Assistant Studies
Medical College of Ohio
Toledo, Ohio

Charles B. Travis, MD
Assistant Professor
Department of Family Medicine
Physician Assistant Program
Medical College of Ohio
Toledo, Ohio

Contents

Preface

The Physician Assistant National Certifying Examination (PANCE) and the Physician Assistant National Recertifying Examination (PANRE) have undergone extensive changes in the recent past. Chief among these changes is the transition to a computer-generated examination.

The resource that you have just purchased has been designed specifically to assist you in your preparation for the PANCE (and also PANRE) examination. Our design closely followed the NCCPA content blueprint in the selection of topics and overall organization to provide a focus for an organized review of the subject matter contained on the PANCE.

This text was designed as an outline review to assist you in your exam preparation. It will provide a concise review that will assist in the identification of areas in your knowledge base where you may want to do more research in one of the standard textbooks of medicine. Content experts wrote each chapter with an eye toward presenting the most important material in a concise and organized fashion to maximize your study time.

In designing a successful overall study plan, this text, in combination with your favorite medical reference, would be particularly effective in combination with Appleton and Lange's Review for the Physician Assistant.

We would like to thank our families and friends, who have provided support throughout the writing of this book. We also wish to thank our contributors for their hard work and dedication to this project, along with the folks at Appleton & Lange and McGraw-Hill, who have provided guidance throughout the process. Good luck on your examination.

Albert F. Simon, MEd, PA-C
Anthony A. Miller, MEd, PA-C

Helpful Hints for Taking the Certifying Exam

CONTENT PREPARATION

✓ Take a refresher course.

✓ Set a weekly schedule for exam preparation: start early, don't try to cram.

✓ If possible, design your review schedule to correlate with your clinical rotation schedule to maximize learning.

✓ Design your reading around the examination content outline.

✓ Remember the PANCE and PANRE exams are primary care oriented.

✓ Select reference books that are up-to-date and easy to read.

✓ Use this outline review to refresh your memory and determine gaps in knowledge; take notes as you review, mark unfamiliar words or phrases, then look them up.

✓ Use practice tests to diagnose strengths and weaknesses.

✓ Practice test-taking to improve speed and proficiency.

✓ Use the practice diskette from NCCPA to familiarize yourself with the test format.

TEST PREPARATION

✓ Register for the exam on time.

✓ Mark your calendar with the assigned date, time, and test center.

✓ Make sure you know how to get to the test center; allow extra time for travel, and be early the day of the exam.

✓ Get plenty of rest the night before.

✓ Be sure you are well nourished, but don't eat a full meal just before the exam.

✓ Dress comfortably in layers, so you can adjust to the temperature of the test center.

✓ Make sure you have an admission card and identification before you leave for the test center.

✓ Keep a positive attitude. Proper preparation helps provide confidence.

DURING THE EXAM

✓ Make sure you are comfortable.

✓ Avoid distractions—concentrate.

✓ Read directions carefully.

✓ Pace yourself to avoid rushing at the end.

✓ Avoid "jumping the gun"—consider all possible answers before selecting.

✓ Don't get discouraged. Some items are designed to be more difficult.

✓ Answer items you are sure of first, then go back to the difficult items.

✓ Don't change your answer unless you are sure you marked incorrectly.

✓ Use the process of elimination to narrow your choices.

✓ Be careful to not select the "common misperception" choice.

✓ Answer all questions.

AFTER THE EXAM

✓ Celebrate!

Dermatology | 1

P. Eugene Jones, PhD, PA-C

[handwritten margin notes: PC, Gir PA 345 / CmD 1299 / 2000]

I. ACUTE EXANTHEMS *(rash)*

A. Varicella (Chickenpox) *Human Herpes virus 3*

► Scientific Concepts

Extremely communicable varicella zoster virus (VZV) disease (a deoxyribonucleic acid [DNA] virus of the herpesvirus family) transmitted by respiratory droplets or direct contact with infected vesicles. Communicable from 1 to 2 days prior to rash onset until all lesions crusted. Average incubation period 14 days. Postinfection immunity is usually lifelong; herpes zoster may later develop by reactivation of latent VZV from sensory ganglia.

► History & Physical

[handwritten margin note: lesions on scalp & mucous membranes / parotid growth is centripetal]

Pediatric prodromal symptoms include fever, headache, malaise just prior to or at onset of cutaneous eruption. Adult symptoms may include chills, malaise, and backache. Lesions begin on trunk, then spread to face and extremities; extent of involvement varies considerably and may be subclinical. New lesions typically appear as "dewdrop-like" vesicles on an erythematous base. Fresh crops occur irregularly for 3 to 5 days, resulting in intermingled papules, vesicles, and crusts. Lesions may also occur on mucous membranes. *[handwritten: All stages simultaneously present]*

► Diagnostic Studies

Viral culture of vesicular fluid; direct fluorescent antibody; Tzanck smear demonstrating multinucleated giant cells (valuable test but does not differentiate varicella from herpes simplex).

► Diagnosis

Characteristic clinical history and appearance is usually diagnostic. May be clinically indistinguishable from disseminated herpes zoster or coxsackievirus viral exanthem. Viral cultures are definitive. Lesions may become secondarily infected; complications can include encephalitis and Reye's syndrome, varicella pneumonia in adults, and higher complication rates in immunosuppressed patients.

► Clinical Therapeutics

Topical: Antipruritic lotions, oatmeal baths, cool compresses, Burow's solution soaks (1:40 dilution).

Systemic: Antihistamines, acyclovir, acetaminophen (no salicylates in children due to risk of Reye's syndrome).

► Clinical Intervention

No clinical procedures indicated. Monitor for complications.

► Health Maintenance Issues

Isolation from seronegative contacts required. Maternal varicella zoster virus infection during pregnancy can result in congenital varicella syndrome with significant embryopathies, disseminated varicella in newborns, and significant morbidity and mortality. Consider use of zoster immune globulin (ZIG), varicella zoster immune globulin (VZIG), *[handwritten: relapse (time) → recrudescence weeks/month days/week]*

[handwritten: PCFsi PA 83]

gamma globulin, acyclovir, vidarabine, or varicella vaccine in selected and appropriate immunocompromised or pregnant candidates.

B. Herpes Zoster (Shingles) *[handwritten: HHV 3 reactivation of varicella]*

► Scientific Concepts

[handwritten: (reactivation] Recrudescence of latent varicella zoster infection presenting as a cutaneous viral infection generally involving the skin of a single dermatome; classically occurring unilaterally. Following chickenpox, the virus remains latent in the sensory dorsal root ganglion cells. Reactivation of latent varicella zoster has been attributed to age, immunosuppression, lymphoma, fatigue, emotional upset, and radiation therapy.

► History & Physical

Cutaneous eruption preceded by several days of pain, presenting as papules and plaques of erythema in a unilateral dermatomal distribution, with vesicular formation often within hours of plaque development. Vesicles become pustular, crust, and heal, usually without scarring. Duration of eruption correlates with patient age, severity of eruption, and presence of immunosuppression, and ranges from 2 to 6 weeks. Preherpetic neuralgia, dermatomal hyperesthesia, fever, headache, and malaise may precede the eruption by several days.

[handwritten: 1) dermatomal spread 2) ? 3) @ only 1 stage]

► Diagnostic Studies

Same as varicella.

► Diagnosis

Characteristic clinical history and appearance is usually diagnostic.

► Clinical Therapeutics

Antiviral therapy with valacyclovir, famciclovir, or acyclovir; nerve blocks; tricyclic antidepressants.

► Clinical Intervention

No clinical procedures indicated. Monitor for complications.

► Health Maintenance Issues

Pain is more severe in elderly; immunocompromised are more likely to have skin necrosis and scarring, postherpetic neuralgia, and disseminated herpes zoster. Herpes zoster ophthalmicus can occur when the ophthalmic division of the trigeminal nerve is involved, with anterior uveitis and keratitis presenting more commonly. Complications include long-term ocular disease and postherpetic neuralgia, reduced by prompt treatment with valacyclovir, famciclovir, or acyclovir.

[handwritten: p 2u 218 T. 16 P.C.M.]

II. OTHER SKIN INFECTIONS *[handwritten: c ADmT 2001 1463]*

A. Candidiasis, Mouth (Thrush) *[handwritten: normal flora]*

► Scientific Concepts

Candida spp. are yeast-like fungal opportunistic organisms that may inhabit the flora of the mouth in the absence of signs or symptoms. Pregnancy, oral contraceptives, antibiotic therapy, diabetes, and factors related to depression of cell-mediated immunity predispose the organisms to become pathogenic. May be the presenting illness for human immunodeficiency virus (HIV)-positive patients, 90% of whom eventually become infected with *Candida*.

▶ History & Physical

The tongue is almost always involved, usually presenting as asymptomatic, white, creamy exudate or flaky, adherent plaques. Chronic infection appears as localized, firmly adherent plaques with an irregular velvety surface on the buccal mucosa. May resemble milk curd or cottage cheese in appearance. Black hairy tongue following broad-spectrum antibiotic administration may be a manifestation of oral candidiasis.

▶ Diagnostic Studies

Potassium hydroxide (KOH) preparation, fungal culture.

▶ Diagnosis

Differentiate from leukoplakia and lichen planus by identifying yeast or pseudomycelia on KOH or by isolating *Candida* on Sabouraud's agar.

▶ Clinical Therapeutics

Amphotericin B lozenges, clotrimazole troches, mycostatin suspension, ketoconazole, itraconazole, and fluconazole tablets.

▶ Clinical Intervention

Due to the potential association with immunodeficiency or endocrinopathy syndromes, recalcitrant or chronic mucocutaneous candidiasis (CMC) may require specialty consultations in infectious diseases, endocrinology, and/or dermatology.

▶ Health Maintenance Issues

Risk factors include underlying disease such as diabetes mellitus or HIV infection. The presence of oral candidiasis does not appear to increase the risk of systemic infection.

B. Candidiasis, Unspecified

▶ Scientific Concepts

Other locations predisposed to candidiasis include the vagina, intertriginous areas, nail beds and nails, and hair follicles.

▶ History & Physical

Vaginal candidiasis typically presents with inflamed pruritic vulva with a white, thick, curd-like discharge, often predisposed during pregnancy. Intertriginous candidiasis typically presents with pruritic erythematous patches with serpiginous, scaly borders and satellite papules and pustules.

Infected nail folds may be tender and painful with purulent inflammation (paronychia). Candidal folliculitis typically resembles tinea barbae and presents with facial scabs and pustules.

▶ Diagnostic Studies
KOH preparation or Sabouraud's agar fungal culture.

▶ Diagnosis
Classic signs and symptoms are highly suggestive; positive KOH or Sabouraud's agar culture is diagnostic. The differential diagnosis list is lengthy and suggests reliance on laboratory data for confirmation.

▶ Clinical Therapeutics
Treatment will vary, depending on host immunocompetence and location and duration of infection. Numerous formulations of the imidazoles, azoles, and polyenes are effective in treating candidiasis.

▶ Clinical Intervention
No procedural interventions are indicated; treatment consists entirely of oral or topical medications combined with patient education regarding predisposing factors.

▶ Health Maintenance Issues
Predisposing factors may include age, immunosuppression, friction, obesity, pregnancy, diabetes, and chronic exposure to water.

C. Cellulitis/Abscess or Other Local Infections

▶ Scientific Concepts
A skin infection typically caused by group A beta-hemolytic streptococci (GABHS) and/or *Staphylococcus aureus*. Organisms typically enter broken skin, then proliferate and spread locally.

▶ History & Physical
Examination reveals edema, erythema, tenderness, and heat at the affected area (typically extremities).

▶ Diagnostic Studies
Cultures of entry sites or aspirate to identify pathogens have a low yield; blood cultures can confirm bacteremia.

▶ Diagnosis
Fever, chills, malaise, and proximally spreading lymphangitis accompanied by lymphadenitis may be seen in erysipelas, a group A strep superficial variant of cellulitis. Differential includes allergic contact dermatitis and urticaria.

▶ Clinical Therapeutics
Clinical recognition of distinctive features requires empiric treatment with a penicillinase-resistant penicillin, a cephalosporin, or erythromycin.

▶ Clinical Intervention
No procedural interventions are indicated. Monitor for hematogenous spread and bacteremia.

[handwritten margin notes: carbuncles = multiple furuncles   Bactroban / furuncle = boil / CDMT 2000 LXX / 2% mupirocin in nose against staphylococcal carrier state]

► Health Maintenance Issues

Recurrent episodes require prolonged antimicrobial prophylaxis and careful history to elicit predisposing factors.

D. Cellulitis/Abscess of Finger/Toe

[handwritten margin note: If a lesion extends into the dermis, there is scarring. Nodules of acne extend into dermis... therefore scarring.]

► Scientific Concepts

Causative organisms of digital cellulitis/abscess (called a parony-chia when the proximal or lateral nail fold is involved) may include bacterial, viral, and/or fungal organisms.

► History & Physical

Repeated exposure to moisture or trauma predisposes individuals to developing a paronychia. Examination reveals tenderness, pain, erythema, and edema of the digit.

► Diagnostic Studies

Drainage or aspirate from infected digit may be cultured to iden-tify pathogens.

► Diagnosis

Differentiate acute versus chronic digital cellulitis/paronychia by speed of onset and occupational predisposition (medical and dental personnel, dishwashers).

► Clinical Therapeutics

Oral antibiotic therapy for 7 to 10 days with appropriate anti-staphylococcal coverage.

► Clinical Intervention

Acute paronychia typically requires incision and drainage in addi-tion to antibiotics.

► Health Maintenance Issues

Hand and foot care instructions with goal of dry environment; glove use when appropriate; avoidance of skin breakdown, trauma, and manipulation.

E. Impetigo

[handwritten margin note: PC & PK / 89-92 / ecthyma is deeper infection of impetigo - caused by GA B-hemolytic streptococci / impetigo - bullous, looks like... / nonbullous - honey colored crust]

► Scientific Concepts

A common, contagious superficial skin infection typically found on the face, caused by staphylococci, streptococci, or both. Manifests as bullous and nonbullous versions.

► History & Physical

Higher rates seen in children in close physical contact; may follow minor skin injury; frequently occurs on intact skin. May present with mild itching and soreness. More common in infants and children, presenting with one or more vesicles that ooze and form a honey-colored crust; regional lymphadenopathy likely.

► Diagnostic Studies

Skin lesion and nasopharyngeal cultures may isolate causative agents.

► Diagnosis

Characteristic clinical history and appearance is usually diagnostic. Clinical appearance may resemble rhus dermatitis, atopic dermatitis, varicella zoster or herpes simplex vesicles, or ecthyma. Complications include poststreptococcal glomerulonephritis, cellulitis, bacteremia, septic arthritis, and osteomyelitis.

► Clinical Therapeutics

Requires topical or systemic antimicrobial coverage against GABHS and *S. aureus.*

► Clinical Intervention

Lesion debridement with warm water soaks.

► Health Maintenance Issues

Monitor infants for life-threatening secondary infections. Predisposing factors include poor hygiene and moist, warm environments. Topical mupirocin bid for 5 days to nares to eliminate carrier state.

F. Mycoses, Dermatophytosis

► Scientific Concepts

Dermatophytes are fungi that typically infect the stratum corneum layer of skin, hair, and nails. Dermatophytes originating from animals and soil may also infect humans. Causal organisms of human predilection include *Epidermophyton, Microsporum,* and *Trichophyton* spp. Predisposing host factors include immune compromise; age; gender; race; geographic location; warm, moist climate; skin occlusion; and trauma.

► History & Physical

In the presence of predisposing historical factors, physical examination typically reveals an erythematous, well-marginated, annual plaque or patch with central clearing and a vesicular, scaly border. Pruritus and burning are occasionally present.

► Diagnostic Studies

KOH looking for translucent, branching, rod-shaped filaments of uniform width (hyphae) in dermatophyte infections, with spores and nonbranching hyphae seen in superficial *Candida* and tinea versicolor infections. Wood's lamp helpful if fluorescence positive; fungal culture diagnostic.

► Diagnosis

The differential diagnosis of papulosquamous lesions is lengthy (see references). Dermatophytosis complications include deep inflammatory infections from zoophilic fungi, secondary bacterial infections, postinflammatory hyperpigmentation, kerion, and generalized infection in the immunocompromised.

► **Clinical Therapeutics**
Topical or oral antifungal agents, depending on severity and duration of infection.

► **Clinical Intervention**
No procedural interventions are indicated.

► **Health Maintenance Issues**
Avoidance of precipitating factors.

III. SKIN ERUPTIONS

10 CPK 107

A. Acne Vulgaris

► **Scientific Concepts**
A disease of the pilosebaceous unit caused by the proliferation and modification of sebum by *Propionibacterium acnes* in predisposed patients with increased sebum production, resulting in cohesive hyperkeratosis and pilosebaceous duct obstruction.

► **History & Physical**
Acne typically affects the face, neck, shoulders, and back, with onset near puberty and lessening as adolescence ends, with varying intensity and duration. Examination of these areas may reveal differing combinations of inflammatory lesions (papules, pustules, and nodules) (Table 1–1) and noninflammatory lesions (open comedones [blackheads] and closed comedones [whiteheads]). Premenstrual flares may occur.

► **Diagnostic Studies**
None.

► **Diagnosis**
Characteristic clinical history and appearance is usually diagnostic; differentiate from steroid acne, occupational acne, acne mechanica, acne cosmetica, and acne rosacea. Complications include treatment

► **table 1-1**

ACNE CLASSIFICATION AND GRADING

Lesion Type	Mild	Moderate	Severe
Papules/Pustules	+/++	++/+++	+++/++++
Nodules	0	+/++	+++

Source: Adapted from TP Habif, Clinical Dermatology: A Color Guide to Diagnosis and Therapy, 3rd ed., St. Louis: Mosby, 1996.

failure, potentially severe psychosocial effects, occupational disability, and disfigurement.

► Clinical Therapeutics

Depending on severity and response, therapeutics can include tretinoin, benzoyl peroxide, drying agents, topical or oral antibiotics, intralesional steroids, acne surgery, and isotretinoin. Consult black box warning in *Physician's Desk Reference* (PDR) before prescribing isotretinoin to women of childbearing age.

► Clinical Intervention

Acne surgery expresses comedones and drains pustules; intralesional steroids rapidly control larger lesions.

► Health Maintenance Issues

Patient education regarding misconceptions; assessment of psychological factors; appropriate follow-up instructions and continuous treatment for optimal results.

B. Insect Bite, Nonvenomous

► Scientific Concepts

Nonvenomous arthropods include fleas, flies, and mosquitoes. Antigen-, toxin-, or enzyme-laden saliva is introduced cutaneously by stylet penetration of the skin, producing varying sensitivity and severity of reaction.

► History & Physical

Depending on individual sensitivity and type of arthropod, patients may experience no response, immediate pain, or delayed hypersensitivity with pruritus or pain. Examination may reveal hypersensitivity bite reactions (papular urticaria), bites in clusters or groups, or pruritic wheals in exposed areas.

► Diagnostic Studies

None.

► Diagnosis

Differential includes cellulitis, contact dermatitis, drug eruptions, and urticaria.

► Clinical Therapeutics

Topical or oral antipruritics/antihistamines, topical or oral corticosteroids may be indicated in some cases.

► Clinical Intervention

Extrication of larvae indicated in cutaneous myiasis.

► Health Maintenance Issues

Risk factors include environmental, previous sensitization, and lack of preventive measures. Repel insects with topical N,N-diethyl-m-toluamide (DEET) or oil of citronella.

C. Scabies

▶ Scientific Concepts

The *Sarcoptes scabiei* mite is responsible for human scabies, a contagious condition arising from skin-to-skin contact with an infected person or from mite-infested bedding or clothing. Fertilized females burrow into the stratum corneum, depositing eggs and fecal pellets (scybala). Hypersensitivity reactions result in characteristic signs and symptoms and may take weeks to develop in first infection.

▶ History & Physical

Onset of minor itching that spreads mites to other areas, resulting in nocturnal pruritus that progresses to intractable, generalized pruritus. Clinical appearance varies, but typical distribution includes linear or serpiginous intraepidermal burrows in the finger web spaces, wrists, lateral aspects of hands and feet, axillae, areolae, genitalia, and buttocks.

▶ Diagnostic Studies

Scabies prep slide (burrow scrapings covered with mineral oil) to examine for mites, eggs, or scybala.

▶ Diagnosis

Typical clinical findings, confirmed by microscopy. Differential includes drug eruption, eczema, psoriasis, or impetigo. Complicated by continuing pruritus up to several weeks following treatment due to mite antigen hypersensitivity reaction.

▶ Clinical Therapeutics

Topical permethrin or lindane; oral ivermectin; antihistamines; topical or oral corticosteroids.

▶ Clinical Intervention

No surgical or procedural interventions indicated.

▶ Health Maintenance Issues

Institutional facilities (nursing homes, prisons) increase risk. Decontaminate environment; examine and treat sexual and household contacts.

D. Secondary Syphilis

▶ Scientific Concepts

A sexually transmitted disease caused by the bacterium *Treponema pallidum*, syphilis is transmitted by direct lesion contact during the primary or secondary stage or during pregnancy or delivery. *T. pallidum* may infect any organ system.

▶ History & Physical

Typically characterized by mucocutaneous lesions, a flu-like syndrome, and generalized lymphadenopathy, clinical signs of secondary syphilis follow the primary (chancre) stage by approximately 6 weeks and may last from 2 to 10 weeks. Typically bilateral and symmetric, the rash of secondary syphilis is polymorphic, with various types of lesions presenting simultaneously. Most patients will develop lesions of the palms and soles.

► Diagnostic Studies

Serologic tests for syphilis include rapid plasma reagin (RPR), Veneral Disease Research Laboratory (VDRL), and fluorescent treponemal antibody-absorption test for syphilis (FTA-ABS).

► Diagnosis

The differential diagnosis of secondary syphilis is lengthy. Similar rashes appear as pityriasis rosea, guttate psoriasis, lichen planus, tinea versicolor, drug eruptions, and viral exanthems. Complications include cardiovascular disease, central nervous system disease, and irreversible multiorgan damage.

► Clinical Therapeutics

Drug of choice is benzathine penicillin G. Consult latest sexually transmitted disease (STD) guidelines for patients sensitive to penicillin.

► Clinical Intervention

No surgical or procedural therapies indicated for secondary syphilis.

► Health Maintenance Issues

Contact local health department to initiate contact tracing. Screen for other concomitant STDs. Advise patient to avoid intercourse until treatment is complete. Safe sex education and condom use.

IV. TUMORS OF SKIN

A. Keratoacanthoma, Acquired

► Scientific Concepts

Thought by some to be a variant of squamous cell carcinoma, keratoacanthomas are common benign epithelial tumors in the elderly, possibly of viral, chemical, or ultraviolet-induced origin. Seen predominantly on exposed skin in older white males. Typically resolves spontaneously over several months.

► History & Physical

A rapidly growing, dome-shaped nodule with a keratinotic central plug.

► Diagnostic Studies

All suspected keratoacanthomas should be biopsied to rule out squamous cell carcinoma.

▶ Diagnosis

Must differentiate from squamous cell carcinoma by biopsy; may resemble verruca vulgaris or hypertrophic actinic keratosis.

▶ Clinical Therapeutics

Nonsurgical intervention includes topical or intralesional 5-fluorouracil, or topical podophyllum resin.

▶ Clinical Intervention

Blunt dissection or electrodesiccation and curettage to ensure complete removal is advised.

▶ Health Maintenance Issues

No risk factors or preventive measures.

B. Lipoma

▶ Scientific Concepts

Etiology and pathogenesis unknown. Lipomas are benign fatty tumors of the subcutaneous tissue, presenting as a lobulated yellow mass surrounded by a thin capsule.

▶ History & Physical

Typically presents as a nontender, freely mobile, soft, palpable subcutaneous mass.

▶ Diagnostic Studies

None.

▶ Diagnosis

Differentiate from sarcoma by histopathology.

▶ Clinical Therapeutics

None.

▶ Clinical Intervention

Elective excision or liposuction.

▶ Health Maintenance Issues

Following diagnosis of initial occurrence, reassurance indicated for subsequent lesions unless symptomatic.

C. Neoplasms

1. Basal Cell Carcinoma

▶ Scientific Concepts

The most common type of skin cancer, basal cell carcinoma (BCC) has a limited capacity to metastasize, but can be locally invasive, aggressive, and destructive. Rare in darker-pigmented persons; susceptibility increases with prolonged sun exposure history.

► **History & Physical**

A bleeding or scabbing lesion that heals and recurs is the most common presenting complaint. Typical lesions are round/ovoid smooth papules or nodules with a pearly translucent rolled border containing thread-like telangiectasias and a depressed/umbilicated center, located on sun-exposed skin. However, BCC can occur in many clinical forms with varying presentations.

► **Diagnostic Studies**

Confirmed by histopathologic examination of lesion biopsy.

► **Diagnosis**

Differentiate from keratoacanthoma, squamous cell carcinoma, and malignant melanoma by biopsy.

► **Clinical Therapeutics**

No adequate medicinal treatment currently available.

► **Clinical Intervention**

Depending on clinical presentation, cell type, and tumor size and location, BCC treatment modalities can include electrodesiccation and curettage, simple surgical excision, or Mohs' micrographic surgery.

► **Health Maintenance Issues**

Because patients with one BCC often develop another, close follow-up is indicated to inspect for new lesions.

2. Squamous Cell Carcinoma

► **Scientific Concepts**

Commonly occurring in sun-exposed areas, squamous cell carcinomas (SCCs) may arise from normal skin, actinically damaged skin, or from underlying actinic keratoses. Those arising from the lip, apparently normal skin, or sites of chronic inflammation are more aggressive.

► **History & Physical**

Unlike BCCs, SCCs are more commonly found on the scalp, dorsal surface of the hands, and superior aspect of the pinnae. Lower-extremity lesions are more common in women. Typical lesions present as indurated, erythematous, yellowish papules, plaques, or nodules in a polygonal, ovoid, or round shape. Crusting, erosion, and ulceration may be present, with a firm elevated margin.

► **Diagnostic Studies**

Confirmed by histopathologic examination of lesion biopsy.

► **Diagnosis**

Differentiate from nummular eczema, psoriasis, Paget's disease, BCC.

► Clinical Therapeutics

No effective oral therapies available.

► Clinical Intervention

Depending on clinical presentation, cell type, and tumor size and location, SCC treatment modalities can include simple surgical excision, Mohs' micrographic surgery, radiation, and chemotherapy.

► Health Maintenance Issues

Risk factors include light skin, poor tanning ability, older age, outdoor occupations, exposure to chemical carcinogens, and geographic area of residence. The lifetime probability of developing SCC varies from 1.5 to 11%, depending on risk factors. BCCs are three times more common that SCCs.

3. Malignant Melanoma

► Scientific Concepts

Malignant transformation of epidermal melanocytes presenting as pigmented lesions, more frequently in fair-skinned patients; etiology predominantly associated with sun exposure. Melanomas present as superficial spreading melanoma (70%), nodular melanoma (15%), lentigo maligna (4 to 10%), and acral lentiginous melanoma (2 to 8%).

► History & Physical

Melanomas typically manifest as pigmented lesions that change in color, symmetry, size, symptoms, or shape over weeks to months in 20 to 40 year olds. Asymmetric lesions greater than 6 mm in diameter with an admixture of colors and an irregular border are highly suspicious.

► Diagnostic Studies

Diagnosis and staging requires complete excisional biopsy or punch/incisional biopsy for larger lesions; curettage or shave biopsies are contraindicated due to inability to accurately stage level of involvement.

► Diagnosis

Differentiate from melanocytic nevus (a benign proliferation of melanocytes), atypical nevus (a benign acquired precursor to melanoma and a marker for melanoma risk), and blue nevus (a benign acquired nevus). Complications include metastatic disease; prognosis based on Breslow thickness.

► Clinical Therapeutics

No effective oral or topical treatment available for primary malignant melanoma; metastatic disease may require a combination of chemotherapy/immunotherapy.

► Clinical Intervention

Complete surgical excision is the treatment of choice for malignant melanoma.

► **Health Maintenance Issues**

Avoidance of sun exposure, sun-protective clothing, liberal use of sunscreen of greater than sun protective factor (SPF) 15, frequent total body examinations following diagnosis.

D. Epidermal (Sebaceous) Cysts

► **Scientific Concepts**

Typically arise from occluded follicles and pilosebaceous units, although epidermal cysts contain cheesy and fetid keratinaceous cellular debris. Epidermal inclusion cysts are lined by keratinizing squamous epithelium and have a similar clinical presentation.

► **History & Physical**

Typically appearing in young to middle-aged adults, epidermal cysts are usually less than 1 cm, firm to fluctuant cutaneous nodules that may regress without treatment but frequently recur unless surgically removed. Common sites include the head, posterior auricular folds, neck, upper trunk, and scrotum; infected cysts are typically larger, erythematous, and more painful.

► **Diagnostic Studies**

None.

► **Diagnosis**

Based on typical history and physical examination.

► **Clinical Therapeutics**

No effective oral or topical therapies available; intralesional steroids can hasten resolution of inflamed but uninfected cyst.

► **Clinical Intervention**

Infected cysts require incision and drainage of purulent material.

F. Viral Warts (Human Papillomavirus)

► **Scientific Concepts**

More than 65 human papillomavirus (HPV) types have been identified and associated with various cutaneous lesions, with the most prevalent being common warts (verruca vulgaris), plantar warts (verruca plantaris), and flat warts (verruca plana). The most common mucosal manifestation of HPV is genital warts (condyloma acuminatum). HPV infections are typically self-limited unless presenting in immunocompromised patients.

► **History & Physical**

Warts may persist for years if untreated. Typically manifesting as papules and plaques, HPV commonly infects keratinized skin.

► **Diagnostic Studies**

Typically made on clinical findings.

► Diagnosis

Although potentially persistent, HPV infections typically resolve spontaneously in immunocompetent patients.

► Clinical Therapeutics

Imiquimod 5% cream (for condyloma acuminatum) and 5-fluoro-uracil (for flat warts) have been used successfully as topical agents; numerous over-the-counter and prescription topical agents containing acetic acid, trichloroacetic acid, salicylic acid, formaldehyde, or podophyllin are available for common warts.

► Clinical Intervention

A variety of therapeutic modalities are used with varying degrees of success, depending on the type and location of warts. Most common are cryosurgery or electrodesiccation and curettage. Unless clinically warranted, aggressive therapies are often painful and may be accompanied by scarring. Condyloma acuminatum and plantar warts warrant more aggressive therapies. Plantar wart therapy must include scar avoidance on weight-bearing areas in the treatment plan.

► Health Maintenance Issues

Condyloma acuminatum HPV types have a major role in the pathogenesis of carcinoma of the anogenital epithelium. HPV can be transmitted to the fetus during delivery, resulting in anogenital warts or recurrent respiratory papillomatosis. HPV also has an important etiologic role in carcinoma of the cervix and cervical intraepithelial neoplasia (CIN).

V. OTHER DISEASES OF THE SKIN/SUBCUTANEOUS TISSUE

A. Decubitus Ulcer (Pressure Ulcer)

► Scientific Concepts

Ischemic tissue necrosis caused by skin compression, shear forces, and friction over bony prominences, typically in bedridden patients.

► History & Physical

Progresses through stages from localized blanching erythema to nonblanching erythema to ulceration of varying depths, resulting in ulceration over bony prominences following prolonged hospitalization or immobility.

► Diagnostic Studies

Based on history and physical examination.

► Diagnosis

Differential includes pyoderma gangrenosum, malignant ulcer, thermal burn, vasculitis ulcer, and infectious ulcer. Complications include osteomyelitis, bacteremia, and sepsis.

► Clinical Therapeutics

Early lesions may respond to topical antibiotics, hydrogels, or hydrocolloidal dressings.

► Clinical Intervention

Surgical management includes debridement, flaps, and skin grafts.

► Health Maintenance Issues

Frequent skin inspection, patient repositioning, massage, skin care, nutritional status monitoring, and early mobilization.

B. Diseases of Nails/Hair

1. Alopecia Areata

► Scientific Concepts

A relatively common, localized area of hair loss (typically the scalp) in a well-demarcated round or oval-shaped lesion without evidence of inflammation or scarring. Etiology remains unknown but suspected to be an autoimmune phenomenon.

► History & Physical

Typically occurs under age 25, may occur in patches of varying stages of hair loss and regrowth. No cutaneous symptoms; predilection for scalp, eyebrows, eyelashes, beard, and pubic hair.

► Diagnostic Studies

None.

► Diagnosis

Based on typical clinical picture.

► Clinical Therapeutics

High-potency topical steroids may be effective; oral steroids induce regrowth, but alopecia recurs on discontinuation and thus should be avoided; oral psoralen plus ultraviolet A (PUVA) (photochemotherapy) may be indicated in extensive cases.

► Clinical Intervention

Intralesional steroids provide effective temporary resolution, especially in critical areas such as eyebrows.

► Health Maintenance Issues

Prepubescent alopecia has greater incidence of leading to repeated episodes and progression to total alopecia.

2. Onychomycosis

► Scientific Concepts

Onychomycosis is an infectious process of the nails caused by a variety of yeasts, molds, and fungi. The subtype tinea unguium is caused by the dermatophyte group of fungi.

► History & Physical
Predominantly on the toenails (particularly the great toe), ony-chomycosis typically presents with a history of marginated streaks or plaques on the nails, with eventual dystrophic thickening and hyper-keratotic debris beneath the nail.

► Diagnostic Studies
Direct microscopic examination via KOH prep; Sabouraud's agar fungal culture to isolate pathogen.

► Diagnosis
Positive KOH or fungal culture is diagnostic. Progressive nail in-volvement occurs if untreated.

► Clinical Therapeutics
Griseofulvin, azoles (itraconazole, ketoconazole, fluconazole), ally-lamines (terbinafine).

► Clinical Intervention
Nail debulking by mechanical means or complete removal may be indicated if thickening precludes ability to wear shoes, etc.

► Health Maintenance Issues
Avoidance of occlusive footwear, overcrowding, communal bathing, and circulatory disturbances.

C. Ulcer of Lower Limbs

► Scientific Concepts
Lower-extremity ulcers typically arise from chronic venous or arter-ial insufficiency or peripheral sensory neuropathy.

► History & Physical
Ulcers secondary to venous insufficiency historically have lower-extremity aching and swelling exacerbated by dependency and allevi-ated by elevation. One typically sees an ischemic blue-red patch fol-lowed by punched-out, irregular-edged ulceration over the malleoli or distal medial calf, often accompanied by lymphedema. If secondary to arterial insufficiency, one may see shiny, atrophic skin with alopecia of lower legs and feet.

► Diagnostic Studies
May require differing studies to determine underlying pathol-ogy/comorbid factors such as sickle cell anemia, diabetes, collagen vascular disease, syphilis.

► Diagnosis
Differential includes vasculitis, infection, trauma, pressure ulcer, pyoderma gangrenosum, sickle cell anemia.

► Clinical Therapeutics

May require systemic antibiotics for secondary infection; treatment of underlying disease states.

► Clinical Intervention

May include corrective surgical debridement, wound therapy, elastic support stockings, systemic antibiotics for secondary infection, and skin grafting.

► Health Maintenance Issues

Avoidance of smoking and control of systemic diseases such as hypertension and diabetes mellitus, correction of anemias or malnourished state, exercise, weight reduction in obese.

VI. BACTERIAL INFECTIONS

► Scientific Concepts

Folliculitis is chemical or microbial inflammation of hair follicles characterized by a follicular papule, pustule, erosion, or crust.

► History & Physical

Grouped lesions on any body surface, more common on scalp, beard area, and limbs, typically appearing as pustules pierced by individual hairs.

► Diagnostic Studies

Consider Gram stain to identify bacteria, KOH to isolate yeast or hyphae, or culture and sensitivity of pustule contents. If recurrent, consider culture of nares to rule out staphylococcal carrier state.

► Diagnosis

Differential includes pseudofolliculitis barbae, keratosis pilaris, contact dermatitis.

► Clinical Therapeutics

Appropriate antimicrobials to cover etiologic agent(s).

► Clinical Intervention

Topical antibacterial cream, soap, or shampoo, as indicated.

► Health Maintenance Issues

Increased personal hygiene, avoid causative factors, suspect immunodeficiency in recalcitrant cases. Risk factors include poor hygiene, hydrocarbon exposure, immunodeficiency, abraded or injured skin.

VII. VIRAL INFECTIONS

A. Herpes Simplex Virus (Nongenital)

▶ Scientific Concepts

Herpes simplex is a DNA virus. Herpes labialis ("cold sore," "fever blister") is due to herpes simplex virus type 1 (HSV-1) in 80 to 90% of cases. Transmission is typically skin-to-skin contact.

▶ History & Physical

Symptomatic primary herpes infection typically includes vesicles at inoculation site with regional lymphadenopathy, fever, malaise, and myalgias. In children, primary herpetic gingivostomatitis is a more common presentation. In recurrent infection, prodrome of tingling, itching, or burning sensation typically precedes skin changes by 24 hours. Vesicles erode to grouped ulcerations.

▶ Diagnostic Studies

Tzanck smear reveals multinucleated giant cells; viral cultures available.

▶ Diagnosis

Differential includes impetigo, aphthous stomatitis, herpes zoster, syphilitic chancre, herpangina.

▶ Clinical Therapeutics

Consider acyclovir, valacyclovir, famciclovir.

▶ Clinical Intervention

No clinical procedures indicated.

▶ Health Maintenance Issues

Avoid contact with neonates and immunocompromised. Frequent hand washing. Increased HSV-1 transmission is associated with crowded and lower socioeconomic conditions. Use of a lip balm with high SPF sunscreen may help prevent recurrences on the lips due to sun exposure.

B. Molluscum Contagiosum

▶ Scientific Concepts

A self-limited epidermal viral infection caused by a poxvirus, occurring in children and sexually active adults.

▶ History & Physical

Lesions typically present as small, discrete, solid, skin-colored papules with a central umbilication, occurring on exposed skin sites in children and genital region in sexually active adults.

▶ Diagnostic Studies

Molluscum contagiosum virus has not been successfully cultured.

► Diagnosis

Based on distinct clinical appearance of lesions. Differential in HIV-infected patients with multiple lesions includes disseminated deep fungal infections.

► Clinical Therapeutics

No oral medications available.

► Clinical Intervention

Curettage or cryosurgery; HIV-infected patients with numerous or large lesions may require electrodesiccation.

► Health Maintenance Issues

Lesions will resolve spontaneously unless patient is infected with HIV. Avoid skin-to-skin contact with molluscum-infected individuals.

VIII. OTHER DERMATOLOGIC/VIRAL INFECTIONS

A. Mumps (Parotitis)

► Scientific Concepts

An acute unilateral or bilateral parotitis caused by a paramyxovirus transmitted by respiratory secretions. Epidemics typically occur in late winter and spring.

► History & Physical

Although 50% may be asymptomatic, mumps may present with a prodrome of fever, nuchal myalgia, and general malaise. Unilateral or bilateral parotid gland pain and swelling usually accompanies Stenson's duct erythema.

► Diagnostic Studies

Typically a diagnosis based on history and physical examination; paramyxovirus may be isolated from saliva, urine, blood, or cerebrospinal fluid if indicated.

► Diagnosis

Differential includes parotitis secondary to influenza and parainfluenza viruses, coxsackieviruses, metabolic diseases, drugs, salivary gland neoplasms, or sialolithiasis with swelling. Complications include encephalitis, postpubertal orchitis or oophoritis, and deafness.

► Clinical Therapeutics

Nonsteroidal anti-inflammatory drugs or acetaminophen for pain and fever; avoid aspirin in children due to potential complication of Reye's syndrome.

► Clinical Intervention

No surgical or procedural interventions indicated.

► Health Maintenance Issues

Frequency decreasing in United States due to two-dose live mumps vaccine; typical cases are without complications; postinfection immunity is permanent.

B. Rubella (German Measles)

► Scientific Concepts

Also known as 3-day and German measles, rubella is a ribonucleic acid (RNA) togavirus typically presenting as a benign childhood exanthemous infection transmitted by aerosolized droplet spray; incidence has diminished 99% since active immunization commenced.

► History & Physical

Fourteen- to 21-day incubation with no specific prodrome; may see conjunctivitis/upper respiratory infection symptoms followed by pink maculopapular rash beginning on forehead and face, spreading to trunk and extremities, typically fading by third day.

► Diagnostic Studies

A clinical diagnosis; confirmed by serology.

► Diagnosis

Differential includes scarlet fever, other viral exanthems, drug eruption.

► Clinical Therapeutics

Symptomatic support

► Clinical Intervention

None.

► Health Maintenance Issues

Congenital rubella syndrome occurs in pregnant women infected during first trimester, resulting in significant fetal anomalies. Rubella is preventable by immunization; titers document immunity.

C. Rubeola (Measles)

► Scientific Concepts

A highly contagious RNA paramyxovirus infection spread by aerosolized droplet spray; outbreaks typically involve unvaccinated children in large urban areas.

► History & Physical

Classic prodromal triad of cough, coryza, and conjunctivitis, followed by appearance of whitish spots on buccal mucosa (Koplik's spots) that precede an erythematous maculopapular rash beginning on the forehead and spreading centrifugally and inferiorly.

► Diagnostic Studies

Virus can be isolated by culture from blood, urine, and pharyngeal secretions; titer increases by serology.

► Diagnosis

Differential includes scarlet fever, other viral exanthems, drug eruption. Complications include otitis media, laryngotracheitis, bronchopneumonia, encephalitis, thrombocytopenic purpura, myocarditis, and pericarditis.

► Clinical Therapeutics

Symptomatic therapy.

► Clinical Intervention

None.

► Health Maintenance Issues

Avoid exposure to other children if infected; active immunization is preventive.

IX. BURNS

► Scientific Concepts

Burns produce thermal skin and tissue injury. Classification by degrees; minor erythema = first degree; blistering = second degree, with pain accompanying first and second degree; third degree = full-thickness burn with charring.

► History & Physical

Assess burn degree and depth, determine etiology and duration of exposure.

► Diagnostic Studies

None; rule of nines estimates extent of burn. Adult values: each leg, 18%; each arm, 9%; front of trunk, 18%; back of trunk, 18%; head, 9%.

► Diagnosis

Based on history and physical examination.

► Clinical Therapeutics

May include fluid and electrolyte resuscitation, burn cleaning and debridement, and grafting.

► Clinical Intervention

Appropriate antibiotics and tetanus toxoid may be required.

► Health Maintenance Issues

Appropriate physical and occupational therapy and rehabilitation may be indicated.

BIBLIOGRAPHY

Arndt KA, Wintroub BU, Robinson JK, LeBoit PE. *Primary Care Dermatology.* Philadelphia: WB Saunders; 1997.

Bondi EE, Jegasothy BV, Lazarus GS. *Dermatology Diagnosis and Therapy.* Norwalk, CT: Appleton & Lange; 1991.

Dambro MR, Griffith JA. *Griffith's 5 Minute Clinical Consult,* 3rd ed. Philadelphia: Williams & Wilkins; 1997.

Epstein E. *Common Skin Disorders,* 4th ed. Philadelphia: WB Saunders; 1994.

Fauci AS, Braunwald E, Isselbacher KJ, et al. *Harrison's Principles of Internal Medicine,* 14th ed. New York: McGraw-Hill; 1998.

Fitzpatrick TB, Johnson RA, Wolff K, et al. *Color Atlas and Synopsis of Clinical Dermatology,* 3rd ed. New York: McGraw-Hill; 1997.

Goldberg JS. *The Instant Exam Review for the USMLE Step 3,* 2nd ed. Stamford, CT: Appleton & Lange; 1997.

Graham-Brown R, Burns R. *Lecture Notes on Dermatology,* 7th ed. Cambridge, MA: Blackwell Science; 1996.

Habif TP. *Clinical Dermatology: A Color Guide to Diagnosis and Therapy,* 3rd ed. St. Louis: Mosby; 1996.

Ear, Nose, and Throat | 2

Rebecca Luebke, MSBS, PA-C, Allan M. Rubin, MD, PhD

I. HEARING IMPAIRMENT

► Scientific Concepts

Hearing loss as a result of auditory disorder may be classified by degree of impairment (mild, moderate, severe) or by type. Classification by type includes conductive, sensorineural, mixed, or central and depends on the site of pathology in the auditory system. **Conductive hearing loss** may be due to disorders in the external or middle ear, resulting in decreased volume for low tones and vowels. Bone conduction usually normal, air conduction abnormal (Rinne test). Tuning fork heard more loudly in ear with conductive loss in Weber test. Conductive hearing loss typically due to middle ear stiffness or middle ear mass. In adults, conductive hearing loss is most commonly due to cerumen impaction or transient eustachian tube dysfunction associated with upper respiratory infection (URI). **Sensorineural hearing loss** may result from disorders of the inner ear, cochlea, or cranial nerve (CN) VIII. Difficulty perceiving high tones common, and equivalent loss of bone and air conduction found. **Mixed hearing loss** involves a combination of conductive and sensorineural hearing impairment, with air conduction usually worse than bone conduction. **Central hearing loss** may or may not appear as hearing loss on pure tone audiogram. Site of pathology is beyond cochlea, anywhere from cochlear nuclei to auditory cortex.

► History & Physical

Careful history, including the following:
1. Family history of childhood hearing impairment
2. Congenital perinatal infection (rubella, herpes, syphilis)
3. Birth weight less than 1,500 grams
4. History of bacterial meningitis, particularly *Haemophilus influenzae*
5. Severe asphyxia
6. Use of ototoxic drugs (aminoglycoside antibiotics, loop diuretics, barbiturates)
7. Exposure to loud noise
8. History of head trauma
9. Complete review of systems

Physical examination includes external ear examination for evaluation of anatomic abnormalities of head and neck, otoscopy, Weber test, Rinne test.

► Diagnostic Studies

Testing done to determine site of lesion and degree of impairment, to aid in determination of nonsurgical rehabilitation, and to determine if further testing is warranted. Pure tone audiometry (air conduction, bone conduction), speech audiometry (speech reception thresholds and speech discrimination score), impedance audiometry (tympanometry and acoustic reflexes).

► Diagnosis

Based on history, physical examination, and diagnostic test results.

► Clinical Therapeutics

Hearing aids, cochlear implants, assistive listening devices, speech reading, auditory training, speech–language training, counseling.

► Clinical Intervention

Possible surgical intervention for cochlear implants.

► Health Maintenance Issues

Avoid loud noises, wear earplugs, avoid overuse of ototoxic drugs.

II. CERUMEN IMPACTION

► Scientific Concepts

The ear canal is generally self-cleaning. Impacted cerumen (wax) can often be attributed to attempts by the patient to clean canals.

► History & Physical

Patient may complain of hearing loss, fullness in the affected ear, ear pressure, or pain in external ear, or be unaware of condition. Patient may also report drainage from the ear. Physical examination includes otoscopic evaluation as well as nose, throat, and neck (lymphadenopathy) to check for possible concomitant infection.

► Diagnostic Studies

Otoscopic visualization.

► Diagnosis

Light to dark brown cerumen filling canal, often impairing visualization of tympanic membrane. May appear dry and hard.

► Clinical Therapeutics

Removal includes eardrops, mechanical means, suction, or irrigation. Irrigate with water at body temperature and only when tympanic membrane is intact! Pretreatment with cerumen softeners may aid in removal. Follow-up for reevaluation may be indicated, particularly to check for development of infection after cerumen removal.

► Clinical Intervention

Usually none.

► Health Maintenance Issues

Avoid use of cotton-tipped applicators and other objects inserted into ears for cleaning or scratching. Clean external canal with warm water and a washcloth over the index finger. Avoid entering ear canal.

III. OTITIS EXTERNA (SWIMMER'S EAR)

► Scientific Concepts

Often follows water exposure or mechanical trauma to ear canal, allowing organism invasion. Usually caused by gram-negative organisms (*Pseudomonas, Proteus*), fungi, or *Staphylococcus aureus.* Tympanic membrane may be involved as its lateral surface is composed of ear canal skin. There may be, however, an acute otitis media present as well.

► History & Physical

Ear pain, pruritus, discharge, lymphadenopathy. Hearing loss if severe. Pain with tragal pressure or auricular traction. External canal erythematous, edematous, with purulent exudate. Edema may obscure tympanic membrane (TM) if severe. TM may appear erythematous but will move normally with pneumatic otoscopy unless there is concomitant otitis media.

► Diagnostic Studies

Direct visualization, palpation, otoscopy, pneumatic otoscopy, culture, Gram stain.

► Diagnosis

Made by examination and identification of causative organisms by culture and/or Gram stain.

► Clinical Therapeutics

Remove superficial debris. Topical antibiotics are most effective, particularly preparations with polymyxin or neomycin. Ciprofloxacin drops are also effective. If canal swelling accompanies infection, use combination antibiotic and steroid drops. Occasionally, oral antibiotics also used if infection extends beyond pinna, pain is severe, cervical lymphadenopathy is present, or patient is febrile.

► Clinical Intervention

Usually none.

► Health Maintenance Issues

Ear canal must be kept dry. Use moldable earplugs if swimming. Prophylactic acetic acid or alcohol drops after swimming, showering for infection-prone patients.

IV. MALIGNANT (NECROTIZING) OTITIS EXTERNA

► Scientific Concepts

Soft tissue infection of external ear (often persistent otitis externa). Typically caused by *Pseudomonas aeruginosa* and found in elderly, diabetic, or immunocompromised. May develop into osteomyelitis of skull base with extension to auricle, scalp, parotid gland, middle and inner ear, and eventually the brain. May cause cranial nerve palsies or destruction, particularly nerves VI, VII, IX, X, XI, and XII. Fatal without aggressive treatment.

▶ History & Physical

Hallmark is deep, boring pain in ear with granulation tissue at bony–cartilaginous junction of ear canal. Otalgia, otorrhea (foul), inflammation, hearing loss, progressive cranial nerve palsies, lymphadenopathy.

▶ Diagnostic Studies

Otoscopic examination, computed tomography (CT), and radionuclide scanning exhibiting osseus erosion. Magnetic resonance imaging (MRI) to evaluate intracranial involvement.

▶ Diagnosis

Culture external auditory canal, CT for determining extent of bony destruction and soft tissue infiltration. MRI more sensitive to evaluate soft tissue involvement. Gallium scan for extent of bony involvement.

▶ Clinical Therapeutics

Long-term (may be several months) intravenous or oral antipseudomonal antibiotics (ciprofloxacin hydrochloride).

▶ Clinical Intervention

Surgical debridement of necrotic tissue and drainage required if severe to prevent progression. Refer to otolaryngologist.

▶ Health Maintenance Issues

Maintain high index of suspicion in high-risk groups (e.g., diabetes mellitus, human immunodeficiency virus [HIV]).

V. OTITIS MEDIA

A. Acute Otitis Media

▶ Scientific Concepts

Middle ear infection most common in infants and children due to short length and horizontal positioning of eustachian tube. Often follows a viral URI that has caused eustachian tube edema. Fluid and mucus accumulate, resulting in a bacterial infection. Most common organisms include *Streptococcus pneumoniae, Haemophilus influenzae, Moraxella catarrhalis, Streptococcus pyogenes,* and *Staphylococcus aureus. Escherichia coli* may be causative organism in infants younger than 6 weeks.

▶ History & Physical

Otalgia, fever, decreased hearing, discharge if tympanic membrane perforates. Erythematous, bulging (when severe) tympanic membrane with decreased mobility by pneumatic otoscopy. Occasional exudate or visible air–fluid levels in middle ear.

► Diagnostic Studies

Otoscopy and culture of any external canal exudate. Tympanocentesis for bacterial and fungal cultures indicated in seriously ill or toxic children, newborns, and immunocompromised patients.

► Diagnosis

Made by symptoms, signs, culture results.

► Clinical Therapeutics

Controversial but generally treated with systemic antibiotics in the United States. Usually, amoxicillin is first-line therapy. Recent studies indicate shorter duration (3 to 5 days) or initial observation may suffice. For resistant organisms or penicillin allergy, use erythromycin, sulfa, cephalosporins, or trimethoprim-sulfamethoxazole. Analgesics and/or oral decongestants may also be needed.

► Clinical Intervention

Refer to otolaryngologist if diagnosis uncertain or treatment fails.

► Health Maintenance Issues

For recurrent infections, consider placement of tympanostomy tubes. Adenoidectomy is also potentially beneficial.

B. Chronic Suppurative Otitis Media

► Scientific Concepts

Chronic middle ear infection due to recurrent or untreated acute otitis media. May follow trauma, other diseases. Causative organisms are different than in acute otitis media and include *Pseudomonas aeruginosa, Proteus* spp., *S. aureus,* mixed anaerobes. Chronic eustachian tube dysfunction with persistent negative middle ear pressure may lead to cholesteatoma (keratin-filled squamous epithelial-lined sac) formation. Leads to local destruction of bone with eventual invasion into cranium or inner ear.

► History & Physical

Tympanic membrane perforation with purulent otorrhea common. Conductive hearing loss due to perforation, interruption of ossicular chain. Pain, fever often absent. Symptoms of meningitis or labyrinthitis possible if cholesteatoma invasion has occurred.

► Diagnostic Studies

Otoscopic examination, culture of purulent otorrhea. Audiogram, tympanogram, CT of temporal bone.

► Diagnosis

Based on history, physical examination, and culture results.

► Clinical Therapeutics

Removal of infected debris from external canal, topical antibiotic drops, earplugs. Systemic antibiotics generally not indicated. Analgesics and/or oral decongestants may be needed. Definitive treatment with tympanic membrane repair.

▶ **Clinical Intervention**
Surgical indications include necrotic bone and cholesteatoma removal.

▶ **Health Maintenance Issues**
Earplugs, early treatment of acute otitis media.

C. Serous Otitis Media (Chronic Otitis Media With Effusion)

▶ **Scientific Concepts**
Fluid in middle ear resulting from prolonged blockage of eustachian tube and negative pressure in middle ear. Results in transudation of fluid. May follow URI, allergies, barotrauma. More common in children.

▶ **History & Physical**
Clear or amber fluid in middle ear, TM retracted, bony landmarks intact. Air bubbles, fluid meniscus may be visible behind TM. TM mobility decreased.

▶ **Diagnostic Studies**
Otoscopic exam, pneumatic otoscopy, tympanometry, audiogram.

▶ **Diagnosis**
Based on history and physical examination findings.

▶ **Clinical Therapeutics**
Usually self-limited. Decongestants, antihistamines if allergic component present. Antibiotics if bacterial involvement suspected.

▶ **Clinical Intervention**
If persistent (> 3 to 4 months) in children, consider myringotomy and/or tubes, and/or adenoidectomy to prevent speech development deficits. Rule out nasopharyngeal tumor in chronic unilateral ear effusion in adults.

▶ **Health Maintenance Issues**
Autoinflation exercises, decongestants prior to flying or diving.

VI. VERTIGO

▶ **Scientific Concepts**
Vertigo/dizziness is difficult to assess because of varying definitions as well as numerous possible etiologies. Descriptions may include "dizziness," "spinning," "imbalance," "lightheadedness," a sensation of "ground moving," "weaving," or "rocking." Possible etiologies

include peripheral or central nervous system defects, cardiovascular disorders, psychiatric disorders, and metabolic disorders. Vertigo, hearing loss, tinnitus, and ear fullness suggest vestibular origin, either central or peripheral.

▶ History & Physical

Vertigo that is sudden in onset and severe suggests peripheral causes, while less severe and vague complaints may suggest central origin. **Peripheral lesions** are usually present with vertiginous complaints. Tinnitus, hearing loss, nausea, vomiting, or diaphoresis may accompany dizziness. Nystagmus in peripheral lesions may be horizontal or rotatory, but not vertical. Symptoms usually severe with sudden onset, lasting minutes to hours. *Benign paroxysmal positional vertigo (BPPV)* may be the etiology if the symptoms are precipitated by certain head movements, particularly when supine or getting up. It is thought to be caused by canalolithiasis in the posterior semicircular canal. BPPV is often found in the elderly. *Ménière's syndrome* involves excessive endolymphatic fluid in the inner ear (endolymphatic hydrops). Accompanying vertigo is fluctuant hearing loss, roaring tinnitus, and ear fullness. Symptoms last minutes to hours, gradually subside, only to return in months to years. Vertigo secondary to *viral labyrinthitis* occurs following a viral URI and involves infection of the cochlea and labyrinth. Hearing loss and tinnitus may also occur. Symptoms generally abate in 3 to 6 weeks. A more serious peripheral cause of vertigo is an *acoustic neuroma* (benign schwannoma of CN VIII). Symptoms may be mild and initially vague, but progress as the tumor enlarges, distinguishing it from other peripheral causes. Patients may report unilateral hearing loss and tinnitus. As the mass impinges on cerebellopontine structures, cranial nerve and brainstem deficits occur, such as facial numbness, gait ataxia, weakness. *Ototoxic drugs* may damage the vestibular portion of CN VIII, eliciting vertigo. Streptomycin and gentamicin are known offenders. Hearing loss typically predominates. **Central lesions** generally present with brain stem symptoms in addition to vertigo. Nystagmus that is vertical or bidirectional suggests central lesion. *Multiple sclerosis* is one cause of vertigo with central nervous system (CNS) etiology. Attacks are difficult to differentiate from peripheral causes as they may be transient, sudden, recurrent, or persistent. Slight facial numbness and voice huskiness may accompany. Another CNS cause is *vertebrobasilar insufficiency.* Initial symptoms may be solely vertigo, but later attacks usually involve brain stem abnormalities (diplopia, sensory loss, dysarthria, dysphagia, hemiparesis). *Sedatives* and *anticonvulsants* may also cause vertigo by suppressing the reticular activating system in the brain stem. **Cardiovascular origins** of vertigo typically due to decreased cerebral perfusion. Etiologies include arrhythmias, fixed or decreased cardiac output, decreased vascular tone, or severe volume depletion. Symptoms usually worsen upon standing and improve supine. Disequilibrium or imbalance may be due to **multiple sensory deficits,** found most commonly in diabetics and/or elderly or in cerebellar disease. Exam findings include gait ataxia and other cerebellar signs. **Psychiatric illnesses** occasionally produce complaints of dizziness, particularly depression, anxiety states, and psychosis. Medications to treat these conditions may also precipitate symptoms. **Metabolic conditions** such as hypoglycemia, hypoxia, hypocarbia, and hypercarbia may cause dizziness that appears similar to that caused by decreased cerebral perfusion.

Physical exam should focus on eye (nystagmus), ear (including hearing acuity), cardiovascular (arrhythmias, bruits), and neurological (including cerebellar function) aspects. Remember that a few beats of nystagmus on extreme lateral gaze is normal. Testing for positional nystagmus (Dix–Hallpike maneuver) aids in diagnosis of BPPV. With the patient sitting on the table, the examiner grasps the patient's head, rotates it to the right, and then transfers him or her to the supine position with the head extended over and dropped 45 degrees below the table edge. Look for rotatory nystagmus with a 1- to 5-second delay in onset. Repeat the maneuver with the head rotated to the left. If the vertigo is due to BPPV, symptoms and nystagmus will occur when patient's head is supine and the involved ear is pointed downward.

▶ **Diagnostic Studies**

Audiologic testing, electronystagmography (ENG), brain stem auditory evoked response testing (if acoustic neuroma suspected), CT, MRI, stapedial reflex testing (indicates abnormal brain stem or CN VIII neurotransmission).

▶ **Differential Diagnosis**

See history and physical above.

▶ **Clinical Therapeutics**

For BPPV, avoid precipitating positions. Repositioning maneuvers may aid in removing the particle from the posterior semicircular canal. Diuretics and low-sodium diet for Ménière's syndrome. Trial of meclizine, diphenhydramine hydrochloride, or dimenhydrinate for viral labrynthitis and other causes. Cardiovascular causes may be treated by adequate hydration, standing up slowly, and discontinuing causative drugs. Those with severe aortic stenosis should be evaluated for surgery. Chronic symptoms may require endolymphatic sac decompression, CN VIII section, labyrinthectomy, or transtympanic canal aminoglycoside injections. Treat underlying disorders accordingly.

▶ **Clinical Intervention**

Referral to neurologist if symptoms persist, are disabling, or if central vestibular disease or acoustic neuroma suspected.

▶ **Health Maintenance Issues**

None.

VII. FOREIGN BODY IN THE EAR

▶ **Scientific Concepts**

More common in children.

► **History & Physical**

Hearing loss, discomfort. Foreign object visible on otoscopic examination.

► **Diagnostic Studies**

Otoscopy.

► **Diagnosis**

Based on history and physical examination.

► **Clinical Therapeutics**

Hook or loop for removal of firm objects. Do not irrigate if TM is perforated or if object is organic in nature (e.g. insects, beans) as water may cause them to swell. Immobilize live insects prior to removal by filling ear canal with lidocaine or mineral oil.

► **Clinical Intervention**

None needed unless object unable to be manually removed or infection ensues. Prophylactic antibiotics may be necessary due to trauma to ear canal and possible late infection.

► **Health Maintenance Issues**

Keep small objects away from young children.

VIII. BULLOUS MYRINGITIS

► **Scientific Concepts**

Infection (often viral) involving the tympanic membrane and deep external auditory canal. Often associated with viral URI and more common in winter. Frequently affects both ears in succession. Causative organism unknown, but *Mycoplasma pneumoniae* has been cultured.

► **History & Physical**

Patients complain of severe otalgia and occasionally decreased hearing. Physical exam reveals erythematous vesicles on the tympanic membrane surface, which enlarge to form bullae. Straw-colored fluid, occasionally tinged with blood, fills the bullae.

► **Diagnostic Studies**

Otoscopy.

► **Diagnosis**

Based on history and physical examination.

► **Clinical Therapeutics**

Treatment consists of topical analgesic drops containing benzocaine or lidocaine, oral analgesics if severe, and systemic antibiotics if bacterial infection suspected or cultured. Oral erythromycin if *Mycoplasma pneumoniae* suspected.

► Clinical Intervention

If otalgia is severe, blebotomy may be performed, which involves opening the blisters with a beveled needle or myringotomy knife.

► Health Maintenance Issues

Usually none.

IX. SINUSITIS

A. Acute Sinusitis

► Scientific Concepts

Usually follows a viral URI. Swelling of the nasal mucosa or mechanical blockage prevents paranasal sinuses from draining. Results in accumulation of mucous secretions in sinuses, which become secondarily infected with bacteria. Maxillary sinuses are the most commonly infected sinuses. Edematous tissue may be due to allergic rhinitis or viral infections, while mechanical blockage may be caused by intranasal foreign bodies or tumors, deviated septum, or nasal polyps. Allergies play large role, particularly in children. Causative organisms include *Streptococcus pneumoniae, Haemophilus influenzae, Staphylococcus aureus, Moraxella catarrhalis, Streptococcus pyogenes.*

► History & Physical

Purulent rhinorrhea, facial pain and pressure (particularly with forward bending) over the cheeks and/or forehead, postnasal drip, maxillary tooth pain. Examination reveals nasal inflammation, tenderness over maxillary or frontal sinuses, decreased transillumination of involved sinuses, purulent rhinorrhea. Drainage may be noted in the posterior oropharynx as well.

► Diagnostic Studies

Ear, nose, and throat examination (including nasal endoscopy); sinus palpation and transillumination, palpate neck for lymphadenopathy. If diagnosis questionable, sinus radiography may show mucosal thickening or air–fluid levels in sinuses. CT scans offer better visualization of both inflammatory changes and bone destruction. MRI if malignancy suspected.

► Diagnosis

Based on history, physical examination, and radiography.

► Clinical Therapeutics

First-line antibiotics include amoxicillin, amoxicillin with clavulanic acid, and trimethoprim-sulfamethoxazole (TMP-SMZ). Cephalosporins also effective. Oral or topical (nasal spray) decongestants, nasal steroid sprays to decrease inflammation and promote drainage. Little evidence to support use of therapies other than antibiotics. Reserve antihistamines, steroids for allergic components as they may dry and thicken secretions. Treatment duration longer than for typical

URI treatment due to limited blood flow to sinuses. Treat for 10 to 14 days minimum.

▶ Clinical Intervention

Referral to otolaryngologist for sinus irrigation indicated when pain is severe and maxillary sinus is not draining. Avoid surgery for acute sinusitis unless infection fails to clear or complications develop. Hospital admission for intravenous antibiotics for persistent infection to prevent intracranial extension.

▶ Health Maintenance Issues

Saltwater nasal sprays help remove nasal crusting and secretions. Warm compresses to face, hot fluids, and inhaling steam improve ciliary function and decrease facial pain and congestion. Remove allergens.

B. Chronic Sinusitis

▶ Scientific Concepts

Usually follows untreated or poorly treated acute sinusitis. Persistent low-grade infection of paranasal sinuses with chronic mucosal thickening. Consider intranasal polyps as contributory factor. Causative organisms include *S. aureus* (20% of cases), *H. influenzae, Pneumococcus,* other streptococci. Anaerobic species include *Streptococcus* and *Bacteroides* spp. Often mixed flora.

▶ History & Physical

Chronic nasal obstruction and/or drainage. Patients may present with thick, purulent discharge in morning and clearing by afternoon. Facial pain, pressure may be persistently present or only during acute exacerbations. Anosmia.

▶ Diagnostic Studies

History, physical examination (including nasal endoscopy), radiography, CT imaging of osteomeatal complex.

▶ Diagnosis

History, physical, radiographic findings. Rule out allergic rhinitis as this may mimic sinusitis. Consider cystic fibrosis in patients with nasal polyps or infection with *Pseudomonas aeruginosa.*

▶ Clinical Therapeutics

First-line antibiotics include augmented amoxicillin, clindamycin, and TMP-SMZ. Prolonged course of treatment. Decongestants (topical for 2 to 3 days, then oral) and intranasal steroids may be used, although extent of benefit questionable.

▶ Clinical Intervention

If recurrent or persistent, referral to otolaryngologist for functional endoscopic sinus surgery. Often restores physiology of sinus aeration and drainage.

► Health Maintenance Issues
Control of perennial allergic rhinitis.

X. ALLERGIC RHINITIS

► Scientific Concepts

Seasonal allergic reactions precipitated by tree pollens in spring, grass in midsummer, and weeds in the fall. Animal dander also allergenic. Perennial conditions often triggered by dust mites, mold. Symptoms from dust mite allergy worse in morning from overnight exposure to furniture, pillows, mattresses harboring large numbers of mites. Poor control may lead to sinusitis, otitis media with effusion, or asthma exacerbation. May aggravate sleep apnea.

► History & Physical

Family history of hay fever, asthma, or atopic eczema. Inquire about pets, smokers, and type of heating system in household. Clear rhinorrhea that is more persistent than found in viral rhinitis. Seasonal variation. Pruritic eyes, nose, and palate; sneezing, tearing, postnasal drainage. Turbinate mucosa pale or violaceous and swollen with excessive crusting. Occasionally nasal polyps, which appear as yellowish boggy masses of hypertrophic mucosa. Allergic shiners (dark discoloration under eyes), allergic salute (crease across nasal bridge from persistently pushing up on nose to wipe secretions and open nasal passages), mouth breathing due to nasal blockage.

► Diagnostic Studies

Smear of nasal secretions reveals eosinophils. Increased immunoglobulin E levels in serum. Eosinophils > 10% of white blood cell count.

► Diagnosis

Based on history, physical examination, nasal smear, serology. Differentiation from viral rhinitis may be sought by color of mucosa (erythematous in viral etiology; pale, violaceous in allergic).

► Clinical Therapeutics

Newer antihistamines less sedating (loratadine, astemizole, cetirizine, fexofenadine). May be combined with decongestants (oral or topical). Intranasal steroid sprays or cromolyn sodium also beneficial. More severe cases may require corticosteroids or immunotherapy.

► Clinical Intervention

For severe cases, skin testing or serum radioallergosorbent (RAST) testing to indicate causative agents. Desensitization another option for treatment. Referral to allergist if symptoms fail to resolve in 3 to 6 months, if complications develop, if quality of life is decreased, or if systemic corticosteroids are required.

► Health Maintenance Issues

Avoid offending allergens. Use air purifiers, dust filters, plastic coverings for pillows, mattresses. Remove dust-collecting objects such as carpet, drapes, bedspreads, wicker. Substitute synthetic materials for animal products.

XI. EPISTAXIS

► Scientific Concepts

Numerous etiologies, the most common being disruption of mucosal blood vessels from trauma (nose blowing, sneezing, digital trauma, foreign bodies). May also be associated with hypertension (usually posterior bleed), ulcerations, repeated cocaine usage, nasal malignancy, bleeding diatheses such as hereditary hemorrhagic telangiectasia (Osler–Weber–Rendu syndrome), and dry mucosa due to low humidity. Bleeding from the vascular plexus on the anterior septum (Kiesselbach's plexus) is most common. Posterior bleeding more serious (may lead to death) because of rapid blood loss and difficulty locating, visualizing bleeding site.

► History & Physical

Anterior bleed usually unilateral and arising from septum. Intermittent, brisk, arterial bleeding with blood in the posterior pharynx generally indicates posterior bleed. Localization of bleeding site necessary. Check oropharynx for blood clots. Review medications for anticoagulants, antiplatelet drugs. Determine pulse, blood pressure.

► Diagnostic Studies

Complete blood count (CBC), prothrombin time, partial thromboplastin time, bleeding time (if recurrent or severe). Toxicology screen if intranasal substance abuse suspected. CT of sinuses only if no site found or bleeding persists.

► Diagnosis

History, physical examination, labs.

► Clinical Therapeutics

Site of bleeding will determine treatment. For all types of bleeds, patient should be sitting with head leaning forward.
Anterior bleeds: Direct pressure of nasal alae, topical nasal decongestants (phenylephrine 0.125 to 1%), topical 4% cocaine as vasoconstrictor and anesthetic. Can substitute topical decongestant (oxymetazoline) and anesthetic (tetracaine) for 4% cocaine. Cauterization of bleeding site with silver nitrate, diathermy, or electrocautery. Anterior nasal packing for refractive bleeding.
Posterior bleeds: Posterior nasal packing and hospital admission.

► Clinical Intervention

Ear, nose, and throat (ENT) referral for recurrent or uncontrolled bleeding episodes.

▶ Health Maintenance Issues

Humidifier, lubrication with petroleum jelly or bacitracin ointment. Avoid vigorous exercise, hot or spicy foods, nasal trauma, excessive nose blowing. Trim children's fingernails.

XII. UPPER RESPIRATORY INFECTION (VIRAL RHINITIS, COMMON COLD)

▶ Scientific Concepts

Acute viral infection resulting in inflammation of nasal, sinus mucosa. Caused by numerous types of adenoviruses, rhinoviruses, other viruses. More common in winter months.

▶ History & Physical

Malaise, fatigue, low-grade fever, chills, sore throat, clear rhinorrhea, postnasal drainage, headache, sneezing, paranasal sinus pressure, plugged ears. Erythematous, edematous nasal mucosa with clear, watery discharge. Purulent discharge suggests bacterial infection.

▶ Diagnostic Studies

CBC with differential reveals increased lymphocytes.

▶ Diagnosis

Based on history, physical examination. Differential includes allergic, vasomotor rhinitis.

▶ Clinical Therapeutics

Oral decongestants (pseudoephedrine) if congested. Topical decongestants (nasal sprays) effective but should be discontinued after 2 to 3 days to prevent rebound congestion, which may be worse than original symptoms. Use antihistamines (loratadine, cetirizine, fexofenadine) for rhinorrhea. Combination decongestants, antihistamines often used. Antipyretics, analgesics, hydration, saline nasal sprays. Usually resolves in 5 to 8 days.

▶ Clinical Intervention

None usually required.

▶ Health Maintenance Issues

To avoid potential drowsiness with older antihistamines (diphenhydramine), choose newer agents (loratadine, fexofenadine, cetirizine).

XIII. NASAL FOREIGN BODY

▶ Scientific Concepts

Foreign object lodged in nasal tissue. More common in children.

► History & Physical

Suspect if unilateral, purulent nasal drainage present. May be malodorous.

► Diagnostic Studies

Usually none needed.

► Diagnosis

Based on history, physical examination.

► Clinical Therapeutics

Mechanical removal if object visible. Avoid irrigation if object is organic as this may cause it to swell.

► Clinical Intervention

Referral to ENT if object not visible or difficult to remove.

► Health Maintenance Issues

Keep small objects away from young children.

XIV. HERPES SIMPLEX

► Scientific Concepts

Herpes simplex virus type 1 (HSV-1) generally responsible for upper body cutaneous disease while type 2 (HSV-2) causes genital infections. Vesicles appear anywhere on face, lips, in mouth. Vesicles quickly enlarge and eventually rupture, forming scabs. Viral shedding lasts 5 to 7 days until crusting over occurs. Trauma, sunlight may precipitate recurrence.

► History & Physical

Prodromal burning, itching, stinging at site where painful vesicles soon appear. Associated fever, malaise, cervical lymphadenopathy may occur. Eventual rupture of vesicles leaves brownish, honey-colored crusting. Recurrent episodes may occur throughout life as fever blisters.

► Diagnostic Studies

Tzanck smear from unroofed vesicles reveals multinucleated giant cells, serology for HSV-1 antibodies.

► Diagnosis

Often based on history, physical examination. Differential includes aphthous stomatitis, impetigo (honey-colored crusted lesions).

► Clinical Therapeutics

Oral acyclovir may decrease severity, duration if initiated during prodromal stage but has little effect once eruption occurs. If recurrences are frequent, daily prophylaxis with acyclovir 200 mg tid or 400 mg bid may be used. Intravenous acyclovir if immunocompromised. Topical acyclovir generally not beneficial.

▶ Clinical Intervention
Suspicion of ophthalmic involvement requires immediate ophthalmology referral.

▶ Health Maintenance Issues
Protection from sunburn, trauma.

XV. ORAL THRUSH (CANDIDIASIS)

▶ Scientific Concepts
Fungal infection of oral cavity. Causative conditions include dentures, diabetes, anemia, debilitation, steroid inhalers, chemotherapy, local irradiation, corticosteroid or broad-spectrum antibiotic use. May also be found in HIV infection.

▶ History & Physical
Painful, creamy-white patches, which are colonies of organisms, on erythematous bases. When removed with tongue blade, leave a raw, red surface.

▶ Diagnostic Studies
Potassium hydroxide wet preparation of scraping reveals spores, possibly nonseptate mycelia. Biopsy shows intraepithelial pseudomycelia of *Candida albicans.*

▶ Diagnosis
Based on history and physical examination. Differential includes leukoplakia, lichen planus that cannot be removed with a tongue blade.

▶ Clinical Therapeutics
Nystatin mouthwash, clotrimazole troches, fluconazole, ketoconazole. Apply Nystatin powder to dentures three to four times per day for several weeks.

▶ Clinical Intervention
Usually none.

▶ Health Maintenance Issues
Rinse mouth after use of steroid inhalers.

XVI. STREPTOCOCCAL PHARYNGITIS

▶ Scientific Concepts
Infection of tonsils by group A beta-hemolytic streptococci.

► **History & Physical**

Severe odynophagia, hemoptysis, weight loss, vocal cord immobility, referred otalgia, fever, anterior cervical lymphadenopathy, malaise. Exam reveals beefy red tonsils, often with exudate, tender adenopathy, scarlatiniform rash.

► **Diagnostic Studies**

Throat culture positive for group A beta-hemolytic strep, CBC with leukocytosis and left shift. Rapid strep test must always be backed up by plated culture due to false-positive rates.

► **Diagnosis**

Based on history, physical examination, culture results. Differential includes sore throat from viruses (exudate absent), *Neisseria gonorrhoeae, Mycoplasma, Chlamydia trachomatis,* mononucleosis, diphtheria (gray tonsillar pseudomembrane).

► **Clinical Therapeutics**

Penicillin, erythromycin (penicillin allergy, *Chlamydia, Mycoplasma*), cephalosporins, other macrolides. Avoid ampicillin if mononucleosis suspected (causes rash). Antipyretics, analgesics, anti-inflammatories.

► **Clinical Intervention**

Antibiotic treatment usually prevents complications such as scarlet fever, rheumatic fever, abscess formation, poststreptococcal glomerulonephritis.

► **Health Maintenance Issues**

Usually none. Tonsillectomy for frequent recurrences.

XVII. ORAL CANCER/LEUKOPLAKIA

► **Scientific Concepts**

Squamous cell carcinoma accounts for ~90% of oral cancers. Tobacco (including smokeless) and alcohol are major contributing factors. Other causes include *Epstein-Barr virus, papillomavirus,* chronic iron deficiency leading to Plummer–Vinson syndrome. Men > women.

► **History & Physical**

Odynophagia, dysphagia, lymphadenopathy, referred otalgia, weight loss. Complete exam of oropharynx including lips, gums, palate, lateral tongue, floor of mouth, buccal mucosa, tonsillar fossae. Leukoplakia (white patch resembling candidiasis but cannot be scraped off with tongue blade) may be premalignant.

► **Diagnostic Studies**

Biopsy of lesions reveals malignant, premalignant changes.

► Diagnosis

Based on history, physical examination, biopsy results. Tumor, nodes, metastases (TNM) staging.

► Clinical Therapeutics

Laser surgical excision for small lesions. Radiation as an alternative, but complications include xerostomia, mandibular necrosis. Combination resection, irradiation for large tumors.

► Clinical Intervention

As above.

► Health Maintenance Issues

Alcohol, tobacco, smokeless tobacco abstinence.

XVIII. EPIGLOTTITIS

► Scientific Concepts

Life-threatening inflammation of epiglottis usually caused by *H. influenzae* (type B). More commonly found in children ages 3 to 5 years, but can occur in adulthood. Incidence decreasing with *H. influenzae* vaccines.

► History & Physical

Odynophagia, high fever, stridor, respiratory distress. Patients often drooling, sitting up, and leaning forward. Direct visualization with tongue blade contraindicated as this may precipitate complete airway blockage.

► Diagnostic Studies

Lateral neck x-ray reveals "thumb sign" or "thumbprinting" (epiglottic edema). Vital signs, blood gases to determine extent of hypoxia/airway obstruction. Blood cultures once airway secured.

► Diagnosis

Based on history, physical examination, radiographic findings.

► Clinical Therapeutics

In addition to intervention (below), third-generation cephalosporins for *H. influenzae* coverage. TMP-SMZ for PCN allergy. Systemic steroids controversial but may decrease inflammation.

► Clinical Intervention

Laryngoscopy in operating room in presence of anesthesiologist and otolaryngologist. Cherry-red, swollen epiglottis seen. Orotracheal intubation is preferred method of treatment. On occasion, tracheostomy may be necessary.

► Health Maintenance Issues

H. influenzae vaccination.

XIX. HOARSENESS

▶ Scientific Concepts

Hoarseness indicates laryngeal involvement. Etiologic factors include viral infections, voice overuse, smoking, inhaled irritants, allergies, benign and malignant neoplasms, recurrent laryngeal nerve damage, gastric reflux, brain stem lesion. Change in voice occurs from inflammation, irritation of vocal cords.

▶ History & Physical

Hoarseness, odynophagia, sore throat, cough, dyspnea. Complete ENT exam, indirect and direct laryngoscopy indicated if symptoms persist > 2 to 3 weeks to rule out neoplasm.

▶ Diagnostic Studies

Indirect and direct laryngoscopy, CT, MRI, throat cultures.

▶ Diagnosis

Based on history, physical examination, diagnostic studies.

▶ Clinical Therapeutics

Acute cases usually resolve spontaneously. Voice rest. Short course of systemic steroids to decrease inflammation.

▶ Clinical Intervention

Chronic cases indicate further workup such as direct visualization and biopsy of any lesions.

▶ Health Maintenance Issues

Smoking cessation, control of gastric reflux.

XX. LARYNGEAL CANCER

▶ Scientific Concepts

Most commonly squamous cell and majority of cases occur in those who use tobacco, smoked or smokeless. Process may be precipitated by tobacco, alcohol, radiation, drugs, diet, pollution, viral infections, and other unknown factors. Tobacco and alcohol have a synergistic effect. Five-year survival is ~50% (75% if detected early, 35% if detected late).

▶ History & Physical

Often, initial presentation is hoarseness, which advances to odynophagia and metastases to cervical nodes. Physical examination includes complete ENT exam, including cervical lymph nodes.

▶ Diagnostic Studies

Indirect mirror exam of the larynx, fiberoptic endoscope.

► Diagnosis

Based on history, physical examination, indirect or direct visualization, and biopsy results if tissue sample obtained.

► Clinical Therapeutics

Radiation therapy, conservation laryngectomy, chemotherapy, or a combination of the three.

► Clinical Intervention

Patients with laryngeal cancer should be followed by an oncologist for life, but more frequently in the first two years when the risk of recurrence is highest. Adequate rehabilitation (physical, functional, psychosocial, occupational) is essential and requires a multidisciplinary approach.

► Health Maintenance Issues

Preventive measures include eliminating or drastically reducing tobacco and alcohol consumption. Although currently inconclusive, other preventive efforts under investigation include antioxidants, particularly vitamin A derivatives.

BIBLIOGRAPHY

Fagnan LJ. Acute sinusitis: A cost-effective approach to diagnosis and treatment. *Am Fam Physician* 58(8):1795–1801; 1998.

Ferri FF. *Ferri's Clinical Advisor: Instant Diagnosis and Treatment.* Chicago: Mosby; 1999.

Goroll AH, May LA, Mulley AG Jr. *Primary Care Medicine: Office Evaluation and Management of the Adult Patient,* 3rd ed. Philadelphia: JB Lippincott; 1995.

Gluckman JL, Farrell M. Head and neck cancer. pp. 722–724. In: Stein JH, ed. *Internal Medicine,* 5th ed. Chicago: Mosby; 1998.

Jackler RK, Kaplan MJ. Ear, nose, & throat. pp. 215–250. In: Tierney LM, McPhee SJ, Papadakis MA, eds. *Current Medical Diagnosis & Treatment,* 37th ed. Stamford, CT: Appleton & Lange; 1998.

Jahn AF, Hawke A. Infections of the external ear. pp. 2787–2794. In: Cummings CW, ed. *Otolaryngology—Head and Neck Surgery,* 2nd ed. Chicago: Mosby; 1993.

Lehrer JF, Poole DC. Diagnosis and management of vertigo. *Comprehensive Ther* 13(9):31–40; 1987.

Lucas BD, Armitage KB, Gross P, Yamauchi T. Respiratory infections: which antibiotics for empiric therapy? *Patient Care* 33(1):76–106; 1999.

Noble J, ed. *Primary Care Medicine,* 2nd ed. Chicago: Mosby; 1996.

Trotto NE, Kaiser HB, Kaliner MA, Slavin RG. Asthma, rhinitis, sinusitis, urticaria. *Patient Care* 33(1):115–139; 1999.

Ophthalmology | 3

J. Dennis Blessing, PhD, PA-C

I. BLURRED VISION

► Scientific Concepts

Blurred vision is a decrease in visual acuity or the inability to distinguish objects clearly. A large number of conditions can cause blurred vision. Vision disturbances can be due to an eye illness or injury, systemic illness or injury, or other organ illness or injury.

► History & Physical

Assess normal condition of eyes including use of corrective lenses, use of contacts; injury, onset (sudden or insidious), duration, pain, tearing, redness, pruritus, discharge (type, color, amount), presence of halos, loss of vision (partial), systemic diseases (hypertension or diabetes) or other health problems, medications, prior history of ocular problems (glaucoma). Examine visual acuity; inspect orbits, cornea, sclera, conjunctiva (palpebral and bulbar), pupils and pupil reaction, extraocular movements, anterior chamber; funduscopic examination. Palpate orbital rims and globes.

► Diagnostic Studies

Fluorescein staining if abrasion or foreign body suspected, slit lamp examination if needed.

► Diagnosis

Determination of cause by history, physical examination, and diagnostic studies.

► Clinical Therapeutics

As indicated by diagnosis.

► Clinical Intervention

As indicated by diagnosis; referral when indicated.

► Health Maintenance Issues

Protection of eyes when potential for injury exists in work and recreational activities; sunglasses in bright sun; treatment of conditions that may have sequelae affecting vision.

II. DECREASED VISUAL ACUITY

► Scientific Concepts

The inability to distinguish objects clearly secondary to an interruption of the light (visual) pathways to the retina.

► History & Physical

Assess normal condition of eyes including use of corrective lenses, use of contacts; onset (sudden or insidious), duration, pain, tearing, redness, pruritus, discharge (type, color, amount), presence of halos, loss of vision (partial), injury, systemic diseases (hypertension or diabetes) or other health problems, medications, prior history of ocular problems, ability to read print and the distance needed to read print. Examine visual acuity; inspect orbits, cornea, sclera, conjunctiva (palpebral and bulbar), pupils and pupil reaction to include the presence of lens opacities (cataracts), extraocular movements, anterior chamber; funduscopic examination. Palpate rims and globes. Examination should concentrate on pathology that would interfere with light projection to the retina.

► Diagnostic Studies

Tonometry if elevated pressures suspected; fluorescein staining if corneal defect or abrasion suspected.

► Diagnosis

Based on findings, some considerations are: need for corrective lenses, presbyopia, corneal opacity, cataracts, failure of pupils to respond, unclear aqueous humor, unclear vitreous humor.

► Clinical Therapeutics

As indicated.

► Clinical Intervention

If corrective lenses needed, then refer to an ophthalmologist or optometrist; emergent conditions (e.g., glaucoma) refer to ophthalmologist; nonemergent conditions are treated as indicated.

► Health Maintenance Issues

Routine eye exam, eye protection, patient education about expected visual changes with age, patient education about complications of systemic diseases including hypertension and diabetes.

III. CATARACTS

► Scientific Concepts

Cataracts are opacities or discoloration of the lens of the eye due to age, disease, injury. It is a common cause of vision loss, particularly in the elderly and usually occurring after age 50.

► History & Physical

Assess normal condition of eyes including use of corrective lenses, use of contacts; injury, onset (sudden or insidious), duration, pain, tearing, redness, pruritus, discharge (type, color, amount), presence of halos, loss of vision (partial or complete), systemic diseases (hypertension or diabetes) or other health problems, medications, prior history of ocular problems. Examine visual acuity; inspect orbits, cornea, sclera, conjunctiva (palpebral and bulbar), pupils and pupil reaction, extraocular movements, anterior chamber; funduscopic examination.

► **Diagnostic Studies**

Usually none unless complicating conditions are suspected.

► **Diagnosis**

By direct examination of lens.

► **Clinical Therapeutics**

Usually none unless complicating conditions are present.

► **Clinical Intervention**

Usually none unless complicating conditions are present. Refer to ophthalmologist for evaluation and possible extraction.

► **Health Maintenance Issues**

Patient education about changes with age or the result of injury to eye and some complications of disease or drug use. Cataracts are one of the most successfully treated problems of vision.

IV. DIABETIC RETINOPATHY

► **Scientific Concepts**

Changes in the retina due to diabetes mellitus are a leading cause of blindness. The longer a person is diabetic, the more likely he or she is to develop diabetic retinopathy; higher incidence in type I diabetics. Three stages of diabetic retinopathy:
1. *Nonproliferative diabetic retinopathy:* Characterized by microaneurysms, hemorrhages, hard exudates, retinal edema.
2. *Preproliferative diabetic retinopathy:* Characterized by retinal nerve infarcts, venous dilation, telangiectasias.
3. *Proliferative diabetic retinopathy:* Characterized by neovascularizations, preretinal and vitreous hemorrhages, fibrous proliferation, retinal detachment.

► **History & Physical**

Visual history, including changes (and progression of changes) in vision, redness, pain, pattern of visual loss, injury to eye, night vision, use of corrective lenses; history of diabetes, including onset, treatment, control, and presence of other complications such as peripheral neuropathy and kidney disease. Presence of other systemic disease such as hypertension; presence of other risk factors such as obesity, medications, and compliance to therapeutic regimens and degree of control. Sudden changes in vision should prompt in-depth evaluation. Examine visual acuity; complete eye exam to include detailed and careful funduscopic examination.

► **Diagnostic Studies**

Funduscopy and angiography (performed by ophthalmologist).

► **Diagnosis**

Usually by direct funduscopy.

► **Clinical Therapeutics**

Referral to an ophthalmologist for evaluation and intervention and recommendations for continuing care.

► **Clinical Intervention**

Control of diabetes and contributing diseases and factors; referral to ophthalmologist for retinopathy evaluation and treatment.

► **Health Maintenance Issues**

Patient education on complications of diabetes and need for reduction of risk factors and control of glucose levels. Patients must understand that, even with good glycemic control, complications may occur. Annual funduscopic examination with dilation by an ophthalmologist is a standard of care.

V. RETINAL DETACHMENT/PUNCTURE

► **Scientific Concepts**

Detachment or separation of the retina from the choroid; retinal detachment can occur as the result of trauma or as a consequence of systemic or ocular disease; occurs more often in men than women; can be caused by ocular trauma; often due to degenerative changes in the retina.

► **History & Physical**

History should include description of symptoms, including onset, duration, trauma, previous condition of the eye, and previous eye problems; acute vision loss usually indicates a large detachment; history may include a "shading" of vision, flashing lights, floaters, and usually in one eye. Examine visual acuity; complete eye exam including funduscopy.

► **Diagnostic Studies**

Usually none except by an ophthalmologist.

► **Diagnosis**

By funduscopy; may reveal elevated retina, retinal folds, grayish discoloration, loss of choroidal background; findings may not be obvious.

► **Clinical Therapeutics**

Refer to an ophthalmologist.

► **Clinical Intervention**

Refer to an ophthalmologist.

► **Health Maintenance Issues**

None.

VI. GLAUCOMA

▶ **Scientific Concepts**

Aqueous humor is continually produced by the ciliary body of the eye; it flows through the pupil, fills the anterior chamber, and is drained through the trabecular network to Schlemm's canal. Any increase in the pressure of any compartment of the eye is spread hydraulically throughout the eye. Glaucoma is an increased intraocular pressure that leads to retinal and optic disk trauma. Two types of glaucoma:

1. *Open-angle glaucoma:* More common (90 to 95% of cases), insidious, less symptomatic.
2. *Closed-angle glaucoma:* Less common, but acute onset and an ophthalmologic emergency. Usually multiple symptoms (see History & Physical below) not found in open-angle glaucoma. Leading cause of blindness in African Americans.

▶ **History & Physical**

Open-angle glaucoma: Usually asymptomatic, but questions should center on vision/eye history, vision problems or symptoms, family history for glaucoma, concurrent disease (particularly diabetes and hypertension). Examination may be normal except for elevated intraocular pressure; may have an increase in physiologic cup to optic disk ratio with displacement of vessels to cup rim (asymmetry to opposite side); may have visual field deficits, but they are often difficult to detect.

Closed-angle glaucoma: Same risk factors as for open-angle glaucoma; onset is usually acute, with pain, red eye, blurred vision, halos around lights, vision loss, nausea (sometimes accompanied by abdominal pain), headache; most commonly unilateral. Pupil dilation is contraindicated. Affected eye may be red, tearing, firm to palpation; fixed mid-dilated pupil (sometimes distorted to oval shape); hazy, cloudy, or steamy cornea; increased physiologic cup to optic disk ratio; shallow anterior chamber; decreased visual acuity; marked increased intraocular pressure.

▶ **Diagnostic Studies**

Tonometry.

▶ **Diagnosis**

Elevated pressure on tonometry; physical findings consistent with glaucoma; must recognize signs and symptoms of closed-angle glaucoma because of the emergent nature of the problem.

▶ **Clinical Therapeutics**

Patients with acute closed-angle glaucoma must be referred immediately to an ophthalmologist. Emergency treatment prior to referral can include topical beta blockers, topical pilocarpine, oral carbonic anhydrase inhibitors, osmotic agents (oral glycerine or intravenous mannitol). Patients with open-angle glaucoma should be referred to an ophthalmologist and treatment based on consultant recommendations.

▶ Clinical Intervention
Referral to an ophthalmologist, emergent basis for closed-angle glaucoma.

▶ Health Maintenance Issues
Periodic checks with tonometry for individuals with a personal and family history of glaucoma and those patients with risk factors; should be part of routine annual examination after age 40. Always screen for glaucoma (history, check depth of anterior chamber, tonometry) before use of mydriatic agents in order to prevent precipitating glaucoma attack.

VII. HYPERTENSIVE RETINOPATHY

▶ Scientific Concepts
Hypertension causes changes in the arterioles of the retina by causing thickening of the walls that result in light reflex changes (copper or silver wiring). Pressure in the arterioles may affect venous pressures at points where veins and arteries cross, thereby compressing the vein, causing dilation in the vein that predisposes it to occlusion. Hypertension also causes changes in the arteriole walls that lead to exudates and hemorrhages, which ultimately will lead to damage affecting vision.

▶ History & Physical
History should center on visual signs and symptoms, other contributing disease (diabetes, thyroid), and eye health, including corrective lenses. Examination may reveal no eye changes, or mild, moderate, or severe changes that include copper wiring, silver wiring, arteriovenous nicking, venous dilation, exudates, cotton-wool spots, flame hemorrhages.

▶ Diagnostic Studies
Refer to an ophthalmologist for evaluation and treatment.

▶ Diagnosis
Findings on funduscopy.

▶ Clinical Therapeutics
Control of blood pressure, periodic checks, complications usually managed by an ophthalmologist.

▶ Clinical Intervention
Refer to an ophthalmologist.

▶ Health Maintenance Issues
Patient education to emphasize the importance of controlling hypertension and other complicating disease; annual funduscopic examination.

VIII. BACTERIAL INFECTIONS

► Scientific Concepts

Bacterial infections of the eye can be serious and have serious sequelae. Corneal infections or infections of corneal ulcerations, such as from contact wear, can cause corneal opacification. Hypopion (pus in the anterior chamber) is an ophthalmologic emergency. Periorbital cellulitis is also considered an ophthalmologic emergency, especially in infants and young children. Infection of the lacrimal ducts (dacryocystitis) is usually unilateral, related to obstruction, and caused by beta-hemolytic *Streptococcus* or *Staphylococcus aureus* in infants and persons over 40 years of age. Less serious infections, such as conjunctivitis (see Other Disorders of the Eye section) and sty can be treated without referral unless there are complications.

► History & Physical

History should include onset, duration, prior vision or visual problems, use of corrective lenses or contacts, history of injury or foreign body sensation, presence of blurred vision or decreased vision, photophobia, halos, loss of vision, pain, fever, discharge or drainage, characteristics of discharge or drainage, treatment by self or health care provider. Examine visual acuity; inspect for redness, discharge, condition of cornea, anterior chamber, pupil, lens, conjunctiva (bulbar and palpebral), sclera, lids; extraocular movements; funduscopy.

► Diagnostic Studies

Fluorescein staining if indicated, tonometry if indicated (usually not done in obvious eye surface infection).

► Diagnosis

Based on history and examination findings. Sty (horedeolum) is a small pustule at the lid margin. Chalazion usually is a small painless mass in the lid. Corneal infections penetrate the corneal layers, and frank pus is present. Hypopion is pus in the anterior chamber; periorbital cellulitis is marked edema, erythema, warmth, and pain of the lids and orbital and periorbital soft tissues. Lacrimal gland infection generally presents with tenderness, swelling, and redness of the upper-outer lid; lacrimal duct infections present as tenderness, swelling, erythema in the nasal corner of the eye; pus can sometimes be expressed from the puncta.

► Clinical Therapeutics

As indicated. Periorbital cellulitis, corneal infections, hypopion must be referred to an ophthalmologist for management. Lacrimal duct and gland infections are managed depending on severity of disease, usually with systemic antibiotics. Sties are treated with frequent warm compresses and topical ophthalmic antibiotic drops. Chalazions are usually asymptomatic and require no treatment. They will resolve with time. Acute infection or inflammation are treated with warm compresses and ophthalmic antibiotic drops. Large chalazions that put pressure on the eye or cause distortion of vision should be referred to an ophthalmologist for excision.

► Clinical Intervention

Referral to an ophthalmologist is indicated for serious infections.

► Health Maintenance Issues

Protecting eyes from exposure to potential infective agents; careful handling of contacts; hand washing before applying contacts.

IX. OTHER DISORDERS OF THE EYE

A. Conjunctivitis

► Scientific Concepts

Common, rarely serious, inflammation of the conjunctiva with dilation of the superficial blood vessels due to allergy, viral infection, or bacterial infection; can be highly contagious, especially among young children.

► History & Physical

Onset over short period of time, usually without pain, photophobia, blurred vision or halos. Discharge in bacterial conjunctivitis is copious, purulent (yellow or green), and may cause eyelashes to mat overnight. Discharge in viral conjunctivitis is moderate and clear. Itching is prominent in allergic conjunctivitis. Presence of foreign body sensations, recent upper respiratory infections, others with disease may help determine cause of conjunctivitis; contact with any toxic substance or known allergens. Note amount and color of discharge, involvement of lids (edema), degree of conjunctival erythema or injection, pupil reaction, visual acuity, and presence of preauricular nodes; Gram stain of discharge may aid in diagnosis. Examine anterior chambers and underside of lids. Presence of preauricular nodes. Examine ears, nose, throat, neck for signs of concurrent disease. (See Table 3–1.)

► Diagnostic Studies

Gram stain of discharge may give indication of type of infection: segmented neutrophils indicate bacterial infection; lymphocytes indicate viral infection; eosinophils indicate allergic reaction; consider gonococcal and chlamydial infections in sexually active individuals.

► Diagnosis

Usually based on history and physical examination; must rule out more serious causes of red eye such as glaucoma, iritis, keratitis, corneal lesions, foreign body.

► Clinical Therapeutics

Bacterial conjunctivitis: Antibiotic drops (no steroids).
Viral conjunctivitis: Artificial tears.
Allergic conjunctivitis: Topical steroids for severe cases (use with care and caution); conjunctivitis in the neonate should be treated with

► table 3-1

SIGNS OF RED EYE

Signs	Acute Conjunctivitis	Acute Iritis	Acute Glaucoma	Corneal Lesions
Conjunctival injection	+/+++	++	++	++
Discharge	+/+++	0	0	0/+
Preauricular lymph node	0/+	0	0	0
Corneal opacification	0/+	0	+++	0/+++
Corneal epithelial disruption	0/+	0	0	+/+++
Ciliary flush	0	++	+	+++
Pupil	N	Mid-dilated irregular	Small/irregular	N/small
Anterior chamber depth	N	N	Shallow	N
Intraocular pressure	N	Low	High	N

+, present; ++, moderate; +++, severe; N, normal; 0, absent.

Source: Goldberg JS. The Instant Exam Review for the USMLE Step 3, *2nd ed., Stamford, CT: Appleton & Lange, 1997, p. 239.*

topical erythromycin (primarily for chlamydial infection), and follow-up should be done.

► Clinical Intervention

Bacterial conjunctivitis: Gentle washing away of exudates, warm compresses to lids, avoid direct sunlight (use sunglasses), follow-up evaluation in 2 to 3 days.

Viral conjunctivitis: Artificial tears, cold compresses to lids, avoid groups (contagious for 2 weeks), wash hands frequently.

Allergic conjunctivitis: Avoid any known allergens, cold compresses to lids. At least one follow-up examination should be done.

► Health Maintenance Issues

Viral and bacterial conjunctivitis are very contagious, especially among young children. Control of known allergens may help in treatment of allergic conjunctivitis. Infected individuals and close contacts should wash hands frequently.

B. Keratoconjunctivitis Sicca (Dry Eye)

► Scientific Concepts

Drying of the eyes can be the result of a number of conditions, both minor and serious. Causes can include systemic disease (e.g., Sjögren's syndrome), disorders of the lacrimal glands/drainage system, medications, eye structure abnormalities, blepharitis, excessive exposure to the elements, and aging.

► History & Physical

History may indicate acute or chronic condition. Attention should be given to both eye and systemic symptoms. Physical examination should include visual acuity, thorough eye exam, and evaluation of suspected systemic findings.

▶ **Diagnostic Studies**

As indicated by history and physical findings.

▶ **Diagnosis**

By history and physical findings.

▶ **Clinical Therapeutics**

Treatment of underlying problems, topically by periodic warm compresses to lids and artificial tears.

▶ **Clinical Intervention**

As above and referral as needed to ophthalmologists or other specialist.

▶ **Health Maintenance Issues**

Avoid prolonged sun exposure and use sunglasses; avoid exposure to other drying elements.

C. Disorders of Optic Nerve/Visual Pathways

▶ **Scientific Concepts**

Loss of vision may be in one eye or both; may be central, temporal, or nasal depending on location of lesion. Vision loss in one eye indicates a lesion of the optic nerve; bitemporal vision loss indicates a lesion of the optic chiasm; homonymous hemianopsia indicates a postchiasm lesion.

▶ **History & Physical**

Very careful delineation of loss or reduced visual acuity, whether one or both eyes, type of defect (central, lateral, medial); pain, halos, injury, systemic disease, other neurologic signs or symptoms. Examine visual acuity; careful examination of the eyes, including visual fields, ophthalmoscopy, complete neurological examination.

▶ **Diagnostic Studies**

Computed tomography (CT), magnetic resonance imaging (MRI) for identification of intracranial lesions.

▶ **Diagnosis**

Based on findings of history, examination, results of special studies.

▶ **Clinical Therapeutics**

Refer to an ophthalmologist, neurologist, or neurosurgeon.

▶ **Clinical Intervention**

Referral as above.

▶ **Health Maintenance Issues**

None.

D. Strabismus

▶ Scientific Concepts

Misalignment of the eyes due to weakness of extraocular muscles; misalignment of the extraocular muscles or impaired innervation of the extraocular muscles; most commonly congenital, but can occur due to trauma, stroke, systemic disease.

▶ History & Physical

Age of onset or when first noted, family history of similar problems, injury, other neurological disorders, visual problems or complaints. Examine visual acuity; thorough eye examination with particular attention to extraocular muscles, other cranial nerve weakness, light reflex, accommodation, cover–uncover test.

▶ Diagnostic Studies

Careful eye examination with ophthalmoscopy; note corneal light reflex; cover–uncover test.

▶ Diagnosis

Based on examination findings; consider concurrent conditions in older children and adults.

▶ Clinical Therapeutics

None.

▶ Clinical Intervention

Refer to ophthalmologist for evaluation and consideration of corrective surgery or other interventions.

▶ Health Maintenance Issues

Eye examination for strabismus should be a part of every routine exam of newborns through infancy and childhood. Early detection may prevent more serious later eye problems.

E. Herpes Simplex

▶ Scientific Concepts

The herpesvirus includes two types: herpes simplex type 1 (HSV-1) and type 2 (HSV-2). HSV-1 is the infecting agent in a vast majority of ophthalmic infections, and the cornea is the structure predominantly affected. Herpes infections of the eye and its structures are rare. The mode of transmission is by direct contact. Herpes simplex and herpes zoster infections of the soft tissues (including the lids) surrounding the eye also occur. Herpes zoster infection of the trigeminal nerve ophthalmic division may involve the cornea. Varicella should also be considered as an etiologic agent.

▶ History & Physical

Initially, a foreign body sensation, followed by increased discomfort, tearing, photophobia, conjunctival injection, decreased visual acuity. May be history of prior infection or recent viral lesions (such as fever blisters). Concurrent sexually transmitted disease (STD) should lead to consideration of HSV-2 infection and other STDs. Examine visual acuity, eyelids, conjunctiva, cornea, anterior chamber, pupils, palpebral conjunctiva of upper and lower lids, regional lymph nodes; funduscopy. Vesicles on the tip of the nose (Hutchinson's sign) may offer a clue to diagnosis and should prompt an immediate referral to an ophthalmologist.

▶ Diagnostic Studies

Fluorescein staining.

▶ Diagnosis

Identification of a branching or dendritic pattern on cornea, occasionally will appear as small punctate lesions on the cornea.

▶ Clinical Therapeutics

Immediate referral to an ophthalmologist for treatment.

▶ Clinical Intervention

Immediate referral to an ophthalmologist for treatment.

▶ Health Maintenance Issues

Avoid transmission to the eye from obvious herpes ulcerations such as fever blisters; frequent hand washing when fever blisters or other herpetic lesions are present. Exposure to sun, ultraviolet light, stress, and trauma may precipitate recurrences.

F. Disorders of the Lids

1. Blepharitis

▶ Scientific Concepts

An inflammatory reaction of the eyelid margins that occurs as a result of infective or noninfective reactions. Infection is commonly due to *Staphylococcus*. Noninfective is commonly a seborrheic reaction due to accelerated skin shedding and sebaceous gland dysfunction. Both can occur concurrently. Both can be chronic.

▶ History & Physical

History may indicate a chronic condition with remissions and exacerbations. The lid margins are usually red, with associated conjunctivitis and mild burning and discomfort. The eye surface may seem to be dry. There may be purulent drainage in bacterial infections. There may be a history of exacerbations with use of eye makeup, exposure to chemicals or the elements, or excessive rubbing. A visual history should be taken. Examination should include visual acuity, which is usually unaffected by the problem. The seborrheic form of the disease is characterized by redness of the lid margins, mild edema, scaling of skin. Persistent signs despite treatment with thickening of the eye margin may indicate skin or sebaceous cyst carcinoma, which needs to be investigated carefully. The infective form of the disease will present in a manner similar to the seborrheic form with purulent material along the lids, crusting, and loss of lashes. Entropion, ectropion, and chronic conjunctivitis may also be present.

▶ Diagnostic Studies
Cultures in atypical cases, biopsy in atypical persistent cases.

▶ Diagnosis
Based on history and physical findings.

▶ Clinical Therapeutics
Eyelid margin scrubs with eyelid cleanser, warm compresses; avoid exposure to eye irritants (including makeup); discontinue contact lens until resolution; topical antibiotic eyedrops for infective form.

▶ Clinical Intervention
Referral to ophthalmologist for persistent cases.

▶ Health Maintenance Issues
Education on good eye hygiene using lid scrubs and warm compresses.

2. Ectropion/Entropion
Ectropion: Eversion or outward displacement of the margin of the lid.
Entropion: Inversion or inward displacement of the margin of the lid.

▶ Scientific Concepts
Inversion or eversion of the lids can have a number of etiologies and may occur as a consequence of aging. The primary problem to the eye is irritation of the eye surface by lashes or drying of the eye surface if lids do not completely close. The lower eyelid is most commonly affected in both conditions.

▶ History & Physical
History should center on eye complaints as well as potential causes from neurologic and systemic diseases. Examination should concentrate on eye and local conditions (inflammation, infection, injury) and systemic and neurologic etiologies (Bell's palsy).

▶ Diagnostic Studies
Usually none for entropion and ectropion alone.

▶ Diagnosis
Based on history and physical examination.

▶ Clinical Therapeutics
Treatment of injury, infection, inflammation or other underlying cause; use of artificial tears, taping eye closed.

▶ Clinical Intervention
Surgical intervention is often needed.

► Health Maintenance Issues
Protect eyes from irritants; keep eye surface moist.

3. Chalazion

► Scientific Concepts
Chalazion occurs when there is blockage or low-grade inflammation of a meibomian gland of the lid, usually resulting in a painless swelling in the lid. May occasionally become acutely infected or inflamed.

► History & Physical
History is a painless, slowly growing mass in the eyelid without other symptoms. Physical examination reveals a small, nontender, firm mass in the lid.

► Diagnostic Studies
Not indicated.

► Diagnosis
Based on history and physical examination.

► Clinical Therapeutics
Antibiotics or other medications are not indicated unless there is acute infection and inflammation (rare).

► Clinical Intervention
Usually resolves without treatment. Warm compresses and eyelid margin washing may help. Large chalazions may put pressure on the globe and distort vision, which requires referral to an ophthalmologist.

► Health Maintenance Issues
Good eyelid hygiene.

4. Sty (Hordeolum)

► Scientific Concepts
Infection/inflammation of a lash or gland of the eyelid margin results in redness, scaling, and irritation. Sties tend to occur in crops. *Staphylococcus* is the most common causative organism, but others do occur. Contact lenses, makeup, and lid margin irritation may predispose to sty formation.

► History & Physical
History is usually that of redness and scaling of the lid. Pain is related to size of the lesion and eye irritation. Examination shows lid margin pustule(s) with localized inflammation and edema, drainage or tearing, and some eye irritation.

► Diagnostic Studies
Usually none indicated.

▶ Diagnosis

Based on history and physical examination findings.

▶ Clinical Therapeutics

Wide range of ophthalmic topical solutions: erythromycin, gentamicin, sulfacetamide.

▶ Clinical Intervention

Frequent hand washing, warm compresses to the eye, daily lid washing. Do not burst pustule; incision and drainage rarely needed.

▶ Health Maintenance Issues

Good eyelid hygiene by washing lids daily.

X. WOUNDS/INJURIES OF THE EYE

A. Cranial or Ocular Injuries

▶ Scientific Concepts

Injury to the head or eye can affect vision and the eye. Intracranial injury may have ocular manifestations.

▶ History & Physical

Time, mechanism, result of injury; changes in signs and symptoms since injury; prior eye history, concomitant injury and symptoms. Initial history may be very directed due to emergent or other overriding conditions (shock, arrest, etc.). Examination may be emergent evaluation, but should include assessment of visual acuity, pupil reaction, and fundi as well as direct indicators of injury (hyphema, laceration, etc.).

▶ Diagnostic Studies

As pertains to the eye; x-ray, CT, MRI as indicated.

▶ Diagnosis

Based on physical and diagnostic findings.

▶ Clinical Therapeutics

As indicated by diagnosis.

▶ Clinical Intervention

Refer to ophthalmologist. In the severely injured patient, the first goal is to save the patient's life and to limit morbidity; eye considerations may need to be secondary to that goal.

▶ Health Maintenance Issues

Protection of eyes during contact sports and in work settings with potential for injury.

B. Burns to the Eye

► Scientific Concepts

Acids and bases that come into contact with the surface of the eye cause chemical burns that can destroy the eye or have lasting vision complications. Eye burns are true ophthalmologic emergencies and require immediate intervention and referral to an ophthalmologist. Base injuries are considered more dangerous because of the continued effect of the base on contacted structures despite irrigation.

► History & Physical

Usually very quick history and limited physical examination of the eye is done as treatment is initiated. Identify offending substance, time since exposure, and emergency treatment should be ascertained.

► Diagnostic Studies

Initially none.

► Diagnosis

By history.

► Clinical Therapeutics

Copious irrigation (at least one liter) with normal saline.

► Clinical Intervention

Emergency referral to an ophthalmologist.

► Health Maintenance Issues

Eye protection for all work and recreational activities that involve toxic substances.

C. Foreign Body in the Eye

► Scientific Concepts

Any number of foreign bodies can lodge on the surface of the eye. The most uncomfortable are those that lodge or abrade the cornea. Some foreign bodies will lodge under the lids. Foreign body sensation may be present with surface ulcerations or injury. Foreign body sensation may persist after removal of a foreign body.

► History & Physical

Activity at time of foreign body, particularly if working around wood or metal such as hammering; onset, duration, associated symptoms, effect on vision; vision history or previous eye or vision problems. Examine visual acuity if possible, cornea, anterior chamber, conjunctiva, sclera, and lids. Retract lower lid down and completely expose; upper lids must be everted and examined for foreign body; carefully examine for penetrating wound, blood in the anterior chamber; examine for fixed or distorted pupils.

► Diagnostic Studies

Fluorescein staining may help identify a foreign body and will demonstrate abrasions from foreign bodies; slit lamp examination will help identify foreign bodies or damage to the eye surface that are difficult to see.

► Diagnosis
Identify the foreign body, but always consider the multiple causes of a red eye.

► Clinical Therapeutics
Prompt irrigation is usually required. Antibiotic eyedrops are usually not indicated for acute foreign bodies, although one-time application after foreign body removal is acceptable. Anesthetic and steroid eyedrops should never be used after foreign body removal. One-time use of a cycloplegic drop may be used to relieve the discomfort following the removal of a foreign body.

► Clinical Intervention
Removal of surface foreign body after topical ocular anesthesia with a cotton-tipped applicator or gentle irrigation; skilled providers may use a small-gauge needle or corneal spoon for removal. Deeply embedded and penetrating foreign bodies must be referred to an ophthalmologist. After foreign body removal, eyes should be patched for 24 to 48 hours. Follow-up should be in 48 hours and the eye observed for complications such as infection or formation of a rust ring.

► Health Maintenance Issues
Eye protection during high-risk activities, particularly hammering, sawing, and where foreign bodies may be created by the activity. Shatterproof lenses should be a must for all corrective eyeglasses. Noncorrective safety glasses should be worn by those who do not need correction or those who wear contacts.

D. Blunt and Penetrating Trauma

► Scientific Concepts
Blunt trauma is defined as trauma to the eye that does not disrupt the continuity of the eye structure. Penetrating trauma is defined as trauma that disrupts the continuity of the eye structure. Injury to the eye can result in short- or long-term problems. Blunt trauma can be as severe as penetrating trauma and must be evaluated as carefully. Initial evaluation and treatment may be key to preserving visual function, as well as cosmetic effect. Generally, evidence of internal eye trauma, disruption of the eye surface, and interference with vision are indications for referral to an ophthalmologist.

► History & Physical
Vision prior to injury, type of injury, mechanism of injury, first aid given, time since injury, changes since injury, concurrent injuries and problem. Careful examination of the eye and surrounding structures, visual acuity if feasible and possible. Examine orbits, lids, conjunctiva, sclera, cornea, anterior chamber, pupils, pupillary response, extraocular movements, and do funduscopic examination. Examination should concentrate on injury and abnormal structures, disruption of

eye integrity, blood in anterior or posterior chamber, retinal injury, presence of foreign bodies, and penetrating injury. Slit lamp examination.

► Diagnostic Studies
As indicated: skull x-rays, CT, MRI.

► Diagnosis
Based on findings.

► Clinical Therapeutics
Usually none since injuries should be referred to an ophthalmologist.

► Clinical Intervention
Refer to an ophthalmologist for penetrating injuries, injuries to any area of the globe and its structures, blood in the anterior or posterior chambers. Injuries to bony and soft tissues surrounding the eye should be handled in a manner that will not harm the eye.

► Health Maintenance Issues
Eye protection during all work and recreational activities that have even a remote possibility of causing eye injury, seat belt use while driving, etc.

BIBLIOGRAPHY

Berson FG. *Basic Ophthalmology for Medical Students and Primary Care Residents,* 6th ed. San Francisco: American Academy of Ophthalmology; 1993.

Goldberg JS, ed. *The Instant Exam Review for the USMLE Step 3,* 2nd ed. Chapter 13. Stamford, CT: Appleton & Lange; 1997.

Moser RL, ed. Ophthalmology. In: *Primary Care for Physician Assistants.* New York: McGraw-Hill; 1998.

Newell FW. *Ophthalmology Principles and Concepts,* 8th ed. St. Louis: Mosby; 1996.

Rakel RE, ed. *Saunders Manual of Medical Practice,* Part II. Philadelphia: WB Saunders; 1996.

Pulmonary Diseases 4

Patricia A. Francis, MS, PA-C, Charles B. Travis, MD

I. ACUTE BRONCHITIS

► Scientific Concepts

Acute bronchitis is characterized by inflammation of the trachea and bronchi. The most common cause is viral. Examples include adenoviruses, influenza, parainfluenza, and respiratory syncytial virus. The most common bacterial species to cause bronchitis include *Streptococcus pneumoniae, Haemophilus influenzae, Moraxella catarrhalis,* and *Mycoplasma pneumoniae.* Exposure to chemical and physical agents can also predispose the patient to bronchitis.

► History & Physical

Usually, there is a preceding upper respiratory tract infection (URI) with fever. Cough is characteristic of acute bronchitis. Cough may be nonproductive, productive, or mucopurulent. There may be pleuritic chest pain. Chest examination may be normal or demonstrate rhonchi.

► Diagnostic Studies

Generally not necessary.

► Diagnosis

Diagnosis is clinical. Differential diagnosis includes influenza, foreign body, and mycoplasma pneumonia. Chest x-rays or bronchoscopy may be necessary to exclude these causes.

► Clinical Therapeutics

Treatment is symptomatic; fluids, rest, antitussive agents and aspirin or acetaminophen. Antibiotics are indicated in patients with chronic obstructive pulmonary disease (COPD), immunocompromised patients, and in patients in whom fever persists for greater than 7 days or whose condition deteriorates. Some prescribe antibiotics for smokers.

► Clinical Intervention

See Clinical Therapeutics.

► Health Maintenance Issues

Smokers should stop smoking. Frequent hand washing and use of handkerchief can reduce spread of infection.

II. INFLUENZA

► Scientific Concepts

Influenza is a respiratory disease usually seen in winter months. Influenza is caused by influenza virus types A, B, and C of the myxovirus group. Transmission is airborne.

► History & Physical

Characteristic symptoms of influenza include cough and systemic symptoms such as fever, chills, myalgias, and headache. The patient appears ill. Conjunctivae may be injected; nasal mucosa boggy; pharynx injected. Chest examination is unremarkable.

► Diagnostic Studies
Not applicable.

► Diagnosis
Diagnosis is clinical. Specific diagnosis requires isolation of virus from pharynx or sputum. Differential diagnosis includes URIs, pharyngitis, bronchitis, and pneumonia. Chest x-ray may be necessary in some cases to rule out pneumonia.

► Clinical Therapeutics
Treatment of influenza is largely symptomatic; fluids, rest, aspirin (avoid in children) or acetaminophen. Amantadine (Symmetrel), may be used for treatment of influenza A infection if begun within 48 hours of beginning of symptoms. Amantadine is also effective for prophylaxis of influenza A infections. Other therapeutic agents are beginning to be released and may show promise because they are effective against influenza A and B (e.g., zanamivir and oseltamivir).

► Clinical Intervention
Patients should stop smoking. Frequent hand washing, use of handkerchief, avoidance of crowds recommended.

► Health Maintenance Issues
Patients over age 65, health care or other workers in contact with the public, immunocompromised patients, and patients with chronic illnesses should receive yearly influenza vaccinations.

III. PNEUMONIA

A. Pneumonia in Adults

► Scientific Concepts
Community-acquired pneumonia in adults is most commonly caused by *Streptococcus pneumoniae*. *Mycoplasma pneumoniae* affects healthy, young adults; influenza virus infects the elderly. Other causes of pneumonia may be other bacteria and viruses, chlamydiae, rickettsiae, protozoa, and parasites. Microbes may enter the lung by inhalation, aspiration, or hematogenous spread from an area of infection.

► History & Physical
Pneumonia may follow viral respiratory infections. Symptoms include high fever, chills, malaise, increased temperature, tachycardia, tachypnea, decreased appetite, weakness, myalgia, pleuritic chest pain, cough, sputum production. Physical examination in bacterial pneumonia may show evidence of consolidation, dullness to percussion, increased vocal fremitus, and crackles or rales. In early pneumonia, chest examination may be normal.

► Diagnosis

A Gram stain and culture of lower respiratory secretions can be obtained. An accurate specimen is characterized by less than five squamous epithelial cells and contain 10 to 15 polymorphonuclear leukocytes per high-powered field—an essential part of the diagnostic workup. Leukocytosis with left shift is usually seen in bacterial pneumonia. Chest x-ray may show segmental, lobar, or diffuse infiltrate with air bronchograms. Blood cultures are positive in 20 to 30% of community-acquired pneumonia.

► Differential Diagnosis

Viral pneumonia is the most common and is seen in the elderly or in patients with chronic heart, lung, or kidney disease. Cytomegalovirus pneumonia is seen in immunosuppressed patients with human immunodeficiency virus (HIV) infection or following organ transplants. Pneumonia from varicella and measles is seen during epidemics. Chest x-ray may show diffuse parenchymal pattern as opposed to lobar consolidation seen with bacterial pneumonia.

Streptococcus pneumoniae is the most common cause of community-acquired pneumonia. Increased susceptibility is seen in persons with sickle cell disease, splenectomy, COPD, leukemia, and alcoholism. Symptoms include fever, chills, cough, and dyspnea. Physical examination of the chest typically shows dullness to percussion, increased vocal fremitus, and crackles or rales over the infected area. Gram stain of sputum will show gram-positive diplococci. White blood count typically shows leukocytosis with shift to the left. Chest x-ray shows lobar consolidation. Most strains of *S. pneumoniae* are sensitive to penicillin G, although there are a few penicillin-resistant strains of streptococcal pneumonia that are sensitive to vancomycin.

Staphylococcus aureus presents like pneumococcal pneumonia. A hematogenous source of infection such as an intravenous (IV) line, septic thrombophlebitis, or endocarditis may be present. Gram stain of sputum shows clusters of gram-positive cocci. Chest x-ray shows multiple nodular infiltrates, which may be associated with abscess formation. Blood cultures are usually positive. Treatment is with a penicillinase-resistant antibiotic such as nafcillin or vancomycin.

Streptococcus pyogenes pneumonia presents like the pneumonias of *S. pneumoniae* and *S. aureus*. Chest x-ray will demonstrate empyema in 30 to 40% of cases. Treatment of choice is penicillin G.

Haemophilus influenzae is the second most common type of pneumonia seen in patients with COPD. Gram stain of the sputum will demonstrate gram-negative coccobacilli. Twenty percent of *H. influenzae* may show resistance due to beta-lactamase production. Treatment therefore requires ampicillin plus a beta-lactamase inhibitor (Augmentin or Unasyn), a second- or third-generation cephalosporin (ceftazidime), or trimethoprim-sulfamethoxazole (TMP-SMZ) (Bactrim or Septra).

Gram-negative bacilli are associated with pneumonia in chronically ill persons and immunocompromised individuals. Gram-negative bacilli are a major source of hospital-acquired pneumonias. Causative organisms are *Klebsiella pneumoniae*, *Escherichia coli*, and *Pseudomonas* *aeruginosa.* Initial treatment with a third-generation cephalosporin (ceftazidime) and an aminoglycoside (gentamicin) is indicated.

Mycoplasma pneumoniae presents with a nonproductive hacking cough. Symptoms may include myalgias, arthalgias, skin lesions, neurologic findings. Erythromycin, azithromycin, and tetracycline are the drugs of choice.

Legionella **pneumonia** presents with dry cough, fever, chills, headache, malaise, confusion, and gastrointestional symptoms such as diarrhea, although nausea and vomiting may be present. Gram stain of sputum shows polymorphonuclear leukocytes. Chest x-ray shows patchy or lobar infiltrate. Diagnosis can be confirmed by direct fluorescent antibody testing of sputum. Treatment is with erythromycin with or without rifampin. Alternative treatments include macrolides such as clarithromycin or azithromycin, the combination of TMP-SMZ and a quinolone such as ciprofloxacin, or a tetracycline such as doxycycline.

► Clinical Therapeutics

Patients with viral and mycoplasma pneumonia can usually be treated as outpatients. Healthy, young patients with bacterial pneumonia may be treated at home provided they are watched by family or friends and have access to a health care provider or hospital. Chronically ill or immunocompromised patients, infants, or the elderly should be hospitalized for close monitoring, IV antibiotics, supplemental oxygen, hydration, aerosol treatments, and chest physical therapy.

► Health Maintenance Issues

Prophylaxis with pneumococcal and influenza vaccines is indicated for patients over 65 years of age, residents of chronic care facilities, those with chronic diseases, health care workers, and people who work with the public.

B. Chlamydial Pneumonia

► Scientific Concepts

Acute respiratory infection that produces patchy inflammatory changes confined to alveolar septum and interstitium of the lung.

► History & Physical

Often, symptoms are confined to fever, headache, muscle aches, and pains. Cough, when present, is dry, hacking, and nonproductive. Seen in previously healthy young adults.

► Diagnostic Studies

Chest x-ray: multiple lobes or segment shows subsegmental infiltrate. Consolidation is rare. Gram stain of sputum (will show polymorphonuclear leukocytes) and culture.

► Clinical Therapeutics

Otherwise healthy adult without respiratory compromise can be managed as an outpatient with appropriate antibiotics (erythromycin or tetracycline), hydration, and symptomatic relief.

▶ Clinical Intervention

Follow-up is important. Patient should return frequently for re-assessment, follow-up chest x-ray 3 to 6 weeks for resolution confirmation.

▶ Health Maintenance Issues

Counsel patient regarding increased risk with exposure to sick children and exposure if residing in a dormitory or barracks.

IV. PULMONARY TUBERCULOSIS

▶ Scientific Concepts

Mycobacterium tuberculosis is transmitted in droplet form from persons with pulmonary tuberculosis. Inhaled bacteria implant in bronchioles, multiply, and disseminate via lymphatics and the bloodstream. Most people infected by tuberculosis develop only a reaction to the Mantoux skin test. There is a higher percentage of tuberculosis in foreign-born ethnic and racial minorities and the poor. Tuberculosis is a major complication seen in acquired immune deficiency syndrome (AIDS) patients. Patients susceptible to the development of symptomatic tuberculosis include infants, children, adolescents, and the elderly. About 5 to 15% of those infected develop disease secondary to delayed reactivation.

▶ History & Physical

Symptoms include mild malaise and fatigue, night sweats, low-grade fever, weight loss, cough, hemoptysis, adenopathy, and apical rales.

▶ Diagnosis

A Mantoux skin test measures induration, not inflammation. Criteria for a positive Mantoux test varies. A tuberculin reaction of 5 mm or more of induration is considered positive for persons who have had recent contact with a person with infectious tuberculosis; persons with chest x-rays with fibrotic lesions that may represent old, healed tuberculosis; and persons with HIV infections. A tuberculin reaction of 10 mm or more is considered positive in persons who have a medical condition that is likely to increase the risk of tuberculosis once infected (silicosis, diabetes mellitus, immunosuppressive therapy, etc.), persons from high-prevalence countries (Asia, Africa, and Latin America), and high-risk minorities (African Americans, Hispanics, and Native Americans). A tuberculin reaction of 15 mm is considered positive in all other persons.

▶ Diagnostic Studies

The chest x-ray shows patchy or lobar infiltrates in the anterior segments of the upper lobes. The Gram stain of morning sputum or gastric aspiration is positive for acid-fast bacteria. The sputum or gastric aspiration culture is positive for *Mycobacterium tuberculosis*.

► Clinical Therapeutics

Combinations of isoniazid, pyrazinamide, rifampin, ethambutol, and streptomycin are used to treat tuberculosis to avoid the development of resistant strains or to treat resistant strains.

Treatment prophylaxis is indicated for the following patients who test positive: persons with HIV infection, close contacts of infected persons, recent skin test converters, persons with abnormal chest x-rays, IV drug users, persons with medical conditions that increase the risk of tuberculosis. Individuals with a positive skin test who are less than 35 years of age without clinical signs of tuberculosis should be treated with isoniazid if they are from countries with high prevalence rate, a minority group with high risk, have low incomes, or are residents of long-term care facilities. Hepatitis is the major complication of isoniazid therapy. The risk of hepatitis increases directly with age from 0% for those persons under 20 years of age to 2.3% for those greater than 54 years of age. Alcohol ingestion increases the risk of hepatitis. Pyridoxine is given with isoniazid to prevent peripheral neuropathy and other central nervous system (CNS) effects in persons with malnutrition, alcoholism, uremia, diabetes mellitus, pregnancy, or seizure disorder.

► Clinical Intervention

Multiple effective drugs must be used to prevent or deal with resistant strains of bacteria. The drugs must be taken as scheduled and for the recommended duration of treatment. Strategies such as flexible clinic hours, observed ingestion of medications, and offering incentives to patients are used to promote compliance. Rest, oxygen, and chest physical therapy are used in conjunction with antibiotics. Patients should be instructed to take the medications for 2 weeks before exposure to the public. Tuberculosis is a reportable disease. Health care workers caring for infected patients should be fitted with an appropriate respiratory filter device.

► Health Maintenance Issues

See above regarding prophylaxis.

V. CHRONIC AIRWAY OBSTRUCTION—EMPHYSEMA

► Scientific Concepts

COPD is a chronic progressive pulmonary disease that affects middle-aged or older individuals. It is characterized by the destruction of intra-alveolar walls, loss of ventilation perfusion areas, and an increase in lung compliance. Cigarette smoking is a major factor in the development of emphysema, although only 10 to 15% of smokers develop emphysema. It is thought that an imbalance between proteases and antiproteases in the lung is the cause of emphysema. A rare cause of emphysema is an alpha-1-antitrypsin deficiency. Bronchospasm is usually present, although less than that found in asthma.

► History & Physical

Patients present with dyspnea on exertion, cough, and sputum production. On physical examination, there are signs of hyperinflation of the lungs, increased anterior–posterior (AP) diameter of the chest, and flattened diaphragms. Increased compliance of the lungs is indicated by decreased breath sounds with increased expiratory phase of respiration and use of accessory respiratory muscles.

► Diagnosis

Chest x-ray shows hyperinflation of the lung fields with an increased AP diameter, flattening of the diaphragm, and a narrow cardiac silhouette. Parenchymal or subpleural bullae may be seen. Pulmonary function tests show a decreased forced expiratory volume in 1 second (FEV_1) and increased residual volume (RV), functional residual capacity (FRC), and total lung capacity (TLC) with poor response to bronchodilators. Arterial blood gases (ABGs) show hypoxia (decreased partial pressure of oxygen [PO_2]) and, in severe cases, hypercapnia (elevated partial pressure of carbon dioxide [PCO_2]). The hemoglobin may be normal or elevated.

► Differential Diagnosis

Asthma, chronic bronchitis, bronchiectasis, senescent lungs, acute bronchitis.

► Clinical Therapeutics

Sympathomimetics (albuterol): Relax bronchial smooth muscle.
Methylxanthines (aminophylline): Relax bronchial smooth muscle less than sympathomimetics, but have a beneficial effect on cardiac and respiratory muscles.
Anticholinergics (ipratropium bromide): Decrease vagally induced bronchospasm.
Anti-inflammatory agents (corticosteroids): Reduce airway inflammation.
Antibiotics (amoxicillin, TMP-SMZ, tetracycline): Treat infection.

► Clinical Intervention

Includes the judicious use of oxygen, hydration, and pulmonary rehabilitation.

► Health Maintenance Issues

Issues to discuss with the patient are smoking cessation, clean air in the home and work environment, and administration of influenza and pneumococcal vaccines where indicated.

VI. CHRONIC BRONCHITIS (WITH AND WITHOUT OBSTRUCTION)

► Scientific Concepts

Chronic bronchitis is defined by a productive cough for 3 of 12 months per year for 3 years. There is an increased resistance to bronchial air flow due to increased mucous production secondary to hyperplasia and hypertrophy of submucosal mucous glands, inflammation, and edema. Mucous plugging may be present. Smoking is the major contributing factor.

► History & Physical

Patients present with chronic cough, increased sputum production, and frequent infections. Chest examination reveals decreased diaphragmatic excursion, crackles, rhonchi, and wheezes.

► Diagnosis

Chest x-ray may show hyperinflation, flat diaphragm, and narrow cardiac silhouette. ABGs may show decreased PO_2 (hypoxia) and increased PCO_2 (hypercapnia) depending on severity of illness. Hemoglobin may be elevated. A peak flow meter will show decreased FEV_1 depending on degree of bronchospasm and obstruction.

► Differential Diagnosis

Acute bronchitis, asthma, bronchiectasis, emphysema.

► Clinical Therapeutics

Sympathomimetics (albuterol): Relax bronchial smooth muscle.
Methylxanthines (aminophylline): Relax bronchial smooth muscle less than sympathomimetics, but have a beneficial effect on cardiac and respiratory muscles.
Anticholinergics (ipratropium bromide): Decrease vagally induced bronchospasm.
Anti-inflammatory agents (corticosteroids): Reduce airway inflammation.
Antibiotics (amoxicillin, TMP-SMZ, tetracycline): Treat infection.

► Clinical Intervention

Supplemental oxygen, pulmonary rehabilitation, influenza and pneumococcal vaccines recommended for specific patient populations.

► Health Maintenance Issues

Stop smoking, clean air at home and work environment.

VII. PNEUMOCONIOSES

A. Silicosis

► Scientific Concepts

Inhalation of silica dust causes an increase in fibrosis of the lung, decrease in lung volume, decrease in compliance, and decrease in diffusion capacity of the lungs.

► History & Physical

Patient's work history reveals exposure to silica (e.g., mining, quarry work, sandblasting). Patients present with dyspnea on exertion and nonproductive cough. Chest examination demonstrates tachypnea and fine crackles.

▶ Diagnosis

Chest x-ray shows eggshell calcifications of hilar and mediastinal nodes. Bilateral nodular densities progress from the periphery to the hilum. Pulmonary function tests show decrease in vital capacity, functional residual capacity, residual volume, and total lung capacity. Diagnosis can be confirmed by open lung biopsy, which will show fibrosis.

▶ Clinical Therapeutics

No successful therapy for this condition except lung transplant.

▶ Clinical Intervention

Associated respiratory distress may be treated with bronchodilators (albuterol), chest physical therapy, and oxygen. Antibiotics (amoxicillin, TMP-SMZ, tetracycline) indicated for superimposed infections.

▶ Health Maintenance Issues

Avoiding inhalation of silica dust by wearing a respirator in mining, quarrying, and sandblasting.

B. Asbestosis

▶ Scientific Concepts

Asbestosis is seen 15 to 20 years after lengthy exposure to asbestos. Pulmonary consequences are similar to those found in silicosis, with interstitial fibrosis and pleural thickening. Increased risk of malignant mesothelioma of the pleura, bronchogenic carcinoma, and tuberculosis with asbestos exposure.

▶ History & Physical

Patient's work history reveals exposure to asbestos (e.g., renovation or destruction of old buildings, ship building). Patients present with fatigue, dyspnea on exertion, nonproductive cough, and pleuritic pain. Physical examination may reveal rales and pleural effusion. There may be clubbing of the fingers.

▶ Diagnosis

Chest x-ray may show interstitial fibrosis, pleural plaques, and pleural effusions. Pulmonary function tests show decrease in vital capacity, functional residual capacity, residual volume, and total lung capacity. A computed tomographic (CT) scan may be necessary to demonstrate parenchymal fibrosis and pleural plaques. Open lung biopsy will confirm the diagnosis.

▶ Clinical Therapeutics

No acceptable therapy except to treat symptomatically.

▶ Clinical Intervention

Associated respiratory distress may be treated with bronchodilators (albuterol), chest physical therapy, and oxygen. Antibiotics (amoxicillin, TMP-SMZ, tetracyclines) indicated for infections.

► Health Maintenance Issues

Avoiding inhalation of asbestos dust by wearing a respirator in ship-yard work, mining asbestos, boilermaking, and building restoration.

VIII. PULMONARY NEOPLASMS

► Scientific Concepts

Benign neoplasms of the lung include the central bronchial ade-noma and the pulmonary hamartoma commonly found in the lung periphery.

Malignant neoplasms of the lung are the principal cause of cancer deaths in men and women. Thirty-five percent of cancers in men and 18% in women are lung cancer. Carcinoma of the lung commonly presents in the 50- to 60-year-old age group. Cigarette smoking is the risk factor associated with most types of lung cancer. Only bron-chioalveolar carcinoma is not caused by smoking. Secondhand smoke is also a risk factor for the development of lung cancer. Asbestos is the second leading cause of lung cancer.

Clinically, malignant tumors of the lung can be divided into two categories:

Small cell carcinomas typically metastasize early and metastases are found on presentation. Small cell carcinoma accounts for 20 to 30% of malignant lung tumors.

Non–small cell carcinoma is composed of squamous cell carcinoma, adenocarcinoma, bronchioaveolar carcinoma, and large cell carci-noma. These neoplasms usually spread locally in the chest before metastasizing to other locations. Squamous cell carcinoma is the most common cell type. Incidence varies from 40 to 70%. Adenocarcinoma has the greatest tendency to metastasize to the liver, brain, bone, adrenals, and lymph nodes. It accounts for 5 to 15% of malignant lung tumors. Bronchioalveolar carcinoma has the best prognosis. Large cell carcinoma is an aggressive type of adenocarcinoma. Inci-dence varies from 1 to 10%.

► History & Physical

Patients may be asymptomatic when the tumor is found on routine chest x-ray or may present with cough, hemoptysis, shortness of breath or dyspnea on exertion, and weight loss. Bone pain from metastasis may be a symptom in patients with small cell carcinoma. Physical examination of the lung may be negative or one may find rales, rhonchi, and wheezes. Adenopathy may also be present.

► Diagnosis

Diagnostic studies include sputum or bronchial cell washings for cytology, chest x-rays, CT of the lung, bronchoscopy and biopsy, fine needle biopsy, thoracentesis, and mediastinoscopy.

► Differential Diagnosis

Bronchitis, pneumonia, pleural effusion, tuberculosis.

▶ Clinical Therapeutics

Therapeutic options are surgery (non–small cell type), chemotherapy, and radiation therapy as indicated by location, presence or absence of metastases, and cell type.

▶ Clinical Intervention

Regular health maintenance, adequate nutrition, and pain control during therapy and after.

▶ Health Maintenance Issues

Stop smoking, avoid secondhand smoke, avoid asbestos dust.

IX. VIRAL INFECTIONS

A. Pleuritis

▶ Scientific Concepts

Pleuritis is characterized by inflammation of parietal pleura. The pleura may be primarily inflamed or inflammation may be secondary to pneumonia.

▶ History & Physical

Patient presents with pleuritic pain (i.e., sharp, localized pain on deep breathing or cough), cough, fever, and dyspnea. On physical examination, there may be rales, bronchial breath sounds, pleural friction rub, and decreased tactile fremitus.

▶ Diagnosis

Diagnosis is clinical; chest x-ray will be negative unless there is underlying pneumonia.

▶ Differential Diagnosis

The differential diagnosis includes costochondritis, shingles, pericarditis, and pneumonia.

▶ Clinical Therapeutics

Analgesics and antitussives are usually adequate treatment.

▶ Clinical Intervention

Heat and temporary splinting when coughing may provide some relief with the caution that splinting may contribute to atelectasis.

▶ Health Maintenance Issues

Stop smoking; influenza and pneumococcal vaccines when indicated.

B. Empyema

▶ Scientific Concepts

Empyema is a pleural effusion that is infected. The infection may be from hematogenous or lymphatic spread or by direct extension from pneumonia or lung abscess. There are three types of empyema: exudative or thin, fibropurulent or thick, and chronic or organized with capillaries and fibroblasts.

► History & Physical

Patient presents with fever, dyspnea, and cough. Chest examination reveals decreased breath sounds, decreased tactile fremitus, and dullness to percussion over affected lung.

► Diagnosis

Diagnosis made by chest x-ray and thoracentesis. Organisms identified by Gram stain and culture.

► Differential Diagnosis

Differential diagnosis includes pleural effusion and pneumonia.

► Clinical Therapeutics

Antibiotics as indicated by Gram stain and culture. Tube thoracostomy used for drainage and evacuation of purulent material.

► Clinical Intervention

Serial thoracentesis, placement of chest tube, or thoracotomy with decortication of fibrous material are clinical options.

► Health Maintenance Issues

Stop smoking; influenza and pneumococcal vaccines.

X. OTHER DISEASES OF THE PULMONARY SYSTEM

A. Asthma

► Scientific Concepts

Defined as reversible airway obstruction, either spontaneous or with treatment. Airway inflammation and increased airway responsiveness to a variety of stimuli are underlying trigger mechanisms. Pathologic changes are characterized by hypertrophy of bronchial smooth muscle, mucosal edema and hyperemia, thickening of epithelial basement membrane, hypertrophy of mucous glands, acute inflammation, and plugging of airways by thick, viscid mucus. About 4 to 5% of the population have asthma. Men and women are equally affected. Until puberty, asthma is twice as common among boys as among girls and reverses between puberty and early adulthood.

► History & Physical

Patients exhibit a wide range of signs and symptoms, including episodic wheezing, feelings of chest tightness, shortness of breath, and cough. More severe attacks associated with use of accessory muscles, distant breath sounds and loud wheezing, anxiety and apprehension. Attacks may occur spontaneously or in response to various triggers, respiratory infections, emotional stress, or weather changes.

Amount of wheezing is not a reliable indicator for severity of episode, and absence of wheezing may be an ominous sign. Pulsus paradoxus, tachycardia, fatigue, and mental status changes may signal severe attack.

▶ Diagnostic Studies

Careful history, physical examination, and laboratory methods are required. Spirometry provides a means for measuring air flow. Level of airway responsiveness can be measured by inhalation challenge tests using metacholine, histamine, or exposure to a nonpharmacologic agent such as cold air.

▶ Diagnosis

Decreased FEV_1 and peak expiratory flow rate (PEFR). Physical signs vary with severity of attack. A mild attack may produce slight increase in respiratory rate, mild wheezing, and cough. More severe attacks are associated with use of the accessory muscles, distant breath sounds, loud wheezing, fatigue, anxiety, apprehension, severe dyspnea, inaudible breath sounds, and diminished wheezing.

▶ Clinical Therapeutics

Nonpharmacologic methods include education, relaxation techniques, controlled breathing, and a program of desensitization. Pharmacologic treatments include bronchodilators (beta-adrenergic agents, ipratropium, theophylline); anti-inflammatory drugs (cromolyn sodium, corticosteroids); aerosol therapy or metered-dose inhaler for delivery of sympathomimetic, anticholinergic, and corticosteroid drugs.

▶ Clinical Intervention

Status asthmaticus management is similar to severe acute asthma, requiring an aggressive multidrug regimen and hospitalization. If progressive, respiratory acidosis develops and may require tracheal intubation and mechanical ventilation.

▶ Health Maintenance Issues

Discuss etiology and expectation of disease. Demonstrate proper use of metered-dose inhaler. Develop a patient treatment plan for severe exacerbations. Counsel patient on need for yearly influenza vaccine and pneumococcal vaccine.

B. Pleural Effusion

▶ Scientific Concepts

Collection of fluid in space between visceral pleura lining the lungs and parietal pleura covering the diaphragm and chest wall. Pleural effusions are classified according to their chemical characteristics into transudates, exudate, chyle, blood, or empyema.

▶ History & Physical

Patients may be asymptomatic or present with dyspnea, cough, and sometimes pleuritic chest pain. Signs on physical examination include decreased chest excursion over the effusion, reduced tactile fremitus, dullness to percussion, and decreased breath sounds.

► Diagnostic Studies

Lateral decubitus chest x-ray showing free fluid in the pleural space. Ultrasound is useful to find the site for thoracentesis. Routine laboratory tests of pleural fluid should include total and differential white blood cell count, protein, lactic dehydrogenase (LDH) and glucose with accompanying values for serum, and Gram stain. Additional tests (culture, acid-fast bacilli, or cytology) may be ordered as required after thoracentesis. Pleural fluid pH is helpful in narrowing differential diagnosis of exudative effusions. The pH is usually 7.4 or greater; pH is commonly below 7.2 when empyema is present.

► Diagnosis

Exudate: absolute protein > 3.0 g/mL, pleural fluid to serum protein ratio > 0.5, pleural to serum LDH > 200 IU/L. Transudates generally require no further search for an etiology and are commonly caused by congestive heart failure, cirrhosis, and hypoalbuminemic states.

► Clinical Therapeutics

Appropriate treatment of pleural effusion depends on underlying etiology.

C. Pleurisy—No Effusion

► Scientific Concepts

Primary infection of the pleura is usually caused by a virus (especially enteroviruses). May also occur as a result of trauma, neoplasm, or any process involving the underlying lung.

► History & Physical

Pain, usually sharp, limited to area in which the pleura is inflamed, worsened by deep breath or cough. Physical examination reveals friction rub over inflamed pleura or pericardium. Aside from low-grade fever and possible friction rub, other findings are usually normal.

► Diagnostic Studies

History, associated symptoms, physical examination, and chest x-ray.

► Diagnosis

It is important to differentiate pleural pain from pain produced by other conditions requiring immediate attention and hospitalization such as pulmonary emboli, empyema, or pneumothorax. Pleurisy is often a diagnosis of exclusion after a normal perfusion lung scan.

► Clinical Therapeutics

Management depends entirely on the underlying diagnosis responsible for the pain. Nonnarcotic pain medications are the initial therapy. Nonsteroidal anti-inflammatory drugs relieve pain and inflammation.

► Clinical Intervention

Occasionally, intercostal nerve blocks with injections of an anesthetic agent are used for refractory pain.

D. Pneumothorax

► Scientific Concepts

Pneumothorax occurs when air enters the pleural cavity, causing partial or complete collapse of the affected lung. Can occur without obvious cause or injury (spontaneous) or as a result of direct injury to chest or major airways (traumatic). Tension pneumothorax is a life-threatening condition of excessive pressure within the pleural cavity.

► History & Physical

Patients present with pleuritic chest pain, increased respiratory rate, asymmetry of the chest, hyperresonant sound to percussion, and decreased or absent breath sounds over the area of the pneumothorax. Deviated trachea, severe tachycardia, hypotension with tension pneumothorax.

► Diagnostic Studies

Confirmed by chest x-ray, which demonstrates a visceral pleural line best revealed on an expiratory film. In tension pneumothorax, chest x-ray shows a large amount of air in the affected hemithorax and contralateral shift of mediastinal structures. Pulse oximetry or ABGs may reveal hypoxia.

► Clinical Therapeutics

Treatment varies with the cause and extent of the disorder. Without treatment in small (10 to 20%) pneumothoraces, the air usually reabsorbs. In large pneumothoraces, needle aspiration or closed drainage system is indicated. Tension pneumothorax treatment involves prompt insertion of large-bore needle or chest tube for decompression.

E. Pulmonary Embolism

► Scientific Concepts

Develops when a blood-borne substance lodges in a branch of the pulmonary artery and obstructs blood flow. The embolism may consist of a thrombus, air, fat, or amniotic fluid. Almost all pulmonary emboli are due to deep vein thromboses.

► History & Physical

Chest pain, dyspnea, and increased respiratory rate are the most frequent signs and symptoms. Can also present with apprehension, cough, hemoptysis, diaphoresis, and syncope (especially with massive pulmonary embolism). Pulmonary infarction causes pleuritic pain, moderate hypoxemia, and blood-stained sputum. Signs include tachycardia, tachypnea, crackles, and accentuation of the pulmonary component of the second heart sound.

► Diagnostic Studies

Blood gases reveal respiratory alkalosis, lung scan (perfusion, ventilation, or both), chest x-ray, electrocardiogram (nonspecific ST changes or right ventricular strain), and, in selected cases, angiography.

► Diagnosis

X-ray may show elevation of a hemidiaphragm and pulmonary infiltration, platelike atelectasis, oligemia in the embolized lung zone (Westermark sign), and prominence of pulmonary artery. A ventilation-perfusion lung scan may be abnormal in other diseases (COPD, asthma, CHF) as well, but an abnormal scan may support the diagnosis. Pulmonary angiography, which can detect emboli as small as 3 mm in diameter, remains the definitive test for diagnosis.

► Clinical Therapeutics

For acute pulmonary thromboembolism, heparin is the anticoagulant of choice. The use of thrombolytic therapy in clinical practice is controversial. Pharmacologic prophylaxis involves use of anticoagulant drugs. Low-dose subcutaneous heparin may be administered to decrease likelihood of deep vein thrombosis, thromboembolism, and fatal pulmonary embolism before and after major surgical procedures. Surgical interruption of the inferior vena cava is indicated with recurrent pulmonary embolism, which can be achieved by ligation, plication, clipping, or insertion of intraluminal filters. Prevention may be accomplished by using physical measures (external pneumatic compression of the legs, early ambulation, elevation of legs for immobilized patients, active and passive leg exercises), low-dose heparin, and antiplatelet drugs in patients at risk.

► Health Maintenance Issues

Identification of people at risk (prolonged bedrest, trauma, surgery, childbirth, obesity, fractures of hip and femur, advanced age, myocardial infarction, congestive heart failure, spinal cord injury); avoidance of venous stasis; early detection of venous thrombosis and hypercoagulability states.

F. Adult Respiratory Distress Syndrome (ARDS)

► Scientific Concepts

Extreme form of noncardiac pulmonary edema as a result of injury to the microcirculation of the lung, including diffuse alveolocapillary injury with increased permeability and abnormal surfactant following a wide variety of systemic or pulmonary insults. The mortality rate associated with ARDS exceeds 50%. If accompanied by sepsis, mortality rate may reach 90%. The major cause of death is multiple organ system failure often with sepsis.

► History & Physical

Progressive respiratory distress, increase in respiratory rate, signs of respiratory failure (labored breathing, tachypnea, intercostal retractions, and crackles).

► Diagnosis

Radiologic findings show extensive bilateral diffuse consolidation of lung tissue. Severe hypoxia persists despite increased inspired oxygen levels. Most patients demonstrate multiple organ failure (kidneys, liver, gut, central nervous system, cardiovascular system).

► Clinical Therapeutics

Treatment goals are to supply oxygen to vital organs and provide supportive care (mechanical ventilation, positive end-expiratory pressure, etc.) until pathologic processes have been reversed and lungs have had a chance to heal.

G. Sarcoidosis

► Scientific Concepts

Multisystem granulomatous disorder of unknown etiology, characterized by exaggerated cellular immune response manifested by noncaseating granulomatous inflammation in affected organs such as the lungs, lymph nodes, eyes, skin, liver, spleen, salivary glands, heart, and nervous system. Young adults are more frequently affected; in the United States it is more common and severe in black patients of African–Caribbean origin.

► History & Physical

Has variable manifestations and an unpredictable course of progression in which any organ system can be affected. Common respiratory symptoms include cough, dyspnea, and chest discomfort. Often presents with bilateral hilar adenopathy and erythema nodosum or uveitis. Nonspecific symptoms are fever, sweating, anorexia, weight loss, fatigue, and myalgia.

► Diagnosis

Almost all patients have abnormal chest x-ray revealing symmetric bilateral hilar and right paratracheal adenopathy, interstitial infiltrates, or both. Diagnosis depends on compatible clinical and radiographic picture and tissue biopsy. Diagnosis usually made using transbronchial lung biopsy, bronchial lavage, the Kveim–Siltzbach skin test, and serum angiotensin-converting enzyme test.

► Clinical Therapeutics

Ninety percent are responsive to corticosteroids and easily controlled on modest maintenance dose when the disease has significant interference with normal life. Review of symptoms, serial radiographs, and serial measurement of ventilatory function and carbon monoxide diffusing capacity usually clearly indicate course of disease.

► Clinical Intervention

Approximately 50% develop permanent pulmonary abnormalities; 5 to 15% have progressive pulmonary fibrosis. Chronic fibrocystic sarcoidosis leads to a clinical picture that resembles bronchiectasis, with chronic productive cough. Hemoptysis can occur and is sometimes life-threatening.

▶ **Health Maintenance Issues**
Pneumococcal and influenza vaccines are recommended.

XI. SYMPTOMS REFERABLE TO THE PULMONARY SYSTEM

A. Cough

▶ **Scientific Concepts**
Neurally mediated reflex that protects the lungs from accumulation of secretions and from entry of irritating and destructive substances.

▶ **History & Physical**
Cough receptors are located throughout the larynx, trachea, bronchi, ear canals, pleurae, stomach, nose, sinuses, pharynx, pericardium, and diaphragm. History should focus on smoking habits, environmental exposures, medications, duration and character of the cough, productive vs. nonproductive, and associated symptoms of respiratory, gastrointestinal, neurologic, and heart disease.

▶ **Diagnostic Studies**
Diagnostic studies are obtained based on history and physical findings such as chest x-ray, spirometry, nasopharyngeal culture, barium swallow, laryngoscopy.

▶ **Diagnosis**
History and physical usually suggest the diagnosis.

▶ **Clinical Therapeutics**
Treatment should be directed at the underlying cause. Cautious use of antitussive agents is warranted. Syrups, lozenges, and topical anesthetics may be helpful. Mucolytics and expectorants are of uncertain value.

B. Dyspnea

▶ **Scientific Concepts**
Generally a sign that pulmonary gas exchange is inadequate. It is a subjective sensation of discomfort associated with difficult or labored breathing.

▶ **History & Physical**
A comprehensive history and detailed physical examination help differentiate cardiac from pulmonary causes.

▶ **Diagnostic Studies**
Chest x-ray, pulmonary function tests, hemoglobin level, thyroid function studies, electrocardiogram, oximetry, and cardiopulmonary exercise testing.

► Diagnosis

A careful, stepwise approach to the complaint will yield a diagnosis.

► Clinical Therapeutics

Relieve the underlying disorder responsible for dyspnea. Supportive and therapeutic use of oxygen and pulmonary training (alter precipitating factors, pulmonary medication compliance, wear mask with cold exposure).

C. Stridor

► Scientific Concepts

Collapse of the upper airways (e.g., laryngomalacia) or increased turbulence of air moving through obstructed airways produces an audible crowing sound called stridor. Impairment above the vocal cords typically produces inspiratory stridor whereas obstructions below will produce mixed or primarily expiratory stridor.

► History & Physical

Usually preceded by URIs that cause rhinorrhea, coryza, hoarseness, and low-grade fever.

► Diagnostic Studies

Chest x-ray and soft tissue neck film.

► Clinical Therapeutics

Usually subsides with exposure to moist air; high, cold humidity; expectorants; antibiotics; bronchodilating agents and antihistamines are not helpful.

XII. FOREIGN BODY IN TRACHEA

► Scientific Concepts

May or may not obstruct the airway and can act as a ball valve. In 20% of cases, the object is in the upper airway; in 80%, it is in the main stem or lobar bronchus. Anatomic variations make it easier for foreign bodies to enter the right main bronchus than to enter the left. Occurs less frequently in adults than in children. The elderly and denture wearers appear to be at greatest risk.

► History & Physical

Classic triad is wheezing, cough, and decreased breath sounds. Other symptoms may include cough, dysphagia, stridor, pain, and dyspnea. History is usually highly suggestive, with a brief asymptomatic interval, then sudden dyspnea, coughing, and gagging after handling a small object.

► Diagnostic Studies

Laboratory evaluation is not helpful. Chest x-ray (expiratory) can be normal or show hyperinflation, atelectasis, infiltrate, or visualization of the foreign body.

► Diagnosis

Lateral neck x-rays for radiopaque foreign bodies in the neck. If lower airway, decubitus films in expiration may reveal more subtle degrees of hyperinflation.

► Clinical Therapeutics

If obstruction is complete and airway clearance maneuvers fail (e.g., Heimlich), remove object by laryngoscopy/bronchoscopy.

► Health Maintenance Issues

Counsel parents on home management. Most airway obstructions occur between the ages of 1 and 5 years. For total obstruction in patients less than 1 year old, back blows and chest thrusts; Heimlich maneuver for all others. Caution parents to keep small objects such as jewelry, toys, pins, peanuts, or candy out of reach.

BIBLIOGRAPHY

Fihn SD, DeWitt DE. *Outpatient Medicine,* 2nd ed., Chapters 19, 54, Section VII. Philadelphia: WB Saunders; 1998.

Rudy DR, Kurowski K. *Family Medicine.* Chapters 11, 12, 30. Baltimore: Williams & Wilkins; 1997.

Saunders CE, Ho MT. *Current Emergency Diagnosis & Treatment,* 4th ed. Chapters 5, 18, 27. Norwalk, CT: Appleton & Lange; 1992.

Stobo JD, Hellmann DB, Ladenson PW, Petty BG, Traill TA. *The Principles and Practice of Medicine,* 23rd ed., Norwalk, CT: Appleton & Lange; 1996.

Tierney LM Jr., McPhee SJ, Papadakis MA, eds. *Current Medical Diagnosis & Treatment.* Chapter 9. Norwalk, CT: Appleton & Lange; 1994.

Cardiovascular Diseases 5

Richard R. Rahr, EdD, PA-C, Salah Ayachi, PhD, PA-C

I. ANGINA PECTORIS

▶ Scientific Concepts

Angina pectoris (AP) is substernal chest pain usually brought on by exertion, stress, eating, sexual activity, emotional stress, or cold weather. Episodes last from 15 to 30 minutes after the causative event, usually relieved by rest. Substernal pain is described as tightness, squeezing, burning, pressing, choking, aching, bursting or "gaslike" pain that radiates to the neck, shoulder, or left arm. The etiology of chest pain is ischemia of the heart muscle due to narrowing of the coronary arteries, usually due to atherosclerosis. However, congenital anomalies, spasms, and aortic stenosis can cause the pain. Usually a family history of coronary artery disease (CAD), diabetes, hyperlipidemia, and hypertension. The risk factors for CAD contributing to chest pain are smoking, stress, inactivity, and high-fat diet. One hallmark of angina pectoris is that pain is relieved in 2 to 3 minutes by administration of nitroglycerin.

▶ History & Physical

The most salient historical finding is the onset of substernal pain with exertion and its rapid relief with rest or nitroglycerin. There is a strong family history of CAD. Patient usually has a profile of risk factors: cigarette smoking, hyperlipidemia, hypertension, obesity and a sedentary lifestyle; a stressful occupation (e.g., airline pilots, air traffic controllers); or a recent period of strenuous activity as is seen in older people. There can be heart murmurs (Table 5–1) and palpitations (Table 5–2). AP is a historical diagnosis with advanced atherosclerosis as underlying disease. Table 5–3 lists cardiac and noncardiac causes of chest pain. The degree of cardiac involvement should be diagnosed with stress testing, angiography, thallium imagery, or exercise echocardiogram.

▶ Diagnostic Studies

Patients will need a baseline electrocardiogram (ECG) and echocardiogram, stress test, and perhaps exercise or stress thallium test.

▶ table 5-1

MURMURS

Type	Location	Radiation	Pitch	Sound
Mitral stenosis	4th–5th ICS, LS	None	Low	Crescendo
Mitral insufficiency	PMI	Axilla	Med–High	Holosystolic
Aortic stenosis	R 2nd ICS	Carotid	Med–High	Crescendo–Decrescendo
Aortic insufficiency	L 3rd–4th ICS	Apex	High	Decrescendo
Tricuspid stenosis	3rd–5th ICS, LS	None	Medium	Crescendo
Tricuspid insufficiency	3rd–5th ICS, LS	None	Medium	Holosystolic

ICS, intercostal space; LS, left sternal border; PMI, point of maximal impulse.

Exercise testing is considered the most useful noninvasive procedure for evaluating angina and to confirm the diagnosis of angina. A complete blood count (CBC), chest x-ray, and Holter monitor can also be useful in confirming the diagnosis. The definitive diagnosis may require coronary arteriograms to identify number and disease state of coronary vessels involved.

▶ Diagnosis

The mainstay of a diagnosis of AP is based on historical findings with laboratory verification of underlying atherosclerosis. There are several other diseases or syndromes that mimic angina that must be considered. Costochondritis (Teitze syndrome) or anterior chest wall pain, vertebral disk disease, lung cancer, pneumonia, rib fracture, pneumothorax, and preeruptive shingles can also be confused for angina. Therefore, a careful history and physical are necessary to pinpoint the exact etiology (see Table 5–3).

▶ Clinical Therapeutics

There are two major approaches to treatment of AP: medical intervention and surgical/radiographic intervention. Medical treatment calls for use of short- or long-acting nitroglycerin preparations (oral tablet, spray, patch) in rapid- or long-acting form to achieve venodilation. Additional drugs, including beta blockers (propranolol, metoprolol, nadolol, atenolol), calcium channel blockers (amlodipine, diltiazem, verapamil), and antiplatelet forming drugs (aspirin), are effective in reducing intensity and severity of pain.

Surgical intervention includes coronary arteriograms, angioplasty with stent placement, coronary artery bypass grafts (CABGs), and atherectomy (shave and laser procedures) to reduce the blockage and improve blood flow. Mortality rate with ejection fractions of 55% or greater is 1 to 3%; with ejection fractions of < 35%, mortality rate increases rapidly. Rate of patency 6 months after CABG is 85 to 90%, whereas with angioplasty restenosis is 30 to 40% for the same period. The major treatment intervention is to reduce smoking and dietary lipids and control blood pressure.

▶ Clinical Intervention

Unstable angina or crescendo angina occurs when chest pain becomes more frequent (requiring more nitroglycerin to relieve the pain), when it occurs at rest, or chest pain lasts longer. Many of these patients are at risk of occlusion of the involved artery because of plaque rupture, ulceration, or hemorrhage. This could lead to an acute myocardial infarction (MI) with full occlusion, and requires immediate intervention with oxygen, bedrest, monitoring, and sedation with benzodiazepines. Patient is treated with heparin or aspirin, nitroglycerin, beta blockers, calcium channel blockers, and thrombolytics. If this does not relieve the pain, coronary arteriography and revascularization are needed. In unstable angina, 10 to 30% of patients will have MI. The one-year mortality rate is 10 to 20%. Stress testing and coronary angiography are needed in most cases to fully assess the patient.

▶ table 5-2

PALPITATIONS

- Normal
- Increased cardiac output
- Increased stroke volume
- Thyrotoxicosis
- Anemia
- Anxiety
- Exercise
- Cardiac arrhythmias—supraventricular tachycardia, ventricular tachycardia

▶ table 5-3

CAUSES OF CHEST PAIN

Cardiac Causes
- Angina pectoris
- Acute myocardial infarction
- Pericarditis
- Myocarditis
- Cardiomyopathy
- Valvular heart disease

Noncardiac Causes
- Lung mass
- Aortic aneurysm
- Disk disease
- Cholecystitis
- Esophageal disease
- Pneumothorax
- Teitze syndrome
- Peptic ulcer disease
- Anxiety states
- Musculoskeletal disease

► Health Maintenance Issues

Patients whose first episode of ischemia is silent may suddenly die. These patients have a history of hyperlipidemia, are overweight, have a strong family history of CAD, have hypertension, smoke cigarettes, and have sedentary and high-stress lifestyles. Screening programs for hypertension, hyperlipidemia, and other risk factors, as well as preexercise programs, are effective in preventing sudden death.

II. ACUTE MYOCARDIAL INFARCTION

► Scientific Concepts

Normal function of the pumping heart requires patent arteries to provide normal blood flow. Therefore, any substantial (75% or higher) narrowing of the arteries causes disruption in this function. When coronary arteries are completely blocked by a thrombus or by severe spasm for a long period of time, an acute MI occurs. The patient who experiences severe substernal chest pain for 30 minutes, unrelieved by three nitroglycerin tablets given at 5-minute intervals, may be experiencing an MI. In 20 to 25% of MI cases, patient may experience no pain. Coronary artery obstruction may be due to thrombosis, vasospasms, vasculitis, dissection aneurysm, or cocaine use. When the left coronary artery is involved, an anterior or septal infarct occurs; involvement of the right coronary artery results in posterior-inferior, septal, or right ventricular infarct. Left circumflex artery involvement results in anterolateral or posterolateral infarct. Underlying pathogenesis is atherosclerosis with marked narrowing of the coronary arteries, which may be seen in families with a history of heart disease or other risk factors (Table 5–4).

► History & Physical

Most patients (80%) present with substernal chest pain that radiates to the jaw, left shoulder, arm, throat, precordium, or retrosternal area. Twenty percent of patients present with no pain. Typically, patients with long-standing AP will have to take three sublingual nitroglycerin tablets without relief. Twenty percent of patients die in the first hour after the onset of pain, before reaching the hospital. About one-third of patients present with symptoms of indigestion. Many pa-

► table 5-4

OTHER FACTORS, MYOCARDIAL INFARCTION

- 30% of patients who undergo cardiac evaluation do not have cardiac disease.
- 25% of cases of myocardial infarction are painless.
- Nitroglycerin is mostly ineffective in ameliorating pain due to myocardial infarction.
- 20% of myocardial infarction cases die before reaching the hospital.

tients present with shock, congestive heart failure (CHF), syncope, or pulmonary edema. Signs of heart failure include jugular venous distention, orthopnea, cough, wheezing, and arrhythmias. Physical findings include edema; cyanosis; S3, S4 gallops; mitral murmur; and possibly edema and fever.

▶ Diagnostic Studies

The ECG is evaluated for S-T segment elevation with transmural infarction and S-T segment depression with subendocardial ischemia, T wave inversion, and Q waves; 30 to 50% of cases do not show Q waves. Serial cardiac enzymes—creatine kinase MB band (CK-MB), alanine transaminase (ALT), and lactic dehydrogenase (LDH)—and troponin T and troponin I levels are the most reliable diagnostic markers. Baseline studies of CBC, electrolytes, chest x-ray (CXR), oxygen saturation, arterial blood gases (ABGs), and creatinine are obtained. Technetium scans, using pyrophosphate (hot spots) or thallium (cold spots), are used to evaluate the size and function of the necrotic tissue.

▶ Diagnosis

The pattern of enzyme elevation diagnostic of infarct entails peaking CK-MB at 12 to 48 hours, ALT at 48 to 72 hours, and LDH at 3 to 5 hours. Troponin T and troponin I peak 3 to 5 days following an MI. The hallmark of diagnosis is either pathologic Q wave on ECG (in cases of transmural infarcts) or elevated isoenzymes. Area of scar tissue is determined by technetium scan. Angiograms often performed to determine location and degree of vascular obstruction.

▶ Clinical Therapeutics

Treatment with tissue plasminogen activator (t-PA), streptokinase, or other thrombolytics within 1 to 3 hours can reduce mortality rates by 50%. A 10% reduction in mortality can be achieved with treatment up to 12 hours after infarction. Thrombolytics should not be used when there is no evidence of S-T segment changes on serial ECGs; they are contraindicated in patients with history of cerebrovascular event, marked hypertension, suspected aortic dissection, or active internal bleeding. Relative contraindications include current use of anticoagulants, recent invasive procedures, and others. All patients are admitted to cardiac care unit and given oxygen, liquid low-salt diet, and morphine for pain. Patients are given nitroglycerin to reduce preload in the acute phase; this is not useful for prophylaxis. If premature ventricular contractions (PVCs) develop, lidocaine can be used to suppress arrhythmia during first 24 hours. However, lidocaine is no longer used for prophylactic suppression of ventricular arrhythmias. Angiotensin-converting enzyme (ACE) inhibitors are frequently used to reduce afterload when ejection fraction is below 35%. Up to 5% of MI patients develop ventricular fibrillation; 80% of these cases develop in the first 24 hours.

▶ Clinical Intervention

t-PA and streptokinase administration, angiography, angioplasty, and CABG reserved for treatment of difficult and refractory cases. In cases of cardiogenic shock, advanced life support becomes necessary.

► **Health Maintenance Issues**

Risk factors for atherosclerosis or CAD must be controlled. Hyperlipidemia, stress, hypertension, lack of exercise, cigarette smoking, and obesity must all be addressed in rehabilitation phase of treatment.

III. PRINZMETAL'S (VARIANT) ANGINA

► **Scientific Concepts**

Clinical syndrome in which chest pain and S-T segment elevation occur secondary to coronary artery spasm. Primarily strikes women under age 50. Affected individuals may awaken from sleep with arrhythmias or conduction disorders usually associated with right coronary artery obstruction. Diagnosis can be made from transient S-T elevation as seen on Holter monitor. Complete workup, including coronary arteriography, is needed to identify fixed lesions.

► **History & Physical**

Patients usually present with intermittent episodes of chest pain and palpitations that occur in early morning hours. Patients tend to be younger than other cardiac patients, and frequently smoke cigarettes or use cocaine.

► **Diagnostic Studies**

Useful diagnostic tests include ECG, use of a Holter monitor, stress test, coronary arteriography, and echocardiography. If lesions are not observed, spasm should be suspected. Ergonovine can be given intravenously (IV) to reproduce arteriolar spasm. IV nitroglycerin is used to reverse spasm.

► **Diagnosis**

Positive ergonovine test, in the absence of fixed lesions and transient S-T segment elevation on Holter monitoring, is diagnostic of Prinzmetal's angina.

► **Clinical Therapeutics**

Nitrates or calcium channel blockers are effective prophylactic agents. Patients with fixed stenosis may benefit from beta blockers.

► **Clinical Intervention**

Surgery may be warranted when spasms are associated with fixed stenoses.

► **Health Maintenance Issues**

Patients should abstain from smoking cigarettes and cocaine use.

IV. CONGESTIVE HEART FAILURE

► Scientific Concepts

CHF is understood to be left heart failure (LHF) in which the left ventricle can no longer forcefully contract to produce an adequate stroke volume, leading to low cardiac output and tissue hypoxia. Symptoms include dyspnea, fatigue, cough, orthopnea, paroxysmal nocturnal dyspnea, and dyspnea on exertion (DOE) (Table 5–5). Physical findings include pulmonary congestion, rales, and gallops (S3, S4).

Right heart failure (RHF) occurs when failure leads to backup of blood, resulting in jugular venous distention, hepatic congestion, dependent edema, and ascites. There is rapid weight gain from fluid accumulation resulting in peripheral presacral edema and ascites (Table 5–6).

A third type of heart failure, referred to as high-output failure, is caused by the inability of the heart to meet demands associated with certain disease conditions, include thyrotoxicosis, anemia, arteriovenous shunting, beriberi, or Paget's disease. This type of heart failure is easiest to correct.

Heart failure can also be described as either systolic or diastolic. Diastolic failure occurs when the atrium becomes stiff and unable to contract or becomes overstretched. May be reversed with ACE inhibitors or vasodilators. Systolic failure results in reduced ejection fraction. Can be managed with diuretics to reduce preload, ACE inhibitors to reduce afterload, and inotropic drugs to increase myocardial contractility.

► table 5-5

CAUSES OF DYSPNEA

Pulmonary Causes
- Airway disease (asthma, chronic obstructive pulmonary disease)
- Lung parenchyma (pulmonary fibrosis)
- Pleural disease (pleural effusion or pneumothorax)
- Respiratory muscle disease (myasthenia gravis)

Nonpulmonary Causes
- Cardiac (congestive heart failure, cardiomyopathy, hypertrophic obstructive cardiomyopathy, angina pectoris)
- Anxiety (hyperventilation syndrome)
- Anemia
- Shock
- Abdominal distention
- Deconditioning
- Hypermetabolic state
- Malnutrition syndrome (hypoalbuminemia)
- Obesity (hypoventilation syndrome)

► table 5-6

CAUSES AND LOCATION OF EDEMA

Causes
- Venous insufficiency
- Nephrotic syndrome
- Premenstrual syndrome
- Congestive heart failure
- Cirrhosis
- Drugs (nonsteroidal anti-inflammatory drugs, calcium channel blockers)
- Malabsorption syndrome (hypoalbuminemia)
- Pre-eclampsia, eclampsia
- Thyroid (hyperthyroidism)
- Renal (glomerulonephritis)

Location
- Pretibial (erect)
- Presacral (bedfast)

Heart failure may be caused by CAD, valvular heart disease, systemic or pulmonary hypertension, MI, or cardiomyopathy, and results in increased end-diastolic volume or preload. Increased preload leads to overstretching of cardiac muscle fibers and decreased stroke volume. Increased catecholamine release, angiotensin production, and increased vascular resistance or afterload early in heart failure further aggravate the condition.

► History & Physical
The major symptoms of LHF are dyspnea, DOE, fatigue, orthopnea, and paroxysmal nocturnal dyspnea. Patients with RHF complain of dependent edema, swollen abdomen, and right upper quadrant pain because of hepatic congestion. RHF patients also present with jugular venous distention, dependent edema, hepatomegaly, and ascites. LHF results in cyanosis, pleural effusions, wheezing, basilar rales, murmurs, and gallops (S3, S4). Cough is a common finding in LHF and in RHF precipitated by LHF.

► Diagnostic Studies
Baseline workup includes thyroid tests, ECG, CXR, electrolytes, CBC, renal function studies, echocardiography, coronary arteriography, and stress testing. If cardiomyopathy is suspected, biopsy is needed to verify underlying cause(s).

► Diagnosis
Heart failure has many causes. Valvular heart disease may be congenital, stenotic, or regurgitant. Infectious processes and chamber dilation may be underlying causes. Myocardial diseases include CAD, MI, and myocarditis. Increased workload may be due to anemia, thyrotoxicosis, septicemia, and systemic or pulmonary hypertension. CHF can be precipitated by volume overload due to excess IV fluids.

► Clinical Therapeutics
The most common therapies include:
1. Place patient on 2.0-g sodium diet.
2. Administer diuretics, usually furosemide (loop diuretic).
3. Administer ACE inhibitor such as captopril.
4. Administer digoxin to patients with systolic failure or low ejection fraction.
5. Use vasodilator such as isosorbide dinitrate or hydralazine to reduce afterload.
6. Consider beta blockers for improvement of heart failure.
7. Avoid calcium channel blockers since they may worsen the condition.
8. Consider anticoagulation in LHF to prevent systemic emboli.
9. Administer antiarrhythmics if patient has ventricular arrhythmias such as frequent PVCs or ventricular tachycardia.

► Clinical Intervention
The prognosis is very poor for patients with CHF, particularly if the ejection fraction is below 20%. In stable patients, the mortality rate is 10%; in unstable patients, 30%.

▶ **Health Maintenance Issues**

Rapid improvement of CHF can be achieved by limiting daily dietary salt intake to 2 g.

V. INFECTIVE ENDOCARDITIS

▶ **Scientific Concepts**

Patients who develop endocarditis usually have organic heart lesions resulting from open heart surgery, IV drug use, artificial valves, or congenital defects (e.g., patent ductus arteriosus). Dental or urologic procedures may precipitate these events. Patients with valvular damage due to rheumatic fever are at higher risk of developing endocarditis. They may develop fever, chills, systemic emboli, and positive blood cultures for organisms most likely to be involved—*Streptococcus viridans* (60% of cases), and *Staphylococcus aureus* (20% of cases). Ten percent of cases result from gastrointestinal procedures. The most common causes of endocarditis are:

- Rheumatic fever
- Mitral valve prolapse
- Ventricular septal defect
- Tetralogy of Fallot
- Aortic coarctation
- Patent ductus arteriosus
- Hypertrophic obstructive cardiomyopathy (formerly idiopathic hypertrophic subaortic stenosis)
- Calcified valves
- Gastrointestinal procedures
- Urologic procedures
- Dental procedures

▶ **History & Physical**

Most patients have fever and chills for about 2 weeks accompanied by cough, dyspnea, arthralgia, diarrhea, and abdominal pain. Physical examination reveals murmurs, petechiae, splinter hemorrhages, Janeway lesions, Roth spots, pallor, Osler nodes, and splenomegaly. CBC shows leukocytosis and anemia. Patients may have hematuria, proteinuria, and renal dysfunction. Serial blood cultures (× 3) are most important to identify organisms over a 24-hour period before initiation of treatment. Fungal cultures are negative 50% of the time. CXR shows pulmonary infiltrates or single-chamber enlargement; echocardiography is used to identify valves involved.

▶ **Diagnostic Studies**

1. Blood cultures—definitive diagnosis
2. CXR—pulmonary infiltrates
3. Echocardiography—infected valves
4. CBC—elevated white blood count, anemia
5. Urinalysis—hematuria, proteinuria

► Diagnosis
Duke University criteria for diagnosing endocarditis:
1. Major criteria:
   • Positive blood culture to identify organism involved
   • Positive echocardiography to show vegetations on valves

2. Minor criteria:
   • Predisposing condition (valve damage)
   • Fever of 38°C or higher
   • Embolic disease
   • Immunologic phenomena (e.g., glomerulonephritis, Osler node, Roth spots, rheumatoid factor)
   • Positive blood culture not meeting major criteria
   • Positive echocardiogram not meeting major criteria

Two major or one major plus three minor, or five minor yield 80% accuracy of diagnosis.

► Clinical Therapeutics
Empiric therapy (before culture results are available), give:
1. Nafcillin, 1.5 g q4h or
2. Penicillin, 2 to 3 million units q4h or
3. Gentamicin, 1 mg/kg q8h or
4. Vancomycin, 15 mg/kg q12h for patients allergic to penicillin
   For cultures positive for *Streptococcus viridans:*
1. Penicillin, 2 to 3 million units IV q4h × 4 weeks or
2. Gentamicin, 1 mg/kg q8h × 2 weeks
   For blood cultures positive for enterococci
1. Penicillin as above or
2. Gentamicin as above
   For *staphylococcus aureus:*
1. Nafcillin, 2 g q4h × 4 to 6 weeks or
2. Oxacillin, 2 g q4h × 4 to 6 weeks

► Clinical Intervention
Surgical intervention for severe valve involvement.

► Health Maintenance Issues
1. Prophylactic antibiotic therapy for the following procedures:
   • Dental procedures
   • Genitourinary procedures
   • Gastrointestinal procedures
   • Cardiac catheterization
   • Pulmonary surgery

2. Prophylactic antibiotic therapy for the following conditions:
   • Prosthetic valves
   • Previous episodes of subacute bacterial endocarditis
   • Congenital heart disease
   • Hypertrophic obstructive cardiomyopathy (HOCM)
   • Mitral valve prolapse
   • Pulmonary shunt

3. Antibiotic treatment—benzathine penicillin, 1.2 million units q4wk

VI. CARDIOMYOPATHY

► **Scientific Concepts**

Cardiomyopathy is a constellation of diseases that affect the cardiac muscle and result in CHF. Major causes include ischemia, hypertension, valvular or congenital defects. Viral myocarditis, toxins, alcohol, nutritional deficiencies, and connective tissue diseases may also be involved.

Cardiomyopathies may be classified into three categories: dilated, hypertrophic, and restrictive. In dilated cardiomyopathy, left ventricle is dilated and associated systolic dysfunction is present. Many dilated cardiomyopathies are idiopathic. Alcohol abuse and myocarditis have been implicated in cardiac fibrosis.

In hypertrophic cardiomyopathy such as HOCM, left ventricle is small and hypercontractile, with associated left ventricular outflow obstruction. There is a genetic element to these cardiomyopathies.

The restrictive cardiomyopathies are rare and characterized by impaired diastolic filling in the face of intact contractile function. Diseases such as sarcoidosis, hemochromatosis, carcinoid syndrome, scleroderma, and amyloidosis result in restrictive cardiomyopathy. May also be a sequela of radiation therapy and open heart surgery.

► **History & Physical**

Dilated cardiomyopathy: The most common symptom is dyspnea. Paroxysmal nocturnal dyspnea (PND), orthopnea, DOE, fatigue, and edema also common findings. Physical examination findings include hypotension, rales, tachycardia, large and displaced point of maximal impulse (PMI), cool extremities, edema, jugular venous distention, ascites. Mitral murmurs and S3 gallops can be found when examining the heart.

Hypertrophic cardiomyopathy: Patient presents with dyspnea, chest pain, syncope with exertion; may experience palpitations and frequent cardiac arrhythmias. It is not uncommon to have young athletes experience *sudden death* after exertion. On physical examination, they are found to have enlarged PMI, S4 gallops, systolic murmurs, and bisferiens carotid pulse.

Restrictive cardiomyopathy: Patients present with dyspnea, fatigue, and findings consistent with right-sided failure. Physical examination reveals edema, jugular venous distention, ascites, and enlarged heart.

► **Diagnostic Studies**

Echocardiography may help to identify valvular damage, ventricular aneurysms, and dilated ventricles. A thallium-201 scan may identify cardiac ischemia. In addition to echocardiography, Doppler ultrasound and cardiac catheterization are used to diagnose hypertrophic cardiomyopathy. ECG and CXR are used to detect LVH, MI, and other cardiac diseases.

ECG and CXR are used to document heart enlargement. Echocardiography may also be used to assess cardiac defects. Appropriate laboratory studies must be performed in order to identify underlying diseases causing cardiomyopathy.

► Diagnosis

Dilated cardiomyopathy: Combine data from ECG, CXR, echocardiogram, catheterization, and thallium scan.

Hypertrophic cardiomyopathy: CXR, ECG, Doppler ultrasound, and cardiac catheterization are needed to measure intracardiac pressures such as left ventricular end-diastolic pressure.

Restrictive cardiomyopathy: In addition to CXR, ECG, echocardiography, and catheterization, a heart muscle biopsy may be used to diagnose this type of cardiomyopathy.

► Clinical Therapeutics

1. Dilated cardiomyopathy:
   - Discontinue alcohol use.
   - Correct any endocrine causes (e.g., thyroid, adrenal medullary, and/or anterior pituitary disorders).
   - Treat autoimmune diseases, if applicable.
   - Treat edema with diuretics or other drugs for CHF.
2. Hypertrophic cardiomyopathy:
   - Beta blocker as initial drug for outflow obstruction
   - Calcium channel blockers
   - Surgical intervention for excision of septum
   - Dual-chamber pacing
   - Implant defibrillator to prevent sudden death
3. Restrictive cardiomyopathy (little useful therapy is available):
   - Diuretic for CHF; overuse can worsen symptoms
   - Steroids for sarcoidosis
   - Transplantation, if possible

► Clinical Intervention

The major intervention involves placement of defibrillator to prevent sudden death. Cardiac muscle biopsy may be needed to identify exact diagnosis.

► Health Maintenance Issues

1. Minimize the use of alcohol and reduce exposure to toxins.
2. Limit salt intake to ameliorate CHF.
3. ACE inhibitors may be used to improve survival and quality of life.

VII. PERICARDITIS

► Scientific Concepts

Acute pericarditis (inflammation of the pericardium) is a common disorder that may be due to any of several disease processes, including uremia, radiation, drug toxicity, hemopericardium, autoimmune syndrome, tuberculosis, human immunodeficiency virus (HIV), varicella, mumps, Epstein–Barr virus, coxsackievirus, echovirus, neoplasms, Lyme disease, and following MI (Dressler's syndrome). The sequelae of pericarditis include pericardial effusion and restriction of diastolic filling. Bloody or serous pericardial effusion and restricted diastolic filling can evolve into a medical emergency because of pericardial tamponade.

► **History & Physical**

Patients with pericarditis present with pleuritic chest pain that is relieved by sitting. Pain may be substernal and radiate to shoulders, back, neck, or epigastrium. They complain of dyspnea, fever, chills, and fatigue. Physical examination reveals a pericardial friction rub, usually heard best along the left sternal border. ECG changes include generalized S-T segment elevation and late T wave inversion. Echocardiography reveals pericardial effusion. CXR shows cardiomegaly. Patient with constrictive pericarditis can present with CHF, jugular venous distention, ascites, edema, hepatic congestion, dyspnea, weakness, fatigue, arrhythmias, and pulsus paradoxus.

► **Diagnostic Studies**
1. ECG—ST-T changes
2. CXR—enlarged (water bottle) heart
3. Echocardiogram—pericardial effusion
4. Magnetic resonance imaging (MRI)—pericardial effusion
5. CBC—leukocytosis

► **Diagnosis**
1. Echocardiography is an excellent tool for diagnosis of pleural effusion and tamponade.
2. Pulsus paradoxus confirmed by blood pressure is important for diagnosis of tamponade.
3. CT and MRI reveal pericardial thickening.
4. CXR shows pericardial calcification in 50% of cases of constrictive pericarditis.

► **Clinical Therapeutics**
1. Viral pericarditis:
   • Aspirin, 650 mg q3–4h or
   • Indocin, 100 to 150 mg qd in divided doses or
   • Short course of steroids in unresponsive cases
2. Pericardial effusion:
   • Pericardiocentesis
   • Pericardiectomy in cases of chronic disease (e.g., uremia, neoplasia)
3. Constrictive pericarditis:
   • Gentle diuresis
   • Pericardiotomy or pericardial window

► **Clinical Intervention**

Cardiac tamponade and constrictive pericarditis may require immediate surgical intervention to evacuate accumulated fluids and/or pericardium.

► **Health Maintenance Issues**

Time is needed for rest and recovery.

VIII. AORTIC COARCTATION

▶ Scientific Concepts

Aortic coarctation is a localized narrowing of the aortic arch just distal to the origin of the left subclavian artery, which results in decreased blood flow to the kidneys, increased release of rennin, and secondary hypertension. Defect is usually congenital and requires surgical repair in childhood years. Narrowing is often located at the level of the ligamentum arteriosum, and may have aortic valve (stenosis, regurgitation) involvement. Resulting increased collateral circulation through intercostal arteries produces "notching" of the ribs seen on CXR.

▶ History & Physical

Classic symptoms are dyspnea, edema, PND, and DOE as seen with heart failure. Major physical findings are significant increases in blood pressure in vessels proximal to defect, blood pressure discrepancy between arms and legs, weak or absent femoral pulses, and harsh systolic murmur auscultable in the back.

▶ Diagnostic Studies

CXR shows left ventricular hypertrophy (LVH), enlarged aortic knob, and lower pulmonary artery and notching (scalloping) of the ribs. ECG shows LVH. Arteriography is used to locate and assess degree of obstruction. Echocardiography is used to identify aortic structures and degree of atrioventricular (AV) involvement.

▶ Diagnosis

Aortography and catheterization are primary methods of diagnosis. Doppler ultrasound can be used to estimate severity of obstruction.

▶ Clinical Therapeutics

Surgical correction is indicated for all patients less than 20 years of age. For patients under 40 years of age, surgical intervention is recommended if there are signs and symptoms of refractory hypertension or if LVH is present. After age 50, balloon angioplasty may be used because surgical mortality is increased. Only 75% of patients show amelioration of hypertension after surgery. Complications of balloon angioplasty may include aortic tears requiring immediate intervention.

▶ Health Maintenance Issues

Salt intake must be carefully monitored. Subacute bacterial endocarditis prophylaxis may be necessary to prevent further valve damage.

IX. CARDIAC ARRHYTHMIAS AND CONDUCTION DISORDERS

► Scientific Concepts

Specialized myocardial fibers make up the conduction system. The sinoatrial (SA) and atrioventricular (AV) nodes are both capable of generating and conducting electrical impulses, normally; the SA node sets the pace (pulse) at 60 to 100 impulses per minute. When it generates impulses at less than 60, sinus bradycardia develops, and when the rate exceeds 100, the condition is called sinus tachycardia. Variation in rate associated with respiratory cycles is termed *sinus arrhythmia*.

If the SA node fails to initiate the impulse, the AV node (junction) becomes dominant and initiates a slower rhythm. Under certain circumstances, an ectopic atrial impulse develops. If transmission of the impulse through the AV node is impeded, an AV block results. AV blocks vary in severity and clinical significance from transient and benign blocks to severe, second-degree AV blocks (type II) and complete heart block, which can be fatal if left untreated.

When the conduction system is damaged at the level of the right and/or left branch of the bundle of His, bundle branch blocks (BBBs) develop. These may be partial (incomplete) or complete. These types of conduction derangement may coexist with other conduction anomalies as well as arrhythmias.

Under certain conditions, when the SA node fails to generate impulses, a focus of activity develops in one of the atria and "paces" the heart at a slightly slower rate than does the SA node. Activity may develop in the same site (focus) in the atria but may also develop in different foci, yielding a wandering atrial pacemaker. In either case, an *atrial escape rhythm* protects against prolonged SA node failure.

When a single impulse arises prematurely in an atrial focus, a premature atrial complex (PAC) develops, which interrupts and resets normal sinus rhythm pattern. PACs may be conducted into AV node and ventricles eliciting early QRS complexes or may be blocked when they reach these structures during their refractory period. As with atrial escape beats, PACs may originate from a single focus or from multiple atrial pacemaker sites.

When three or more PACs occur consecutively, there is atrial tachycardia, which may last a few seconds or may be sustained for hours or days. One of two processes may be responsible for this tachyarrhythmia: (1) enhanced automaticity by physiologic disturbances or (2) impulse reentry, both of which suppress SA node pacemaking activity.

► History & Physical

Sinus bradycardia is a normal finding in physically well-conditioned persons, but may also be the result of pathologic processes. Similarly, sinus tachycardia is a normal response both to physiologic and pathologic conditions. Its etiology must be determined. Individuals with first-degree AV blocks (P-R interval > .20 sec and constant) are often asymptomatic until the block is aggravated by drugs, such as digitalis, or by vagotonic influences, at which time patient may complain of dizziness or lightheadedness.

Patients with Wenckebach (Mobitz type I) AV block may develop lightheadedness, weakness, and fatigue, and may require pharmacologic and/or electronic therapy. Mobitz type I may be seen in patients with acute myocardial infarction or myxedema, either singly or in conjunction with other conduction disturbances, but may also be seen in individuals with increased vagal tone who are otherwise normal.

Patients treated with drugs such as digitalis, procainamide, quinidine, lidocaine, propranolol, or tricyclic antidepressants such as amitriptyline (Elavil), all of which depress conduction, may be at risk of developing Mobitz type II AV block due to interference with conduction. Mobitz type II can develop into complete (third-degree) AV block. Patients may present with lightheadedness and syncopal episodes.

Patients with supraventricular tachycardia (i.e., rhythms driven by pacemakers above common bundles) may complain of palpitations (see Table 5–2) and lightheadedness, and may experience syncope.

▶ Diagnostic Studies

The ECG provides important clues in identifying the various impulse generation and/or conduction disorders. The His bundle electrogram is a record of electrophysiologic events in the conduction pathways and offers additional insights into these processes. His electrography is an invasive procedure.

▶ Diagnosis
See Table 5–7.

▶ Clinical Therapeutics

Therapeutics should treat underlying condition(s). Pathologic conditions that produce sinus bradycardia include decreased metabolic activity (myxedema, hypothermia) and increased intracranial pressure (cerebral edema, subdural hematoma). Conditions that produce sinus tachycardia include hyperthyroidism, fever, anemia, heat exposure, shock, CHF, acute MI, pulmonary emboli, hypoxia, hypercapnea, smoking, pain, anxiety, adrenergic agonists, and vagolytic agents.

A first-degree AV block that accompanies MI, myocarditis, drug intoxication, or other cardiac problems of recent onset should be evaluated thoroughly. Second-degree AV blocks develop with more severe depression of AV nodal conduction because of disease or by vagotonic influences (i.e., carotid pressure, vomiting) causing failure of some impulses to traverse the AV node or reach and activate the ventricles. The result is missed beats and an atrial rate higher than that of ventricles. Wenckebach (Mobitz type I) is usually transient and reversible, but may progress to more severe block. Type II AV block differs from type I in that, in addition to AV node block, there is an intermittent block in one bundle branch and a complete block in the other. This form of AV block can progress to third-degree AV block or asystole re-

▶ table 5-7

ELECTROCARDIOGRAPHIC EVALUATION

Atrioventricular Blocks (AVBs)

AVBs	PR Interval	Dropped Beat(s)	P:QRS Ratio
1°	> .20 sec	No	1:1
2° Type I	Normal to prolonged	Yes	Variable (ex: 3:2, 4:3, 5:4)
Type II	Normal, constant	Yes	
3°	Variable	Yes	Variable

Complete Bundle Branch Blocks (C-BBBs)

Type	PR Interval	QRS Interval	QRS Shape	Check in Lead(s)
C-RBBB	normal	> 0.12 sec	"M" shape	V_1
C-LBBB	normal	> 0.12 sec	"Rabbit ears"	V_5 and V_6

Premature Complexes

Type	P Wave	QRS	Compensatory Pause	Cause(s)
PAC	Abnormal	Normal	No	Smoking, caffeine, alcohol, stress
PJC	None, inverted	Normal	No	Diseases, enhanced automaticity
PVC	None	Abnormal	Yes	Drugs, toxins, electrolyte disturbance

Arrhythmias

Type	Rate Beats/Min	Rhythm	P Wave	QRS
PAT	150–250	Regular	Upright	Normal
SVT	150–250	Regular	None	Normal
PJT	150–250	Regular	Inverted Retrograde	Normal
Aflutter	250–350	Usually Regular	Sawtooth Baseline	Normal
Afib	> 350	Irregular	Undulating Baseline	Normal
PVT	150–250	"Regular"	—	Abnormal pattern
Vflutter	Irregular	Irregular	—	None identifiable

PAC, premature atrial complex; PJC, premature junctional complex; PVC, premature ventricular complex; PAT, paroxysmal atrial tachycardia; SVT, supraventricular tachycardia; PJT, paroxysmal junctional tachycardia; Aflutter, atrial flutter; Afib, atrial fibrillation; PVT, paroxysmal ventricular tachycardia; Vflutter, ventricular flutter (between tachycardia and fibrillation).

quiring transcutaneous pacing. In third-degree AV block, there is complete dissociation between atria and ventricles; atrial rate (usually normal) exceeds ventricular rate, which may be in the 40 to 60 range, if there is a junctional escape beat, or 30 to 40 if ventricular pacemaker is below AV junction. This condition requires immediate electronic pacing.

Tachyarrhythmias require suppression of the "irritable" focus with antiarrhythmic drugs; in emergent cases, electrocardioversion may be required. However, in cases of arrhythmias due to reentry phenomena, surgical ablation of the anomalous bypass tract may ameliorate the condition. Carotid massage can be used to distinguish AV nodal reentrant tachyarrhythmias.

► Health Maintenance Issues

A number of conduction problems may be attributed to hyper-responsiveness to physiologic stimuli; others are due to pharmacologic agents and/or ischemic, inflammatory, and degenerative processes. While some of these are not amenable to modification, judicious use of pharmacologic agents goes a long way toward preventing some of these problems.

X. PERIPHERAL VASCULAR DISEASE

► Scientific Concepts

Peripheral vascular disease (PVD) is narrowing of arteries supplying blood to upper and lower extremities. Lower-extremity disease is more common with decreased blood flow due to narrowing of aorta, iliac, and femoral arteries. The disease manifests itself by cramping, affecting calf muscles upon walking two blocks or less. PVD affects males more than females, is due to atherosclerosis, and is aggravated by smoking.

► History & Physical

The onset of PVD is gradual. Over time, patients have thinning of skin and loss of hair on lower extremities. There is elevation pallor and dependent rubor of lower legs. Later findings included ulceration and gangrene of one or both lower legs. In severe cases, patients experience pain at rest during the night.

If calf pain develops after walking two blocks, disease is considered mild; it is considered moderate and severe when pain develops after one and one-half blocks, respectively. Severe disease calls for immediate surgical intervention. Calf pain is relieved by rest. In later stages of the disease, dorsalis pedis pulses may not be palpable and need to be verified by Doppler.

► Diagnostic Studies

Doppler studies, with and without exercise, may be used to measure blood flow. Arteriograms are used to locate areas of blockage if bypass or angioplasty procedures are contemplated.

► Diagnosis

Diagnosis of blockage or narrowing can be achieved by using Doppler or arteriograms.

► Clinical Therapeutics

Medical treatment involves use of aspirin, 325 mg qd, and pentoxifylline, 400 mg tid to ameliorate blood flow. Patients may undergo bypass surgery; 75 to 80% of grafts remain patent after 5 years. Laser, thermal, mechanical, or balloon angioplasty with stent placement can be used to improve blood flow. Lumbar sympathectomy has been used in a few cases to increase flow.

► Clinical Intervention

Patients who experience pain at rest or at night are at high risk for gangrene. These individuals are candidates for immediate surgical intervention. Seven to 10% of graft patients undergo amputation after 5 years.

► Health Maintenance Issues

Abstinence from tobacco products tends to allow development of collateral blood flow. Similarly, exercise and lowering of dietary fat reduce risk of arteriosclerosis.

XI. AORTIC ANEURYSM

► Scientific Concepts

Pathologic dilation of a blood vessel is an aneurysm. Most common area is abdominal or thoracic aorta. The principal cause is arteriosclerosis. However, syphilitic aortitis, media necrosis, and bacterial infections can cause the defect. True aneurysm involves all three layers—intima, media, and adventitia—whereas a pseudoaneurysm usually involves intima and media, but spares the adventitia.

Aortic aneurysm classification is based on location (abdominal vs. thoracic) and pattern of dissection (ascending vs. descending). Untreated, an aneurysm of 6 cm or greater carries mortality risk of 50% in 2 years. Surgery is recommended for aneurysms > 6 cm in diameter.

► History & Physical

The pain of thoracic aneurysm has a tearing quality and radiates to the back. Patient may experience syncope, weakness, tracheal deviation, hoarseness, claudication, and CHF. The mediastinum may appear wide in the presence of a thoracic aneurysm. Patients with abdominal aneurysms have a pulsatile mass and almost always have an abdominal bruit.

► Diagnostic Studies

The usual labs include ECG, CXR, transthoracic and transesophageal echocardiography, and ultrasonography; the latter is the most cost effective. CT and MRI are also useful. In some instances, an aortogram is obtained before surgery.

► Diagnosis

Diagnosis is established when aorta diameter is ≥ 4 cm. Surgery is performed if diameter is smaller and patient is symptomatic. Aortic dissection with tearing pain is a life-threatening condition.

► Clinical Therapeutics

In high-risk patients, treatment may include use of beta blockers when aortic diameter is 4 to 6 cm.

► Health Maintenance Issues

Since underlying cause of all aneurysms is arteriosclerosis, patients need to be counseled to control blood pressure, lower dietary fat, abstain from smoking, and increase physical activity.

XII. THROMBOPHLEBITIS

► Scientific Concepts

Thrombophlebitis refers to partial or complete occlusion of veins in upper or lower extremity by inflammatory processes. Predisposing factors include trauma, surgery, bedrest, pregnancy, hypercoagulopathic states, and neoplasms, especially of lower-extremity veins. Thrombophlebitis may result in sudden death because of embolization of clots into lungs.

► History & Physical

Patients with thrombophlebitis complain of tender, hot, and visible calf veins. In more extensive cases, pain may involve entire leg, including the thigh. Those who present with dyspnea, hemoptysis, syncope, tachycardia and pleuritic chest pain may have pulmonary emboli. Patients with CHF, on oral contraceptive agents, or with history of varicose veins have higher incidence of thrombophlebitis.

There are 800,000 new cases of thrombophlebitis each year; 80% involve deep calf veins and 25% popliteal and femoral veins. Fixed splitting of S_1 and supraventricular arrhythmias are common with pulmonary emboli.

► Diagnostic Studies

Doppler ultrasound, phlebography, and venography are used to evaluate blood flow. Prothrombin time (PT), partial thromboplastin time (PTT), and international normalized ratio (INR) are used to measure clotting time to detect hypercoagulopathic states. Ventilation-perfusion scans are used to detect pulmonary thromboemboli. Special tests can be performed to detect deficiencies or excesses of antithrombin II, fibrinolytic proteins C and S, lupus anticoagulant, and homocystinuria. PTT is used to measure effectiveness of heparin in treating venous stasis.

► Diagnosis

Differential diagnosis of thrombophlebitis includes cellulitis, muscle strain, ruptured Baker's cyst, and obstruction of lymphatics.

► Clinical Therapeutics

Treatment of deep and superficial thrombophlebitis is often a judgment call. Following are guidelines for deep and superficial thrombophlebitis. All patients who are anticoagulated need to be observed carefully for bleeding.

Superficial thrombophlebitis: If disease process is localized and not near saphenous femoral vein junction, local heat and bedrest with elevation are usually effective in limiting the thrombosis. A nonsteroidal anti-inflammatory drug can be used to relieve the symptoms. If the process is extensive or begins to involve the saphenous vein junction, or if the junction is involved initially, ligation of saphenous vein at saphenofemoral junction is indicated. Removal of the involved vein could result in more rapid recovery. Anticoagulation therapy is usually not warranted unless thrombophlebitis is rapidly progressing.

Deep vein thrombophlebitis: All patients with extensive thrombophlebitis are placed on bedrest and leg elevation (10 to 15 degrees) to level of heart. Rapid intravenous infusion (bolus) of heparin at 5,000 to 10,000 units followed by continuous infusion of 1,000 to 1,500 units qh until PTT is two times normal over 7 to 10 days may be used. A second option is to give IV heparin by heplock at 5,000 units over 8 to 12 hours for 7 to 10 days until PTT is two times normal. Warfarin is given 4 to 5 days before termination of heparin treatment and continued for 6 to 12 months. To prevent venous stasis, patient may be treated with aspirin, 80 to 325 mg qd.

▶ Clinical Intervention

In cases of severe pulmonary embolization resulting in significant hemodynamic changes, surgery may be necessary. In cases of recurrent emboli, vena cava filter or plication may be indicated to prevent embolization.

▶ Health Maintenance Issues

Patients with varicose veins should be encouraged to participate in reasonable exercise activities, and to wear thromboembolic disease hose to prevent venous pooling and reduce risk of embolization.

XIII. RHEUMATIC FEVER

▶ Scientific Concepts

Rheumatic fever is a very rare disease in the United States due to screening and treatment of beta-hemolytic streptococcal pharyngitis. The disease usually strikes children aged 5 to 15 years. Pharyngitis usually precedes rheumatic fever by 1 to 3 weeks. Valvular heart disease is common when condition is not treated. Mitral valve is affected in 75 to 80% of cases, aortic valve is affected 30% of the time, and tricuspid and pulmonary valves are affected 5% of the time.

▶ History & Physical

Patients with rheumatic fever present with major physical findings, including carditis (rigidity of valve cusps, fusion of commissures, shortening and fusion of chordae tendinea, valvular stenosis, valvular cusp lesions, pericarditis, pericardial friction rub, prolonged P-R interval on ECG, cardiomegaly, CHF, hepatomegaly, sinus tachycardia, erythema marginatum, subcutaneous nodules, Sydenham's chorea, and migratory polyarthritis. Minor physical findings include fever and polyarthralgia. Laboratory findings include P-R prolongation on

► table 5-8

JONES CRITERIA FOR DIAGNOSIS OF RHEUMATIC FEVER

Major Findings	Minor Findings
Carditis	Arthralgia
Polyarthralgia	Fever
Chorea	Elevated sedimentation rates
Erythema marginatum	C reactive protein
Subcutaneous nodules	Prolonged P-R interval on electrocardiogram (lead II)

ECG, elevated erythrocyte sedimentation rate (ESR), and positive and rising streptococcal titers. Two major findings or one major and one minor finding are required for the diagnosis of rheumatic fever. Patients with long-standing CHF can present with rales, ascites, edema, jugular venous distention, orthopnea, PND, and DOE at two blocks. Final diagnosis is made using Jones Criteria (Table 5–8).

► Diagnostic Studies

In the acute phase of the disease, the following are observed: rise in antistreptolysin-O (ASO) titer and ESR, cardiomegaly and heart failure signs, prolonged P-R interval, arrhythmias, and pericarditis changes on ECG. Diagnosis is established when two major or one major and one minor Jones criteria are met. Both ASO titer and ESR must be elevated in the acute phase as well. The differential includes rheumatoid arthritis, osteomyelitis, endocarditis, systemic lupus erythematosus, and Lyme disease.

► Clinical Therapeutics

Patients are treated with bedrest; aspirin, 600 to 900 mg q4h; and penicillin, 1.2 million units IM qd × 10 days. Patients with penicillin allergy may be treated with erythromycin, 250 mg PO tid × 10 days. Patients with associated severe pericarditis and CHF are also treated with 40 to 60 mg corticosteroids × 2 weeks, then tapered. The immediate mortality rate in acute treatment is 1 to 2%.

► Clinical Intervention

Patients are followed and treated for CHF. As with subacute bacterial endocarditis, antibiotic prophylaxis is given for genitourinary, dental, surgical, and obstetric procedures.

► Health Maintenance Issues

Acute sore throats with cervical lymphadenopathy require rapid strep screen and treatment. Patients are advised to complete the entire course of antibiotics.

BIBLIOGRAPHY

Andreoli TE, Bennett JCM, Carpenter CJC, Plum F. *Cecil Essentials of Medicine,* 4th ed. Philadelphia: WB Saunders; 1997.

Barry MM, Amidon TM. Heart. In: Tierney LM Jr., McPhee SJ, Papadakis MA, eds. *Current Medical Diagnosis & Treatment,* 37th ed. Stamford, CT: Appleton & Lange; 1998.

Bickley LS, Hoekelman RA. *Bates' Guide to Physical Examination and History Taking,* 7th ed. Philadelphia: JB Lippincott; 1999.

DePilippi CR, Runge MS. Evaluating the chest pain patient: Scope of the problem. *Cardiol Clin* 17:307–326; 1999.

Dershewitz RA. *Ambulatory Pediatric Care,* 2nd ed. Philadelphia: Lippincott-Raven; 1993.

Johnson PA, Goldman L, Sacks DB, et al. Cardiac troponin T as a marker for myocardial ischemia in patients seen at the emergency department for acute chest pain. *Am Heart J* 137(6):1137–1144; 1999.

Martina B, Bucheli B, Stotz M, et al. First clinical judgment by primary care physicians distinguishes well between nonorganic and organic causes of abdominal or chest pain. *J Gen Intern Med* 12:459–465; 1997.

Massie BM. Systemic hypertension. In: Tierney LM Jr., McPhee SJ, Papadakis MA, eds. *Current Medical Diagnosis & Treatment,* 37th ed. Stamford, CT: Appleton & Lange; 1998.

Skillings J. Therapeutic options in angina pectoris. *Clinical Advisor for Physician Assistants,* June 1999; 29–37.

Gastroenterology and Nutrition 6

Tonya Babbitt, PA-C, Albert F. Simon, MEd, PA-C

I. ESOPHAGUS

A. Esophagitis

▶ Scientific Concepts

Most commonly due to gastric acid reflux but may be secondary to infection (*Helicobacter pylori*, viral) or medication irritation. Results from prolonged or too frequent relaxation of or decreased lower esophageal sphincter (LES) tone, obesity, caffeine, fats, and pregnancy. Ulceration, erosion, and stricture formation are complications. Barrett's esophagus is considered a premalignant lesion.

▶ History & Physical

Heartburn, substernal chest pain, regurgitation, water brash, cough, hoarseness, dysphagia, odynophagia, asthma.

▶ Diagnostic Studies

Upper endoscopy (esophagogastroduodenoscopy [EGD]) with biopsy if Barrett's suspected, 24-hour pH monitoring, manometry, barium swallow, and upper gastrointestinal (UGI) radiography.

▶ Diagnosis

Often made on visual inspection; biopsy important if Barrett's suspected; abnormal number of reflux events on 24-hour monitoring or decreased LES tone on manometry.

▶ Clinical Therapeutics

Antacids offer effective relief of reflux symptoms but are costly and inconvenient. Histamine (H_2) blockers (e.g., cimetidine, ranitidine) reduce acid, but proton pump inhibitors (e.g., omeprazole, lansoprazole) most effective. Use of prokinetic agents (e.g., metoclopramide, cisipride) increase LES tone and are sometimes used in combination, though this is controversial.

▶ Clinical Intervention

Antireflux surgery for refractive cases, periodic endoscopic exam for screening in patients with Barrett's.

▶ Health Maintenance Issues

Weight loss if obese; reduce fat, caffeine, chocolate and alcohol; eliminate peppermint; stop smoking; elevate head of bed. Nothing by mouth (NPO) for 2 to 3 hours prior to bedtime.

B. Motor Disorders

▶ Scientific Concepts

May result from stroke, multiple neurologic disorders, aperistalsis, achalasia (failure of LES to relax), diffuse esophageal spasm, or scleroderma.

▶ History & Physical

Dysphagia (solid and/or liquid), sticking sensation, odynophagia, chest pain, heartburn, hoarseness.

► **Diagnostic Studies**

Manometry to demonstrate peristalsis, force, and function of LES; upper endoscopy; barium swallow.

► **Diagnosis**

Disordered peristalsis, increased LES pressures on manometry.

► **Clinical Therapeutics**

Prokinetic agents, anticholinergics, nitrates, calcium channel blockers, or beta agonists are effective in approximately 50%.

► **Clinical Intervention**

Balloon dilation, injection of botulinum toxin, surgical myotomy, and treatment of underlying conditions as indicated.

► **Health Maintenance Issues**

Long-term prognosis dependent on cause of motor disturbance. Prognosis with achalasia and diffuse esophageal spasm is promising.

C. Neoplasm

► **Scientific Concepts**

Adenocarcinoma and squamous cell carcinoma occur in equal numbers. U.S. population at low risk. Predisposing factors include smoking, alcohol, geography, vitamin deficiency, history of lye ingestion, achalasia, Barrett's esophagus. Diagnosis usually late, after metastasis/extension.

► **History & Physical**

Dysphagia initially with solids, then liquids; weight loss; anorexia; pain secondary to extension. Bleeding rare.

► **Diagnostic Studies**

Upper endoscopy with biopsy, UGI barium study, ultrasound, computed tomography (CT) to evaluate for extension into adjacent structures.

► **Diagnosis**

By pathology on biopsy specimen.

► **Clinical Therapeutics**

Esophageal cancers are resistant to chemotherapeutic agents. They are of little or no benefit either primarily or adjuctively.

► **Clinical Intervention**

Surgical resection for tumors of distal third, followed by radiation; radiation alone for proximal lesion. Stents may be useful to maintain lumen.

► **Health Maintenance Issues**

Prognosis poor, 5 to 10% survival at 10 years.

D. Injury/Hemorrhage

▶ Scientific Concepts

External or iatrogenic trauma may rupture (Boerhaave syndrome), foreign body may obstruct trachea, caustic ingestions will produce scarring, motility disturbances, and predispose to cancer. Severe vomiting may cause Mallory–Weiss tear in mucosa with brisk bleeding.

▶ History & Physical

History of trauma or instrumentation, alcoholism, portal hypertension. History of large meal followed by forceful vomiting.

▶ Diagnostic Studies

Urgent upper endoscopy.

▶ Diagnosis

Evaluate extent of injury, identify bleeding points, locate foreign body.

▶ Clinical Therapeutics

Fluid and transfusion as indicated to prevent circulatory collapse.

▶ Clinical Intervention

Extraction of foreign body, endoscopic sclerotherapy of varices. Most Mallory–Weiss tears stop bleeding spontaneously. Vomiting should not be induced.

▶ Health Maintenance Issues

Long-term follow-up after caustic ingestion; alkali causes worse damage.

II. STOMACH

A. Gastritis/Duodenitis

▶ Scientific Concepts

Acute or chronic inflammation, localized or generalized, caused by drugs (nonsteroidal anti-inflammatory drugs [NSAIDs], aspirin, alcohol), caustic substances, stress related to severe illness, burns, postsurgical, or infection (most commonly *H. pylori*).

▶ History & Physical

Epigastric pain, nausea, vomiting, hematemesis, 30% asymptomatic.

▶ Diagnostic Studies

Upper endoscopy with biopsy is most sensitive.

► Diagnosis

Gastritis is not a clinical diagnosis. Is made when histological changes are seen.

► Clinical Therapeutics

H_2 blockers, or proton pump inhibitors (PPIs) which are more effective.

► Clinical Intervention

Remove or discontinue offending agents. If NSAID cannot be stopped, add misoprostol in non–childbearing age patients. Fluids and/or blood transfusion may be indicated in acute conditions.

► Health Maintenance Issues

Periodic endoscopic screening in chronic conditions; stop smoking.

B. Peptic Ulcer Disease

► Scientific Concepts

Ulceration occurs when mucosal barrier to acid is broken with resulting direct injury to underlying mucosa. Hemorrhage, perforation, penetration, and peritonitis can occur. *H. pylori*, smoking, some medications, and alcohol are contributing factors. Stricture, pyloric stenosis, and obstruction are late consequences. Gastric ulcers have malignancy potential, duodenal do not. Hemorrhage can be rapid and fatal when ulcer erodes arterial vessel.

► History & Physical

Periodic epigastric pain radiating to back or left upper quadrant, often at night; nausea, vomiting, hematemesis, melena. Pain may be exacerbated or relieved with food. Abrupt increase in pain signals perforation. Most NSAID ulcers are painless.

► Diagnostic Studies

Upper endoscopy with biopsy of ulcer margins. Barium UGI studies less sensitive and unable to provide tissue specimen.

► Diagnosis

Often made by history, but definitive diagnosis can be made only by visual exam.

► Clinical Therapeutics

If hospitalized, intravenous (IV) H_2 blockers with or without antacid. For outpatient setting, PPIs are more effective and have better compliance. Recommendations for *H. pylori* eradication are many, but all include antibiotics and acid suppression.

► Clinical Intervention

NPO, possible nasogastric (NG) suction, fluids, transfusion, endoscopic sclerotherapy for active bleed, surgery for rebleed. Significant nonhemorrhagic ulcer may need hospitalization for bowel rest and IV

H_2 blockers. Consider pH monitoring. Outpatients may be managed with twice-daily PPIs, antacid for breakthrough pain, and avoidance of evocative foods (e.g., caffeine, alcohol, citrus).

► Health Maintenance Issues

Aggressive prophylactic IV H_2 blockade in severely ill/intensive care unit patients; remove offending agents; stop smoking. Contribution of psychosocial stress is controversial. Rescope in 6 to 8 weeks to document healing of gastric ulcers. Bland/milk diets no longer indicated. Some evocative foods may need to be eliminated during healing.

C. Nonulcer Dyspepsia

► Scientific Concepts

Functional disorder with great deal of overlap with irritable bowel syndrome. Certain medications, diet, and many psychosocial factors involved. Patients have lifelong functional complaints interfering with work and social life. Typically, there are periods of resolution and exacerbation.

► History & Physical

Symptoms may be indistinguishable from peptic ulcer disease. Patient will have intermittent upper abdominal pain, gnawing, burning, and aching, with bloating, belching, and nausea, especially after meals. Nighttime pain rare.

► Diagnostic Studies

Upper endoscopy, UGI barium studies.

► Diagnosis

Diagnosis is one of exclusion. Endosopy will rule out structural versus functional cause.

► Clinical Therapeutics

All medications used in ulcer disease have been used with varying success. Prokinetic agents show some promise.

► Clinical Intervention

Avoid overevaluation and treatment once diagnosis is made.

► Health Maintenance Issues

Maintaining trust between patient and provider is key; reassurance and allaying fears (e.g., cancer) is therapeutic.

D. Neoplasm

► Scientific Concepts

Appears to be a genetic link, so family history is important. Tobacco use, consumption of overly processed foods and nitrites contribute to risk. Premalignant conditions include gastric polyp, pernicious anemia, atrophic gastritis, previous gastrectomy.

► **History & Physical**

Abdominal pain, early satiety, weight loss, anorexia, and vomiting. Bleeding rare.

► **Diagnostic Studies**

UGI endoscopy with biopsy.

► **Diagnosis**

On pathology, all gastric ulcers need biopsy and follow-up.

► **Clinical Therapeutics**

Chemotherapy effective for lymphoma but of little/no use in adenocarcinoma.

► **Clinical Intervention**

Surgery with follow-up radiation is therapy of choice.

► **Health Maintenance Issues**

Five-year survival with adenocarcinoma approximately 12%. Disease is diagnosed late after spread or extension. Prognosis with lymphoma better.

III. SMALL BOWEL

A. Small Bowel Obstruction

► **Scientific Concepts**

May be due to mechanical obstruction from adhesions forming postsurgically or after infection, secondary to hernia, stricture, tumor, endometriosis, volvulus, or intussusception. Adynamic or paralytic ileus occurs following open abdominal surgery, peritonitis, pancreatitis, cholecystitis, or pneumonia. Exacerbated by narcotics.

► **History & Physical**

Symptoms depend on location. Proximal obstruction presents with diffuse abdominal pain, nausea, and protracted vomiting. Pain is more crampy and distention greater the more distal the lesion. Mechanical obstructions produce hyperactive bowel sounds that will become absent late in the course and is an ominous sign. Bowel sounds characteristically absent in ileus. Dehydration and obstipation may occur.

► **Diagnostic Studies**

Plain abdominal films; acute abdominal series, kidney, ureter, bladder (KUB); UGI series with small bowel follow-through. When possible, the cause should be identified, but often these resolve spontaneously with decompression (these obstructions most often due to adhesive bands compressing small bowel).

► Diagnosis

Plain film with multiple air–fluid levels, dilated proximal loops, and lack of air in rectum. Barium studies to document transit time to cecum.

► Clinical Therapeutics

Fluid replacement, electrolyte correction with mechanical obstruction. Discontinue narcotics and anticholinergics with ileus.

► Clinical Intervention

Bowel rest, NG decompression, barium studies may be therapeutic as well as diagnostic. Urgent surgical correction of persistent mechanical obstruction prior to intestinal ischemia leading to necrosis, perforation, and peritonitis.

► Health Maintenance Issues

Prompt presentation to health care provider with onset of symptoms.

B. Irritable Bowel Syndrome

► Scientific Concepts

Classified as a functional disorder with no organic component to the symptom complex. Reporting of symptoms varies by age, gender, and ethnic group. Often misdiagnosed and is responsible for significant work loss and cost to society. The individual patient's perception of gut function, psychological factors, and diet all relevant.

► History & Physical

Intermittent abdominal pain relieved/altered by defecation, stools looser and more frequent, mucus, feeling of incomplete evacuation, and abdominal distention. Physical examination essentially normal, though some with mild tenderness to palpation.

► Diagnostic Studies

With careful history, few studies required. Younger patients need flexible sigmoidoscopy; those over 40 or with family history of cancer require full colonoscopy. Lactose challenge may be helpful. Evaluate for depression and anxiety disorders.

► Diagnosis

Physical examination and endoscopic examination normal.

► Clinical Therapeutics

No pharmaceuticals reliably effective except antidepressants in patients with coexisting depression.

► Clinical Intervention

None required or appropriate.

► Health Maintenance Issues

Dietary fiber must be increased gradually, often recommending supplements. Reassurance, avoidance of overtesting and medicating. Address any psychiatric or psychological disorder.

C. Infectious Gastroenteritis

▶ Scientific Concepts

Most enteric infections result from oral–fecal transmission. The toxins are either preformed, in which the illness occurs within hours after ingestion, or toxins form after adherence or penetration into bowel wall. Symptoms then occur after several days.

▶ History & Physical

Travel, food, concurrent household illness, and sexual history important. Acute, crampy abdominal pain with watery diarrhea, occasionally with blood.

▶ Diagnostic Studies

Stool culture, *Clostridium difficile* titer, colonoscopy with biopsy when indicated.

▶ Diagnosis

Often made by history, stool culture for enteric pathogens and/or biopsy.

▶ Clinical Therapeutics

Avoid empiric antibiotics with *Salmonella* in immune competent adult. Travelers' diarrhea, cholera, pseudomembranous colitis, *Campylobacter*, and all sexually transmitted infections require appropriate therapy. Fluid replacement, oral or IV, necessary in most cases.

▶ Clinical Intervention

None required.

▶ Health Maintenance Issues

Education regarding food-borne organisms and necessity of proper hand washing, food handling, and cooking. Adequate community sanitation. Prophylaxis is recommended when traveling to some endemic areas (e.g., cholera). However, it is generally not recommended for common travelers' diarrhea.

D. Inflammatory Bowel Disease (IBD)

▶ Scientific Concepts

IBD refers to both regional enteritis (Crohn's disesase [CD]) and ulcerative colitis (UC). There are many similarities but treatment and prognosis differ; thus, it is important to make correct diagnosis. Etiology uncertain but both probably immune/autoimmune disorder with familial and environmental factors. Important to rule out infectious causes as source of chief complaint.

Crohn's is transmural granulomatous disease affecting any part of GI tract from mouth to anus. Nearly all patients have involvement of terminal ileum. Extraintestinal manifestations (skin, eye, joint) are common and may be presenting complaint. "Skip areas" of normal GI tissue are characteristic. Complications include fistulae, perianal disease, stricture, malnutrition, growth retardation, and carcinoma.

Ulcerative colitis is inflammatory disease of mucosa and submucosa only. Usually develops in a continuous pattern, with rectum nearly always involved. Islands of pseudopolyps seen on endoscopy and destruction of haustral markings on x-ray (leaving colon appearing flat) are characteristic. Complications include toxic megacolon, hemorrhage, perforation, and rarely stricture. Cancer even more prevalent than with Crohn's disease.

► History & Physical
CD presents with colicky right lower quadrant (RLQ) pain and diarrhea with fever and weight loss. Physical examination finds tender RLQ and possibly perianal disease. Bleeding rare. UC patients present with bloody diarrhea, crampy abdominal pain, and tenesmus; fever and weight loss variable. Symptoms may be present for months prior to presentation.

► Diagnostic Studies
Stool culture, ova and parasite exam, other labs (complete blood count [CBC], electrolytes, erythrocyte sedimentation rate [ESR], C reactive protein [CRP]) nonspecific but reflect severity of disease, inflammation. Barium studies and colonoscopy are indicated and have characteristic findings as above, but must be avoided when patient is acutely ill.

► Diagnosis
Stool with mucus, blood, and/or white blood cells; edematous, friable colonic mucosa. On x-ray, cobblestoning, and string sign with CD; loss of haustral markings with UC.

► Clinical Therapeutics
Sulfasalazine, 5-aminosalicylate acid enemas, steroid enemas, systemic steroids, methotrexate, antibiotics, antidiarrheals.

► Clinical Intervention
Total colectomy in UC for refractive cases and cases of toxic megacolon. In CD, local resection with correction of fistula/stricture and colectomy are of no use and are to be avoided.

► Health Maintenance Issues
Psychosocial aspects are many, support groups widely available, family counseling may be needed. All patients with active IBD require yearly colonoscopy to screen for cancer.

E. Ischemic Bowel Disease

► Scientific Concepts
Mesenteric ischemia occurs both acutely and chronically in patients over 50 with history of arteriosclerosis, coronary artery disease, myocardial infarction, peripheral vascular disease, or after stroke or

abdominal aortic aneurysm repair. Ischemic colitis occurs in patients with similar profile but develops due to hypoperfusion of smaller vessels of intestinal wall. Focal ischemia often results from episodes of hypotension. Intestinal angina occurs with repeated bouts of ischemia. Infarction followed by perforation may result.

► **History & Physical**

Classically "pain out of proportion" to physical findings. Severe, crampy abdominal pain, often worse postprandially. May also present with fever, nausea, vomiting, and hematochezia. Initially, abdominal examination may be normal or include decreased bowel sounds, mild distention, and tenderness progressing to a rigid, acute surgical abdomen.

► **Diagnostic Studies**

CBC, amylase, lipase, lactic acid, and Doppler ultrasound. Arteriography is the gold standard.

► **Diagnosis**

High index of suspicion for diagnosis because specific signs and symptoms do not often appear. Increased white blood count (WBC), amylase, and lactic acid. Evidence of significant narrowing/occlusion of vessels on imaging. Diagnosis often made at laparotomy.

► **Clinical Therapeutics**

Bowel rest, fluids, antibiotics.

► **Clinical Intervention**

Most require urgent laparotomy.

► **Health Maintenance Issues**

Vigilance is required in patients with vascular disease presenting with abdominal pain.

F. Neoplasm

► **Scientific Concepts**

Malignant tumors rare, with carcinoid most common. Typically diagnosed late after significant metastasis. Lymphoma has better prognosis. Benign lesions include lipoma, leiomyomas, and adenomas.

► **History & Physical**

Often asymptomatic. Symptoms include obstruction, GI bleed (occult or frank), dysphagia. Characteristic symptomatic carcinoid presents with facial flushing and diarrhea.

► **Diagnostic Studies**

UGI with small bowel follow-through, abdominal CT, EGD for proximal lesions.

► **Diagnosis**

Histological exam of surgical specimen.

▶ **Clinical Therapeutics**
Lymphoma responds to chemotherapy.

▶ **Clinical Intervention**
Surgical resection and staging.

▶ **Health Maintenance Issues**
None.

IV. COLON/RECTUM

A. Constipation

▶ **Scientific Concepts**
Symptom of delayed transit time and reduced water content in stool. Often due to lack of exercise, inadequate fiber in diet, pregnancy, tumor, volvulus, intussusception, obstruction, hypothyroidism, medications, or psychiatric disorder. May result in laxative abuse with lifelong dependence.

▶ **History & Physical**
Bowel movements occur infrequently (less than every other day), are overly hard, and are difficult and painful to pass.

▶ **Diagnostic Studies**
Colonoscopy, barium enema to rule out structural abnormality. Thyroid function testing if hypothyroidism suspected.

▶ **Diagnosis**
Constipation is a symptom, not a disease; therefore, it is not a diagnosis and underlying causes often need investigation.

▶ **Clinical Therapeutics**
Increase fluid and fiber, fiber supplements if necessary, occasional stool softener or laxative. Treat underlying disorder.

▶ **Clinical Intervention**
If severe, soap suds (or alternative) enema, or manual disimpaction providing that obstruction requiring surgical intervention has been ruled out.

▶ **Health Maintenance Issues**
Attention to adequate diet and fluids, increase physical activity, discontinue offending medications. Reassure that bowel function is not identical for all individuals and that some variation is to be expected.

B. Appendicitis

▶ **Scientific Concepts**
Inflammatory condition secondary to obstruction, followed by bacterial proliferation, edema, and vascular compromise. If untreated,

necrosis, perforation, and peritonitis may occur. Age of occurrence is bimodal at 10 to 30 and over 60, with equal male/female prevalence.

► History & Physical

Initially, periumbilical pain migrating to RLQ (McBurney's point) over several hours, nausea, vomiting, anorexia, and fever. Physical examination reveals, tender RLQ, diminished or absent bowel sounds, guarding and rebound as peritonitis develops. Pain with flexion of iliopsoas or rotation of obturator muscles and exacerbation of pain with rectal exam also supports the diagnosis of appendicitis.

► Diagnostic Studies

Careful history, avoid reliance on "no way I could be pregnant" statements. Lab studies to include CBC, urinalysis, urinary chorionic gonadotropin. CT becoming gold standard; abdominal ultrasound to rule out gynecological source for RLQ pain (most critically, ectopic pregnancy).

► Diagnosis

Most often, clinical diagnosis is made on history and physical and confirmed in operating room. Diagnosis more difficult in pregnant females, patients on steroids, and elderly, who may not have pain, fever, or elevated WBC. Mortality is increased in the elderly. The differential diagnosis of right lower quadrant pain includes many causes (Table 6–1).

► Clinical Therapeutics

Preoperative antibiotics, fluids.

► Clinical Intervention

Strictly surgical disease, no role for nonsurgical treatment. May be performed as traditional open procedure or laparoscopically.

► Health Maintenance Issues

None.

► table 6-1

DIFFERENTIAL DIAGNOSIS OF RIGHT LOWER QUADRANT PAIN

Gastrointestinal	Gynecological	Genitourinary	Vascular	Other
Appendicitis	Endometriosis	Ureteral calculi	Leaking aneurysm	Psoas abscess
Intestinal obstruction	Ectopic pregnancy	Pyelonephritis	Abdominal wall	Hernia
Crohn's disease	Ovarian cyst/torsion	Renal pain/spasm	hematoma	Peritonitis
Diverticulitis	Salpingitis	Seminal vasculitis		Pneumonia
Cholecystitis	Mittelschmerz			(especially in
Perforated				elderly)
peptic ulcer				Herpes zoster

C. Diverticular Disease

► Scientific Concepts

Common disorder of Western civilization with low-fiber diet. Not true diverticula, formed only of mucosa and submucosa where blood vessels penetrate colon wall. Most prevalent in narrower sigmoid colon. Complications include progression to diverticulitis with microperforation, bleeding, abscess, peritonitis, and fistula formation to bladder/vagina.

► History & Physical

Often asymptomatic. Crampy lower abdominal pain, usually left lower quadrant (LLQ), with alternating constipation/diarrhea. With diverticulitis, fever and pain become more constant, lower gastrointestinal (LGI) bleed becomes more likely.

► Diagnostic Studies

Barium enema, colonoscopy, sigmoidoscopy. Avoid these studies in acute phase or if perforation is suspected. CT is preferred study.

► Diagnosis

Diverticula easily seen on x-ray or endoscopy. Will see blood and/or pus as signs of inflammation with diverticulitis.

► Clinical Therapeutics

High-fiber diet, bowel rest. Add antibiotic if diverticulitis diagnosed. Quinolones, broad-spectrum penicillins with metronidazole most commonly used.

► Clinical Intervention

Surgical resection for abscess, stricture, fistula, or persistent blood loss.

► Health Maintenance Issues

Maintain proper bowel function with adequate fiber, fluid, and exercise.

D. Colon Carcinoma

► Scientific Concepts

Currently second leading cancer in males and females in the United States. Contributing factors include low-fiber, high-fat/red meat diets; exposure to environmental toxins; and prolonged exposure to bile acids. Risk factors include advancing age; personal or family history (first-degree relative) of colon, genital, or breast cancer; familial polyposis; > 10-year history of IBD. Most tumors are thought to arise in an adenomatous polyp.

► History & Physical

Adequate history taking important to establish risk factors and initiate screening since signs and symptoms are often vague and occur late. Lower gastrointestinal bleeding (either occult or frank), weight loss, change in bowel habits or stool caliper, change of appetite, malaise. Occasionally, palpable mass felt on physical examination. Right-sided lesions, though less common, present even later.

► Diagnostic Studies

Flexible sigmoidoscopy, barium enema, followed by complete colonoscopy. Synchronous lesions not uncommon. If symptoms are suspicious or patient is high risk, proceed with formal colonoscopy. Initial labs include CBC, liver function test, and, if lesion confirmed, carcinoembryonic antigen, and CA19-9.

► Diagnosis

Apple-core lesion on x-ray, mass on endoscopy biopsied and confirmed by pathology. Extent of disease and prognosis determined by Duke's classification.

► Clinical Therapeutics

Chemotherapy dependent on Duke's stage of disease.

► Clinical Intervention

All require surgical intervention either with resection or, in some cases of lower rectal tumors, ablation with yttrium aluminum garnet laser. Radiation often adjunctive.

► Health Maintenance Issues

Decrease fat and red meat in diet, increase fiber and antioxidants (beta carotene; vitamins A, C, E; and estrogen all reduce risk). Avoid constipation. Participate in recommended screening procedures dependent on age and risk factors. Guidelines suggest yearly occult blood testing after age 40 and periodic sigmoidoscopy or colonoscopy after age 50 in the low-risk individual. When risk factors such as family history, ulcerative colitis, or familial polyposis exist, screening must begin earlier and be more aggressive. Occult blood testing can be misleading, with many false negatives and positives, yet still an inexpensive and somewhat useful initial approach.

E. Hemorrhoids

► Scientific Concepts

Arise secondary to increased pressure exerted on anus from straining, obesity, lifting, with pregnancy when hormone changes exacerbate, or with alcoholism secondary to cirrhosis. Internal hemorrhoids occur above dentate line and originate from superior hemorrhoidal vessels; they may bleed but are not painful unless prolapsed or thrombosed. External hemorrhoids arise from inferior hemorrhoidal venous plexus and are typically more symptomatic.

► History & Physical

Bright red rectal bleeding with bowel movement, pain, sense of fullness, pruritus, mucus in stool. Will appear purple with or without erosion when thrombosed.

► Diagnostic Studies
Visual exam, anoscopy.

► Diagnosis
Friable, edematous, tender, rectal mass with or without erosion, maceration.

► Clinical Therapeutics
Steroid creams, suppositories, sitz bath.

► Clinical Intervention
Thrombosed hemorrhoids require urgent evacuation and excision. Partial or complete hemorrhoidectomy if refractive or recurrent as indicated.

► Health Maintenance Issues
Proper bowel function requires adequate fluid, fiber, and exercise. Avoid straining. Some patients may require stool softeners.

F. Anal Fissure

► Scientific Concepts
Tearing of anoderm secondary to straining with hard stool results in fissure. Sphincter now exposed and goes into spasm, which fails to relax with next defecation, so injury becomes more extensive and may lead to anal ulcer. Occurs at the anterior and posterior midline position; if found elsewhere, consider Crohn's, tuberculosis, malignancy, abscess, or sexually transmitted infection.

► History & Physical
Abrupt-onset, intense rectal pain with bowel movement, blood on tissue; constipation often follows due to fear of recurrent pain.

► Diagnostic Studies
Visual examination, anoscopy often difficult if unanesthetized.

► Diagnosis
Observation of linear tear.

► Clinical Therapeutics
Bulk agents, stool softeners, hydrocortisone suppositories/cream, sitz bath.

► Clinical Intervention
Occasionally require sphincterotomy.

► Health Maintenance Issues
Maintain good bowel function with fluid, fiber, and exercise.

G. Anorectal Abscesses and Fistulae (Fistula-in-Ano)

► Scientific Concepts

Perianal abscesses result from obstruction, stasis, and finally infection of cryptoglandular tissue. Hard stool, diarrhea, foreign bodies, and anal intercourse may all be traumatic and begin this process. Fistulous tracts are inflammatory, orginate in the abscess, and communicate to skin. Proper history is important to rule out underlying contributory conditions (e.g., diabetes, IBD, engagement in anal sexual activity).

► History & Physical

Acute pain and swelling worsening with ambulation and defecation. Pus drains from fistulous ostia. Fever and chills may accompany. Urgent problem in the diabetic and immunocompromised patient.

► Diagnostic Studies

Visual examination, palpation of tender, red mass; anoscopy, transrectal ultrasound (generally requires anesthesia).

► Diagnosis

By inspection on physical examination.

► Clinical Therapeutics

Broad-spectrum antibiotics, IV are often required.

► Clinical Intervention

Surgical drainage done urgently, preferably in operating room. Fistula-in-ano requires excision of fistulous tract; not emergent condition.

► Health Maintenance Issues

Avoid rectal trauma; seek prompt attention in patient with diabetes or malignancy or immunocompromised patient.

H. Pilonidal Disease

► Scientific Concepts

May occur congenitally due to malformations in sacrococcygeal area. Sinus formation and small skin pits develop. Hair (after puberty) invades and acts as foreign body creating draining sinus.

► History & Physical

Pain, swelling, and purulent drainage from ostia in gluteal cleft. Most always found with embedded hairs. Does not communicate with anorectum, which differentiates it from fistula-in-ano.

► Diagnostic Studies

None.

► Diagnosis

Inspection on physical examination.

► Clinical Therapeutics

Antibiotic to cover skin flora.

► Clinical Intervention

Sitz bath, surgical incision, drainage with either primary closure or marsupialization. May recur when primarily surgically closed.

► Health Maintenance Issues

Patient may need to keep area shaved to prevent recurrence once treated.

V. GALLBLADDER

► Scientific Concepts

Cholecystitis occurs both acutely and chronically as result of inflammation of gallbladder lining secondary to obstructive stones/sludge or infection. When stones are present, most are composed of cholesterol, having precipitated out of an inadequate bile salt pool. Factors predisposing to stones include multiple pregnancies, rapid weight loss, oral contraceptives, ileal disease (Crohn's), and genetics. The remaining stones are pigmented of bilirubin from excessive hemolysis. Except in the diabetic, asymptomatic stones do not require therapy.

► History & Physical

Patients complain of epigastric to right upper quadrant (RUQ) sharp, wavelike pain, which may radiate around and into the back, often with nausea and vomiting. Episodes last approximately 3 hours. On palpation, patient may stop inspiration abruptly and involuntarily guard (Murphy's sign). Attacks frequently begin postprandially. May present with fever, chills, and ileus.

► Diagnostic Studies

Gallbladder ultrasound preferred. If negative but clinically suspicious, nuclear scan (hepato-iminodiacetic acid [HIDA]) may be added. Some centers do oral cholecystograms. Both studies add cholecystokinin to stimulate contraction and image gallbladder function. WBC and liver function profile (LFP: alanine transaminase [ALT], aspartate transaminase [AST], alkaline phosphatase, bilirubin).

► Diagnosis

Labs may all be modestly elevated. Presence of stones, sludge (thickened bile is semiobstructing), thickened gallbladder wall, dilated cystic/common duct, grossly enlarged bag, and/or reduced contraction support diagnosis.

► **Clinical Therapeutics**

Oral bile acid therapy (ursodeoxycholine) appropriate only in patients completely unfit for surgery due to limited efficacy. IV antibiotics and fluid resuscitation preoperatively in acute setting. Antispasmodics may be helpful in the less acute patient awaiting surgery.

► **Clinical Intervention**

Cholecystectomy—vast majority done laparoscopically.

► **Health Maintenance Issues**

In the mildly symptomatic, low-fat diet and antispasmodics will provide temporary relief. In general, gallbladder disease cannot be prevented.

VI. PANCREAS

A. Pancreatitis

1. Acute Pancreatitis

► **Scientific Concepts**

In the industrialized world, 70 to 80% is due to alcohol abuse or gallstones. Other etiologies include trauma, drugs, hyperlipidemia, post endoscopic retrograde cholangiopancreatography (ERCP)/surgery, hypercalcemia, infection, and tumor. Severity ranges from mild, isolated, self-limited to severe, life-threatening condition with massive hemorrhage and autodigestion of abdominal contents.

► **History & Physical**

Sharp, continuous, periumbilical pain, may be severe with radiation to back. Nausea, vomiting, fever often present. Tachycardia, tachypnea, and hypotension when severe.

► **Diagnostic Studies**

Serum amylase, lipase, liver function tests (LFTs), CBC, plain abdominal films, abdominal ultrasound, CT, ERCP.

► **Diagnosis**

Amylase and lipase elevated in majority, but levels do not correlate with severity. Elevated 6-hour urinary amylase is the gold standard. Alkaline phosphatase and bilirubin elevated with biliary obstruction. Plain film shows isolated air–fluid level near pancreas (sentinel loop); ultrasound will identify ductal dilatation and stones. CT may define pancreatic changes.

► **Clinical Therapeutics**

Aggressive fluid replacement, IV antibiotics, pain control avoiding morphine (elevates ampullary pressure), and hyperalimentation in some cases.

► **Clinical Intervention**

Bowel rest with or without NG tube drainage, ERCP for stone extraction. Vigilant monitoring of status and development of complications, including pancreatic pseudocyst and progression to hemorrhagic pancreatitis.

► **Health Maintenance Issues**

Sobriety is mandatory for alcohol-induced disease. Discontinue offending medications and treat hyperlipidemia.

2. Chronic Pancreatitis

► **Scientific Concepts**

Ninety percent due to chronic alcohol ingestion, anatomical anomalies (pancreas divisum) familial, ductal obstruction from previous scarring, fibrosis, or stent placement. Ten to thirty percent of cases are idiopathic.

► **History & Physical**

Periodic or continuous periumbilical pain radiating straight through to back, malnutrition, weight loss, steatorrhea, and diabetes mellitus.

► **Diagnostic Studies**

ERCP, ultrasound, CT, plain abdominal films. Labs may or may not be useful.

► **Diagnosis**

Calcifications may be seen on plain films or ultrasound. CT delineates inflammatory changes; ERCP reveals ductal dilatation/stricture.

► **Clinical Therapeutics**

Analgesia, usually requiring opioids, replacement of pancreatic enzymes, insulin if hyperglycemic.

► **Clinical Intervention**

Celiac plexus block for pain control. Partial pancreatectomy in severe cases. Surgery may also be required for complications, most commonly pseudocyst drainage.

► **Health Maintenance Issues**
Sobriety is mandatory to halt progression.

B. Pancreatic Neoplasm

► **Scientific Concepts**

Nearly all tumors are adenocarcinomas, being dense, firm, fibrotic, thus easily able to invade adjacent structures. These characteristics are usually responsible for presenting symptoms. Advanced age, male sex, smoking, chronic pancreatitis, and exposure to dichloro-diphenyl-trichloro-ethane (DDT) are risk factors.

► History & Physical

Few characteristic signs of primary disease. May complain of vague, dull, upper abdominal pain, weight loss, anorexia, diarrhea, and jaundice. Painless jaundice is presumed to be pancreatic cancer until proven otherwise.

► Diagnostic Studies

CT, magnetic resonance imaging (MRI), ERCP, CT-guided percutaneous biopsy, exploratory laparotomy may be necessary. CA19-9 and 242 tumor markers are reasonably specific.

► Diagnosis

Confirmed only by histologic examination of biopsy specimen.

► Clinical Therapeutics

Chemotherapy and radiation for palliation only. No curative therapeutics.

► Clinical Intervention

Less than 15% amenable to surgical resection (Whipple procedure); even those have poor 5-year survival. Aggressive pain control with permanent IV catheter, nerve block.

► Health Maintenance Issues

Measures are supportive and palliative. Tumors are aggressive, fast growing, and fatal.

VII. LIVER

A. Hepatitis

► Scientific Concepts

Inflammatory condition of liver parenchyma leading to necrosis. Causes include viral types A–E, alcohol, drugs, toxins, autoimmune and hereditary disorders, cytomegalovirus, Epstein–Barr virus, and not-yet-identified non-A non-B virus. A type G has been described, which may account for some. Types A and E are endemic in underdeveloped countries and are spread via oral–fecal route. They cause only acute hepatitis and do not become chronic or exist in carrier state. Types B and C are spread parenterally. IV drug users, promiscuous individuals, homosexual males, and health care workers exposed to blood/blood products are at risk. Hepatitis B and C may result in acute, chronic, or asymptomatic carrier states and may progress to cirrhosis and hepatocellular carcinoma. Type D only coexists with type B as a "superinfection," increasing morbidity and mortality. Alcohol alone is generally not a causative factor when consumed at levels less than 80 g/d in males and 40 g/d nonpregnant females. However, other coexisting conditions (e.g., viral hepatitis, drug use, malnutrition) may accelerate alcoholic fatty liver and proceed to fulminant hepatitis. Drugs may present direct hepatotoxins with predictable necrosis, based on dosage, indirectly by interfering with normal metabolism or via immune response. Hemochromatosis (common), Wilson's disease (rare), and alpha-1-antitrypsin deficiency all may result in hepatitis.

▶ History & Physical

History to include age, gender, race, travel, immunizations, occupation, sexual preferences/behaviors, IV drug use, medications, and family history. Presenting symptoms nonspecific, often flulike, malaise, fatigue, fever, arthralgia, arthritis, rash, jaundice, dark urine, pale stools, upper abdominal fullness/pain. Physical findings may not be present or, depending on severity, include hepatosplenomegaly, lymphadenopathy, ascites, and, when appropriate, stigmata of chronic alcoholism.

▶ Diagnostic Studies

LFP including alkaline phosphatase, bilirubin, ALT, AST, and gamma-glutamyl transpeptidase (GGT). CBC, viral serology, alcohol/drug (illicit and legitimate) screen. Liver biopsy often indicated.

▶ Diagnosis

ALT and AST measures, both absolute levels and their ratios can help identify likely cause. Alcoholics often with depleted protein stores, anemia, macrocytic and target red blood cells, elevated GGT. Elevated bilirubin and alkaline phosphatase indicate either biliary or intrahepatic obstruction. Appropriate viral serology can identify the specific virus and status of infection. Rapid return to normal LFP following withdrawal of offending drug confirms chemical hepatitis. Biopsy specimen can demonstrate progression to cirrhosis.

▶ Clinical Therapeutics

Supportive care, adequate fluid and nutrition, avoidance of liver toxins mainstay of therapy for all types of hepatitis. No additional measures needed for viral types A and E. Interferon is effective in reducing severity, complications, and long-term sequelae in types B and C. Must be instituted early. If infection becomes fulminant, patient will require protein restriction and lactulose to prevent hepatic encephalopathy, high-dose corticosteroids, and an exchange transfusion. Autoimmune hepatitis responds to steroids. Hemochromatosis and Wilson's disease require long-term chelation therapy and phlebotomy. Nonimmunized individuals with accidental or inadvertent exposure to blood/body fluids should receive hepatitis B immune globulin immediately. Infants exposed perinatally, household contacts, and sexual partners should also be offered postexposure prophylaxis when not previously immunized.

▶ Clinical Intervention

Liver transplantation is mandatory if patient fails to respond to aggressive therapy and continues to deteriorate.

► Health Maintenance Issues

Appropriate immunizations for patients traveling to endemic areas for types A and B. Type A vaccine also indicated for military personnel, lab workers, homosexual males, IV drug users, day care workers, and primate handlers. Type B vaccine to all infants, health care workers, patients on dialysis, those with high-risk behaviors, regular recipients of blood products, and inmates. Avoidance of occupational and environmental toxins (e.g., organic solvents). Moderate alcohol consumption is permitted in the nonalcoholic individual; however, strict abstinence is mandatory in the alcoholic. Proper nutrition with vitamin supplementation also helpful.

B. Cirrhosis

► Scientific Concepts

Defined as presence of fibrosis with creation of excessive extracellular matrix. This interferes with normal blood flow through liver, impairing nutrient/metabolite exchange and reducing synthesis of hepatic products. Initially, liver enlarges, firm nodules form, liver then gradually becomes shrunken. Most frequent causes are alcohol consumption and viral hepatitis. Others include drugs, toxins, autoimmune complexes, biliary obstruction, congestive heart failure, and some metabolic or genetic abnormalities. Ultimate complications of portal hypertension, GI hemorrhage, and liver failure are fatal.

► History & Physical

History suspicious for any type of hepatitis or family history. Complaints nonspecific with malaise, fatigue, weakness. On examination, ascites, jaundice, stigmata of chronic alcoholism, hepatomegaly with mild tenderness. Liver may be enlarged, firm, or shrunken and nonpalpable. Splenomegaly, muscle wasting, mental confusion/encephalopathy are late manifestations. When advanced to portal hypertension, signs include hemorrhoids, caput medusa, esophageal varices, and splenomegaly. No clinical findings are diagnostic.

► Diagnostic Studies

LFP, 5'nucleotidase, albumin, protime, bleeding time, viral hepatitis panel, serum ammonia, abdominal ultrasound, CT, ERCP, ultimately liver biopsy will confirm diagnosis. EGD may demonstrate esophageal varices. Because of the increased risk of coagulopathy, the biopsy is best done with laparoscopic direct visualization.

► Diagnosis

Mild elevation of hepatocellular enzymes, decreased albumin and coagulation proteins. (Prothrombin time is reliable monitor of liver function.) Definitive diagnosis made by pathologic examination of biopsy specimen.

► Clinical Therapeutics

All therapy aimed at treating sequelae of cirrhosis. Sodium and fluid restrictions combined with low-dose diuretics can reduce ascites.

Encephalopathy can be treated with protein restriction and lactulose (reduce ammonia). Nonselective alpha blockade to reduce portal pressures.

► Clinical Intervention

Sclerotherapy/banding of esophageal varices, placement of Laveen or Denver shunt to drain ascites (controversial, last-ditch effort at palliation), placement of transjugular intrahepatic portosystemic shunt (TIPS) (connects hepatic and portal veins). All are palliative and are not predictably effective. Liver transplantation may be appropriate for the alcohol-abstinent patient.

► Health Maintenance Issues

Treatment for alcoholism if appropriate; avoid alcohol in all cirrhotic patients; eliminate offending drugs/toxins; address high-risk behaviors; limit acetaminophen. With early intervention, fibrosis may be halted, thus avoiding the ultimately fatal complications.

C. Hepatocellular Carcinoma (Hepatoma)

► Scientific Concepts

Uncommon primary tumor in United States, accounts for 50% of malignancies in parts of South Africa and Asia. Etiology is unknown, but preexisting cirrhosis secondary to chronic type B or C viral hepatitis, alcoholism, hemochromotosis, and alpha-1-antitrypsin deficiency are all significant risk factors. Others include long-term treatment with exogenous androgens, schistosomiasis, and clonorchiasis. Unlike primary hepatoma, metastatic liver disease is common. In non–third world countries, 50% of patients dying with malignancies will have liver metastases. Benign hepatic cysts and hemangiomas are common and require no treatment unless painful due to size or bleeding.

► History & Physical

History of cirrhosis or other risk factors. Patient presents with fatigue, malaise, rapid weight loss, abdominal pain. Ascites may be bloody; enlarged liver may be tender and firm. Bruit heard over liver is highly suggestive. Jaundice is uncommon finding.

► Diagnostic Studies

LFP, alpha-fetoprotein, gallium scan, CT, angiography, and cautiously performed liver biopsy. Tumors are highly vascular, and patient often has coexisting coagulopathy.

► Diagnosis

Abrupt increase in alkaline phosphatase in previously stable cirrhotic patient, increased alpha-fetoprotein, filling defect on gallium scanning, tumor blush on angiogram.

► Clinical Therapeutics

No effective treatment currently available. Prognosis poor, with life expectancy generally less than 6 months.

► **Clinical Intervention**

Surgery rarely indicated and only when confined to one lobe.

► **Health Maintenance Issues**

Avoidance of risk factors for cirrhosis. Proper immunizations, early identification and treatment of hemochromatosis and alpha-1-antitrypsin deficiency. Careful follow-up in patients with chronic hepatitis B and C.

D. Abscess

► **Scientific Concepts**

Pyogenic abscesses most commonly are secondary to biliary disease (e.g., acute cholecystitis, ascending cholangitis). The bacteria, frequently gram negatives and anaerobes, may also gain entry from contiguous organs or penetrating trauma. *Entamoeba histolytica* is the only parasitic pathogen and is spread via fecal–oral route. Persons at high risk are institutionalized individuals and homosexual males. Asymptomatic carriers found in the United States. *Candida* is a source of liver abscess in the immunocompromised patient.

► **History & Physical**

History of risk factors, surgical history. Presenting complaints of malaise, right upper quadrant (RUQ) pain, fever/chills, mild hepatomegaly. Jaundice found in 25%.

► **Diagnostic Studies**

LFP, CBC, blood culture, chest x-ray, abdominal ultrasound, CT with IV contrast, serology (immunoglobulin M enzyme-linked immunosorbent assay [IgM ELISA]) if parasitic infection is consideration.

► **Diagnosis**

Elevated white blood count, mildly elevated LFP, increased gamma-glutamyl transpeptidase (GGTP), blood culture positive in 50%. Round/oval defects on ultrasound, air–fluid levels within liver. Amebic abscess more typically single than multiple.

► **Clinical Therapeutics**

Broad-spectrum IV antibiotics to cover for gram negatives and anaerobes in pyogenic abscess. Metronidazole followed by iodoquinol (intestinal amebicide).

► **Clinical Intervention**

In absence of coagulopathy or ascites, CT-guided percutaneous drainage of pyogenic abscess is indicated. Open surgical drainage may be required when primary treatment fails. Therapeutic aspiration indicated when amebic abscess large and in danger of rupture with resulting pulmonary and anaphylactic complications.

► **Health Maintenance Issues**

Good sanitation, avoid high-risk behaviors, prompt treatment of acute biliary disease.

VIII. HERNIA, EXTERNAL

▶ Scientific Concepts

Hernias occur wherever a defect appears in a supporting structure (commonly abdominal wall) allowing its contents to protrude. The most common types are direct and indirect inguinal, umbilical, and incisional. Femoral, obturator, and Spigelian occur rarely. The groin hernias occur more frequently in males and are described depending on their anatomic location in reference to the inferior epigastric and femoral vessels. Both groin and umbilical hernias may be congenital or acquired. When acquired, they are due to greater intra-abdominal pressures than the strength of the abdominal wall, allowing the defect to enlarge. Small or large bowel, omentum, or bladder then protrudes through the defect. Severity can range from an easily reducible and painless hernia (these are usually large defects) to incarcerated (unable to reduce) to strangulated. With strangulation, obstruction occurs, the blood supply is lost and necrosis then ensues. Urgent surgical correction is required. Incisional hernias can occur through fascia wherever previous incision has been made. They may result from inadequate surgical technique in the closure or, more often, a wound infection.

▶ History & Physical

The patient describes sudden or gradual onset of a bulge in the groin, scrotum, or umbilicus. However, often a bulge is not apparent and the patient complains of dull, throbbing pain radiating to thigh, scrotum, and lower back. The pain is made worse with activity and improves with rest. A sudden increase in pain, change to a colicky nature, nausea, or vomiting with decreased bowel sounds indicates an obstruction regardless of location.

On examination, the umbilical hernia will protrude when the patient coughs or lifts head while supine. The defect is palpable. Groin hernias often visible but may be detected only by placing the index finger up to the external ring, having patient cough or bear down, then feeling bulge of soft tissue pressing against the examining finger. Perform with patient upright or supine.

▶ Diagnostic Studies

None usually required, though some obscure types (e.g., obturator, internal, paraesophageal) may need CT or barium studies.

▶ Diagnosis

A physical examination will detect the hernia, although the clinician will not necessarily be able to distinguish among the types of groin hernias until surgery.

▶ Clinical Therapeutics

There is no role except for temporary pain management until repair can be made.

► Clinical Intervention

There are several surgical approaches to groin hernias, most commonly using mesh reinforcements in some manner. Laparoscopic repair is an alternative but is controversial due to greatly increased cost, increased risks, and possible greater recurrence rate. Incisional and umbilical hernia repairs may or may not require mesh. In the patient unsuitable for surgery, a truss may provide some support and pain relief.

► Health Maintenance Issues

Infant groin hernias should be identified and corrected as early as possible. Use of good body mechanics in heavy work can reduce incidence of groin hernia. Umbilical hernias in adults are often secondary to or aggravated by obesity. Weight loss and improved abdominal wall strength will benefit these patients. Surgical repair is recommended for most to avoid complications. The small, painful hernia is the one at greatest risk and is easier to repair early on.

IX. NUTRITIONAL REQUIREMENTS AND ASSESSMENT

► Scientific Concepts

Despite the large number of different tissues in the body, only a small number of nutritional elements are essential to maintain health. Essential elements are those that cannot be synthesized by the body to be used in the metabolic process.

► Essential Nutritional Elements

The following are required for normal nutritional functioning:
- Water
- Energy source (i.e., carbohydrates)
- Water-soluble vitamins
- Fat-soluble vitamins
- Essential amino acids
- Minerals
- Essential fatty acids

► Daily Requirements

How much of a particular element is needed is defined by the recommended daily allowance (RDA). RDA levels have been established by the Food and Nutrition board of the National Academy of Science to express the amount of a nutritional item needed to maintain a healthy state. The RDAs in many cases are two standard deviations above the mean requirement estimated necessary for much of the population. Many factors may influence the specific nutritional requirements of an individual, including the composition of a diet, various disease states, and physiologic factors (i.e., pregnancy).

▶ Levels of Specific Nutrients

Vitamins are a group of organic compounds needed to conduct metabolic functions. Vitamins are divided into water-soluble and fat-soluble categories. Fat-soluble vitamins can accumulate and cause toxic syndromes. Deficiencies of both water- and fat-soluble vitamins cause specific syndromes that will be discussed later in this chapter. Safe and adequate levels for all vitamins can be found in any standard textbook of nutrition or medicine. See Table 6–2 for a summary of selected vitamin functions and sources.

Minerals are inorganic compounds needed for proper metabolic function. The minerals are divided into major and minor mineral groups by the amount needed each day.

Protein is needed to provide for structural integrity and function. The nine essential amino acids are needed to synthesize other needed proteins. Supplemental nitrogen should be available to provide for proper protein synthesis. Amount of protein needed in diet depends in part on quality of protein consumed. Animal sources provide the highest-quality protein, followed by legumes and other plant sources.

Fat provides the densest calorie source available to the body for energy. However, the primary role for dietary fat is to provide essential fatty acids (specifically linolecic acid needed for prostaglandin synthesis).

Carbohydrate should supply most of the energy requirements in

▶ table 6-2

SUMMARY OF VITAMIN ACTIONS AND SOURCES

Vitamin	Type	Important Action	Sources
A	Fat soluble	Retinal function, wound healing; under investigation for prevention of cancer/heart disease	Pigmented vegetables
D	Fat soluble	Acceleration of phosphorus and calcium absorption in gastrointestinal tract	Sunlight, fresh fruits, milk
E	Fat soluble	Thought to protect cell membranes and structures as antioxidant, ? role in prevention of cancer, heart disease and cataracts	Vegetables, seed oil
K	Fat soluble	Promotes hemostasis by assisting in function of coagulation factors; synthesized by bacteria in intestine	Leafy green vegetables
Thiamine (B$_1$)	Water soluble	Cofactor in carbohydrate oxidation	Meat, milk, eggs
Riboflavin (B$_2$)	Water soluble	Cofactor in oxidation-reduction reactions	Meat, dairy products, fish
Niacin	Water soluble	Involved in oxidation reduction reactions, can be used to lower blood lipids	Cereals, vegetables, dairy products
Pyridoxine (B$_6$)	Water soluble	Metabolism of amino acids	Meat, starchy vegetables
C (ascorbic acid)	Water soluble	Synthesis of collagen, antioxidant, wound healing, absorption of iron	Fresh fruits and vegetables

the average American diet. Sources of carbohydrate include simple sugars, complex carbohydrates (starches) and indigestible carbohydrates. Insoluble dietary fiber can assist in lowering levels of cholesterol and improving colonic function. Aside from assuring adequate energy levels, the body has no specific requirement for carbohydrate per se.

► History & Physical

To ascertain nutritional status of patient, it is necessary to employ history, physical examination, and laboratory investigations. Goal is to identify patients at nutritional risk or those who already have clinically recognizable disease.

History questions should be directed at what meals are eaten each day and general composition of meals. Specific attention should be directed toward groups that are at traditionally high risk for nutritional deficiency: pregnant and nursing women, the poor, the elderly, and adolescents. Patient-generated food intake records may be kept for 24 hours or longer periods (several days) in attempt to provide a more accurate diet history.

The targeted physical examination is directed at observation of muscle mass, detection of muscle wasting, and recognition of clinical syndromes of nutritional excess or deficiency (see vitamin deficiency and protein calorie malnutrition sections). Observation of body habitus to detect such conditions as obesity is also performed at this time. Standard reference charts giving "ideal height–weight guidelines have been produced by actuarial organizations. For more detailed analysis of body composition, anthropomorphic measurements are available. Most commonly performed anthropomorphic measurement is skin fold thickness analysis of triceps and arm muscle circumference. Currently, there are several sophisticated options available to conduct anthropomorphic measurements. Most are expensive and require specialized equipment to perform.

► Diagnostic Studies

Serum albumin has long been used to serve as a marker for protein calorie malnutrition. While it is true that malnutrition will cause abnormally low levels of albumin, other diseases (e.g., liver disease) will also suppress levels of this protein. Other protein markers can be measured but are no more specific than albumin.

Lab workup for nutritional assessment often includes measures of immune function. Total lymphocyte count and reactions to common skin antigens (e.g., purified protein derivative and strep) are usually employed for this assessment.

Serial weights can be measured by nursing personnel, and dieticians can perform calorie counts to more objectively monitor elements of nutritional intake. Other investigations for specific deficiencies (e.g., vitamin B_{12}) will be discussed in other sections.

► Diagnosis

While laboratory investigations may provide some helpful clues to diagnosis, most are nonspecific and one must keep in mind that other nonnutritional processes may be responsible for alterations in laboratory values.

▶ Clinical Therapeutics
None.

▶ Clinical Intervention
None.

▶ Health Maintenance Issues
Health care providers should encourage patients to eat a balanced diet following recommendations set in the "Food Guide Pyramid," as established by the U.S. Department of Agriculture. "Fad diets" whose concepts are not founded on clinically proven data should be avoided. Patients should be cautioned that excessive consumption of some vitamins and minerals might be harmful.

A. Protein Calorie Malnutrition

▶ Scientific Concepts
Adequate energy and protein supplies are necessary for normal physiologic functioning. Shortages of both or either of these elements will result in protein calorie malnutrition. Two distinct syndromes are classically described in relation to malnutrition, kwashiorkor syndrome (deficiency of protein) and marasmus (both protein and energy deficiency). Primary causes of these deficiencies (due to shortage of food intake) are rare in industrialized nations. In the United States, most causes of malnutrition are secondary, related to another disease process. The following factors may play a role in development of secondary malnutrition.
• Increased utilization of calories (e.g., burns)
• Decreased intake (e.g., oral trauma)
• Malabsorption (e.g., diarrhea)
Malnutrition effects virtually every organ system. Chief clinical effects may include decreased production of proteins by liver and decreased cardiac contractility resulting in electrocardiographic shifts. Wound healing is impaired due to defective immunologic functioning.

▶ History & Physical
Clinician should seek history of unintentional weight loss, poor dietary intake, or history of clinical circumstances that may produce malnutrition from secondary cause.
Most obvious finding on physical examination would be weight loss in adult patient. Children will manifest failure to thrive. Skin will usually be dry and hair thin. Edema may be present from low protein levels. In more extreme cases, face and extremities will exhibit loss of fat stores ("sunken eyes," etc.).

▶ Diagnostic Studies
No specific laboratory findings. Look for decreases in serum albumin level and lymphocyte count.

► Diagnosis

Watch for development of risk factors in susceptible patients. Do not overlook diagnosis in patients who are hypermetabolic. They may not manifest significant weight loss.

► Clinical Therapeutics

Correct underlying deficiencies in electrolytes and infections first. Then begin process of replacing energy and proteins. Advance calories and protein intake slowly while observing patient carefully. Most adults can tolerate 30 kcal/kg and 0.8 g of protein. Later, advance patient to 40 kcal. Vitamins and minerals can be added initially. Most texts recommend holding fat calories until later in recovery.

► Clinical Intervention

Patients may need parenteral feedings if enteral is not available. Enteral feedings always preferable if that route is available.

► Health Maintenance Issues

Being alert to which patients are at risk. Providing adequate nutritional support to hospitalized patients may prevent development of protein calorie malnutrition.

B. Vitamin Deficiencies

► Scientific Concepts

Vitamins serve as cofactors to allow metabolic reactions to occur. Clinically, most vitamin deficiencies occur as part of protein calorie malnutrition or in concert with other vitamin deficiencies rather than as single entity. Table 6–2 on page 140 summarizes important basic functions of each vitamin (vitamin B_{12} and folate are discussed in Chapter 14, "Hematology and Oncology").

1. Vitamin A Deficiency

► History & Physical

Seek history of concurrent malabsorption, alcoholism, or laxative abuse. Night blindness symptoms should also be sought. Sometimes patients complain of loss of taste. Vitamin A deficiency most common cause of blindness in many developing countries. Physical examination may reveal evidence of poor wound healing, xerosis, and hyperkeratosis of the skin. Small white spots may appear on conjunctiva (Bitot's spots). More serious ocular findings such as blindness are late findings.

► Diagnostic Studies

Serum levels for vitamin A.

► Diagnosis

Usually obvious in the appropriate clinical setting. Night blindness may be only finding in early disease.

► **Clinical Therapeutics**

Treat with vitamin A, 30,000 IU/d × 1 week. Higher doses may be needed for more advanced disease.

► **Clinical Intervention**

None needed.

► **Health Maintenance Issues**

Encourage proper diet to minimize risk of developing deficiency. Recognize patients at risk.

2. Vitamin D Deficiency

► **History & Physical**

The classic deformities from vitamin D deficiency, rickets, is uncommon in the United States today. Features include skeletal deformities such as genu valgus and varum. Other abnormalities include enlarged spleen, liver, and skull, along with thoracic deformities. Today, patients at risk for vitamin D deficiency are urban elderly, particularly those who live in cold, northern climates. Lack of sunlight, staying indoors, and diet poor in vitamin D–enriched products and calcium add to the risk. Certain anticonvulsants are also efficient in converting vitamin D to inactive compounds. Other anticonvulsants may interfere with calcium absorption.

► **Diagnostic Studies**

Serum calcium and phosphate levels, possibly radiography in severe cases.

► **Diagnosis**

Vitamin D deficiency should be considered in patients with hypocalcemia of moderate to severe degrees. One must also determine reason for vitamin D deficiency, such as malabsorption or resistance to action of vitamin D.

► **Clinical Therapeutics**

Administration of vitamin D and calcium.

► **Clinical Intervention**

None needed.

► **Health Maintenance Issues**

Importance of vitamin D and calcium supplementation to patients at risk.

3. Vitamin E Deficiency

► **History & Physical**

Seek history of malabsorption, cystic fibrosis, or cholestatic liver disease. Physical examination may reveal absence of reflexes. May also discover a sensory neuropathy consisting of proprioception and vibration changes. Gait disturbances may occur as well.

► **Diagnostic Studies**
Serum vitamin E levels should be measured.

► **Diagnosis**
Typical clinical symptoms with low levels of serum vitamin E.

► **Clinical Therapeutics**
Controversy still exists about the correct therapeutic dose of vitamin E for replacement therapy. Has been given at up to 80 times recommended daily dose without apparent harmful effect.

► **Clinical Intervention**
None required.

► **Health Maintenance Issues**
Observe patients at risk for development of clinical deficiency.

4. Vitamin K Deficiency

► **History & Physical**
Because body stores of vitamin K are small, deficiency may develop quickly. Patients who have received broad-spectrum antibiotics may hamper the production of vitamin K by intestinal bacteria. Patient with history of poor dietary intake also at risk. No specific findings on physical examination.

► **Diagnostic Studies**
Abnormally prolonged prothrombin time (PT) (partial thromboplastin time [PTT] only slightly prolonged, or at least less so than PT).

► **Diagnosis**
Patient with risk factors and typical pattern of coagulation abnormalities. Therapeutic trial of vitamin K when diagnosis is in question.

► **Clinical Therapeutics**
Subcutaneous vitamin K at 15 mg.

► **Clinical Intervention**
None required.

► **Health Maintenance Issues**
Recognize patients at risk; ensure proper diet.

5. Thiamine (Vitamin B₁) Deficiency

► **History & Physical**
Alcoholic patients are at particular risk to develop thiamine deficiency. Early complaints may include muscle cramps and paresthesias. Patients are prone to develop heart failure and may complain of dyspnea on exertion. Physical examination findings are most prominent on examination of cardiovascular and neurologic systems. Classic signs of heart failure may be present. On neurologic examination,

search for peripheral sensory neuropathy that is more marked on the arms than the legs. Patients with advanced disease may develop one of the two classic syndromes associated with thiamine deficiency. Wernicke's encephalopathy consists of confusion with ophthalmoplegia. Korsakoff's syndrome includes amnesia and confabulation.

▶ Diagnostic Studies

Usually no diagnostic tests are done since the assays for thiamine deficiency are expensive. The clinical response to a trail of thiamine is usually diagnostic.

▶ Diagnosis

Consider thiamine deficiency in alcoholic patient with typical symptoms.

▶ Clinical Therapeutics

Administer thiamine parentally, approximately 50 to 100 mg/d for several days. Follow with oral thiamine at 5 to 10 mg/kg. Most clinicians treat with concomitant administration of other water-soluble vitamins in addition to thiamine replacement.

▶ Clinical Intervention

None needed.

▶ Health Maintenance Issues

Attempt interventions in alcoholic patients aimed at abstinence from alcohol and proper diet to prevent development of thiamine deficiency.

6. Riboflavin (Vitamin B$_2$) Deficiency

▶ History & Physical

Most patients have a concurrent condition that causes riboflavin deficiency. Seek evidence of alcoholism, medication interaction, or any other cause of malnutrition. Clinical examination should look for evidence of cheilosis, angular stomatitis, or glossitis. Dermatitis also common finding.

▶ Diagnostic Studies

Riboflavin deficiency is usually treated empirically.

▶ Clinical Therapeutics

Administer oral preparation at 5 to 15 mg/d.

▶ Clinical Intervention

None needed.

▶ Health Maintenance Issues

Maintain proper diet for patient to prevent deficiency; treat coexisting nutritional problems.

7. Niacin Deficiency

► History & Physical

Niacin deficiency presents with combination of dermatitis, diarrhea, and dementia. In classic form, deficiency is referred to as *pellagra*. Dermatitis is symmetric and characterized by appearance of desquamated and hyperpigmented lesions. Any diarrhea that is present may also accompany stomatitis or glossitis. Dementia is nonspecific, manifested by loss of memory, hallucinations, and finally psychosis.

► Diagnostic Studies

No specific lab tests will confirm.

► Diagnosis

Typical clinical syndrome and response to therapeutic trial.

► Clinical Therapeutics

Oral niacin (10 mg/d) in conjunction with adequate tryptophan.

► Clinical Intervention

None needed.

► Health Maintenance Issues

Maintenance of balanced diet. Pellagra was once believed to be linked to diet in which corn supplied most of the calories. Although there is a relationship, interplay of intake of corn and development of pellagra is now recognized to be more complex.

8. Pyridoxine (Vitamin B$_6$) Deficiency

► History & Physical

A history of ingestion of isoniazid, penicillamine, or oral contraceptives is important as interactions with medications is one of the most common causes of pyridoxine deficiency. Alcoholism can also be a contributing factor. Physical examination may reveal cheilosis, stomatitis, and dermatitis. More significant deficiency may result in sensory neuropathy.

► Diagnostic Studies

Measure pyridoxine phosphate levels in the blood.

► Clinical Therapeutics

Treat with vitamin B$_6$ orally in doses of 10 to 20 mg/d. Vitamin B$_6$ is routinely prescribed when patients are receiving medications that interfere with metabolism of this vitamin.

► Clinical Intervention

None needed.

► Health Maintenance Issues

See Clinical Therapeutics above.

9. Ascorbic Acid (Vitamin C) Deficiency

▶ **History & Physical**

Patients at risk for vitamin C deficiencies are those who smoke cigarettes, are poor, or have chronic illnesses. Scurvy will develop in patients who have moderate or severe deficiency of vitamin C. Classic findings in scurvy are perifollicular hemorrhage, petechiae, and purpura. As disease progresses, hemorrhages occur into gums, joints, and even intracerebrally. Mild vitamin C deficiency may manifest only lethargy and fatigue. Wound healing also impaired.

▶ **Diagnostic Studies**

Diagnosis is made on clinical grounds or by using plasma ascorbic acid levels.

▶ **Diagnosis**

Made from typical clinical appearance.

▶ **Clinical Therapeutics**

Begin treatment with 300 to 1,000 mg/d of ascorbic acid.

▶ **Clinical Intervention**

None needed.

▶ **Health Maintenance Issues**

Counseling about proper nutrition.

C. Obesity

▶ **Scientific Concepts**

Defined as a weight in excess of 20% of ideal body weight (although some definitions vary). Ideal weights can be read off a table prepared that relates to gender, frame size, height, and weight. Body mass index (BMI) is a newer, useful tool to relate height and weight in a clinically useful way. A BMI of 20 to 25 kg/m^2 is considered healthy. Once BMI increases to a value of 30 kg/m^2, obesity is present. It is now recognized that many factors may play a role in development of obesity. Genetic factors, environmental factors, and dietary intake all play a role to some extent in development of obesity. Obesity increases risk of developing many diseases, including gallbladder disease, joint problems, diabetes mellitus, cardiovascular disease, and several forms of cancer.

▶ **History & Physical**

Dietary histories relayed by patients tend to underreport calorie ingestion. Food intake logs kept by patient over a period of days may help to portray intake more accurately. Take drug history, seeking medications associated with weight gain, such as steriods. Be alert for congenital syndromes associated with obesity that may be present and recognizable from physical examination (e.g., Prader–Willi), although in practice these syndromes are rare. Measure the BMI to confirm clinical assessment of body fat. Ascertain waist circumference. If circumference is > 100 cm in men and 90 cm in women, there is associated risk of low high-density lipoprotein (HDL) levels and high trigylcerides.

▶ Diagnostic Studies

Measurement of blood lipids, serum glucose, etc., for comorbid conditions.

▶ Diagnosis

Diagnosis is made from clinical presentation and determination of BMI.

▶ Clinical Therapeutics

Use of medications to treat obeisty should be reserved primarily for patients who have a BMI > 30 kg/m². There are many appetite suppressants currently available to clinicians. Two major categories of medications are serotonergic agents and noradrenergic agents. Use of amphetamine for weight loss is no longer advisable.

▶ Clinical Intervention

Nonphamacologic therapies to assist obese patient may help to induce or maintain weight loss. Exercise is an important adjunct to assist patient in maintaining normal weight. Behavior modification therapy may provide assistance in initial weight loss and eating behavior. Diet therapy may also be used to reduce overall fat and calorie intake. More frequent, small feedings with high-carbohydrate and fiber-containing foods will help maintain satiety. Patient must also be aware that location of eating may promote consumption of high-fat foods or excessive intake. This includes buffet style or cafeteria settings.

Surgery is a consideration for those with BMI of 40 kg/m² or 35 kg/m² (or greater) with significant comorbidity factors. Recommended procedure is the Roux-en-Y anastomosis.

▶ Health Maintenance Issues

Weight regain is a significant issue to the obese patient who has been successful in losing weight. A regime of exercise and supportive environment will be helpful to maintenance of more desirable weight for the patient.

BIBLIOGRAPHY

Greenfield L. *Surgery, Scientific Principles and Practice*. Philadelphia: Lippincott-Raven; 1997.

Grendell JH. *Current Diagnosis and Treatment in Gastroenterology*. Stamford, CT: Appleton & Lange; 1996.

Haubrich WS. *Bockus Gastroenterology*, 5th ed. Philadelphia: WB Saunders; 1995.

Isselbacker K. *Harrison's Principles of Internal Medicine*, 13th ed. New York: McGraw-Hill; 1994.

Rakel R. *Conn's Current Treatment,* 50th anniversary ed. Philadelphia: WB Saunders; 1998.

Sabiston S. *Textbook of Surgery, The Biological Basis of Modern Surgical Practice,* 14th ed. Philadelphia: WB Saunders; 1991.

Schwartz S. *Principles of Surgery,* 6th ed. New York: McGraw-Hill; 1994.

Tierney L. *Current Medical Diagnosis and Treatment 1994.* Norwalk, CT: Appleton & Lange; 1994.

Renal Diseases | 7

Brenda L. Jasper, PA-C

I. RENAL FUNCTION

► Scientific Concepts

The nephron is the functional unit of the kidney, with 1.0 to 1.3 million nephrons per kidney. Responsible for fluid and electrolyte maintenance, excretion of waste products of metabolism, and secretion of hormones.

A. Measurement of Renal Function

► Scientific Concepts

Blood urea nitrogen (BUN): Produced from metabolism of amino acids in the liver. Increased in states of increased tissue breakdown (gastrointestinal [GI] bleeding, corticosteroids), high dietary protein intake, and prerenal azotemia. Decreased in malnutrition and liver disease.

Creatinine: Produced from metabolism of creatine in skeletal muscle. Daily production is fairly constant. As the glomerular filtration rate (GFR) decreases, the creatinine increases. A doubling of serum creatinine represents loss of one-half of the GFR (i.e., rise in plasma creatinine from 1.0 mg/dL to 2.0 mg/dL represents 50% loss of renal function, and subsequent doubling of plasma creatinine represents an additional 50% loss of the remaining renal function).

GFR: Direct measure of renal function based on filtration of plasma across the glomerulus.

Creatinine clearance (CrCl): Clinical measurement of creatinine filtered across glomerulus and secreted by tubule. A direct measure of GFR is not clinically feasible; therefore, CrCl is used to estimate the GFR. CrCl is calculated by obtaining a 24-hour urine collection for creatinine and measurement of serum creatinine using the following formula:

$$CrCl = \frac{urine\ creatinine \times volume\ (mL/min)}{plasma\ creatinine}$$

Normal creatinine clearance in men is 120 ± 25 mL/min; women, 95 ± 20mL/min; decreases by 1 mL/min/y over the age of 40. Estimation of CrCl by serum creatinine:

$$CrCl = \frac{(140 - age) \times weight\ in\ kilograms}{plasma\ creatinine \times 72}$$

In women, multiply result by 0.85 due to decreased muscle portion of body weight.

B. Urinalysis

1. Hematuria

► Scientific Concepts

Detection of hemoglobin in urine, gross or microscopic. May originate from any site in the urinary tract.

► History & Physical

Evaluate for gross hematuria, recent illness such as upper respiratory infection (postinfectious glomerulonephritis, immunoglobulin A [IgA] nephropathy), urinary symptoms suggestive of infection or stones, other systemic illnesses (systemic lupus erythematosus, vasculitis, bleeding disorder, sickle cell trait or disease), family history of kidney disease (hereditary nephritis, polycystic kidney disease), and prostatic disease. Rule out hematuria secondary to menstrual bleeding in women.

► Diagnostic Studies
Urinalysis: Two red blood cells per high-power field in centrifuge urine specimen. Red sediment with clear supernatant indicates hematuria. Heme-positive red supernatant indicates hemoglobinuria (intravascular hemolysis) or myoglobinuria (muscle damage). Heme-negative red supernatant indicates porphyria, ingestion of beets, or phenazopyridine use. Cells are dysmorphic in glomerular bleeding and of uniform size and shape in nonglomerular bleeding.
Other diagnostic studies: Intravenous pyelogram (IVP), renal sonogram, cystoscopy, urine cytology; computed tomographic (CT) scan may detect small tumors; renal angiography to detect arteriovenous malformations. If no cause identified, follow and reevaluate.

► Diagnosis
Identify site of bleeding as either glomerular or extraglomerular. A three-tube test may help determine source of bleeding. Hematuria may be transient or persistent, with transient hematuria most common; source not found in most cases. Tumors of genitourinary (GU) tract, infections, and benign prostatic hypertrophy (BPH) should be ruled out as causes.

► Clinical Therapeutics
Treat infection or underlying disease if identified.

► Clinical Intervention
Renal biopsy can identify form of glomerulonephritis associated with hematuria (IgA nephropathy, hereditary nephritis, or membranoproliferative glomerulonephritis) but reserved for those cases associated with deterioration in renal function, proteinuria, or unexplained hypertension.

► Health Maintenance Issues
Microscopic hematuria is a common finding and can be transient; careful history and appropriate testing should be done on all older patients due to increased risk of malignancy.

2. Proteinuria

► Scientific Concepts
Increased permeability of glomerular capillary wall to albumin or low-molecular-weight proteins; normal protein excretion < 150 mg protein per day.

► History & Physical
Identify any history of systemic illness associated with proteinuria (diabetes mellitus, systemic lupus erythematosus, etc.), past history of

poststreptococcal glomerulonephritis, or family history of renal disease.

▶ Diagnostic Studies

Random urine specimen: Urine dipstick sensitive for albumin; sulfosalicylic acid detects all proteins including nonalbumin proteins such as immunoglobulin light chains. Three separate specimens to confirm. If under age 25, rule out orthostatic proteinuria.

24-hour urine for protein excretion: < 1 g/d usually benign form of isolated proteinuria, > 2 g/d indicative of serious renal disease, and > 3.5 g/d indicates nephrotic range proteinuria.

Renal sonogram or IVP to rule out structural lesions. Renal biopsy reserved for those with evidence of abnormal renal function, > 2 g/d proteinuria, or associated hematuria.

▶ Diagnosis

Benign orthostatic (postural): Increased protein excretion when upright, normal protein excretion when supine. Usually seen in adolescents, rare over age 30. Proteinuria often disappears over years and is not generally associated with renal damage.

Transient (intermittent): Most commonly seen. Benign form that often resolves on repeat exams. Can be seen with exercise, fever, and acute illness.

Persistent: Ongoing protein excretion of 1 to 2 g/d. More likely associated with underlying renal disease. Prognosis better in those under age 25.

▶ Clinical Therapeutics

Treatment of underlying glomerular disease, if present, is key. Angiotensin-converting enzyme (ACE) inhibitors work by lowering efferent arteriolar resistance and have effect on glomerular capillary permeability. Nonsteroidal anti-inflammatory drugs (NSAIDs) occasionally used, but only when renal function is not severely impaired because they lower GFR and can lead to acute renal failure or hyperkalemia.

▶ Clinical Intervention

Dietary protein restriction (in select patients, 0.6 to 0.8 g/kg/d plus protein added to match urinary protein losses), reduction in blood pressure.

3. **Cells**
   - *Red cells:* Can be present from any site in urinary tract. Red cell morphology can help identify site. Cells are dysmorphic in glomerular bleeding, uniform shape in nonglomerular bleeding.
   - *White cells:* Pyuria indicative of infection; eosinophils may be clue to interstitial nephritis.

4. **Casts**
   - *Hyaline:* Mucoprotein composition; not associated with renal disease. Can be seen in volume depletion and with diuretic use.
   - *Red cell:* Indicative of glomerular disease, usually glomerulonephritis or vasculitis.

- *White cell:* Seen in pyelonephritis and other tubulointerstitial disorders.
- *Broad/waxy:* Form in tubules which have been dilated; seen in chronic or advanced renal failure.

5. Osmolality

- Urine osmolality can vary under influence of antidiuretic hormone (ADH) released from the posterior pituitary gland. Useful in clinical settings of hypernatremia, hyponatremia, polyuria, and when differentiating prerenal disease from acute tubular necrosis.

6. Volume

- *Anuria:* Urine volume less than 50 mL/d.
- *Oliguria:* Urine volume less than 500 mL/d.
- *Polyuria:* Urine volume exceeding 3 L/d.

II. INFECTIOUS DISEASES AND INFLAMMATORY CONDITIONS OF THE KIDNEY/URINARY TRACT

A. Urinary Tract Infections (UTIs)

▶ Scientific Concepts

Uncomplicated UTI: Not associated with anatomic or structural deformity in urinary tract, recent surgery involving urinary tract, catheters, or other GU procedures. Community-acquired infections mostly seen in females, rare in males. Eighty percent are secondary to *Escherichia coli*. Long-term sequelae are rare.

Complicated UTI: Associated with anatomic abnormalities, obstructive uropathy, or abnormal bladder function. Risk factors include catheters, renal calculi, GU procedures, and pregnancy. More common in infants (anatomic abnormalities) and the elderly (BPH, obstruction, catheters, nosocomial infections). *E. coli* is the most common organism, but many other organisms are seen and are often more resistant to antibiotics. Duration of therapy is 7 to 21 days.

1. Lower Urinary Tract Infections (Bladder, Prostate, Urethra)

▶ History & Physical

Symptoms include frequency, urgency, dysuria, voiding small amounts, suprapubic pain, cloudy urine, occasional hematuria.

▶ Diagnostic Studies

- Microscopic exam of urine for pyuria, hematuria, and Gram stain.
- Urine culture colony count of 100,000 colony-forming units of bacteria per milliliter of urine. Urine should be midstream specimen in sterile container after proper cleaning of external genitalia. *E. coli* most common organism in uncomplicated UTIs. *Proteus* organisms seen in patients with staghorn calculi. *Pseudomonas* and *Candida* common in patients with indwelling catheters.
- Prostate secretions for white blood cells (WBCs), bacteria, and culture.

- Urethral or cervical discharge for Gram stain and culture (bacterial or viral) to identify organism; gram-negative intracellular diplococci in gonococcal urethritis; Tzank test for herpes simplex virus; rapid monoclonal immunofluorescent antibody detection in *Chlamydia.*
- Radiodiagnostics are not indicated for uncomplicated cystitis or urethritis in women. Cystoscopy, voiding cystourethrogram (VCUG), and IVP reserved for complicated or chronic cases and should be considered in infants or males with first infection.

► Diagnosis

Cystitis: Symptoms generally sudden in onset. Patient may present with any symptoms of lower UTI. Risk factors include gender (mostly female), age (18 to 40), sexual intercourse, delayed postcoital voiding, and pregnancy. *E. coli* is most common organism.

Urethritis: Often presents with dysuria, pyuria, or urethral discharge. Urine culture shows low bacterial count or no bacteria. Often associated with sexually transmitted diseases (STDs) such as *Chlamydia trachomatis, Neisseria gonorrhoeae,* or herpes simplex virus.

- *Chlamydial urethritis:* Asymptomatic or symptoms of urethritis, cervicitis, or pelvic inflammatory disease. Discharge usually clear or mucoid and watery. Undetected or untreated chlamydial infections are one of the leading causes of female infertility in the United States. In males, chlamydial infections may cause epididymitis or prostatitis.
- *Gonococcal urethritis:* Usually associated with urinary symptoms, purulent urethral discharge, and gram-negative intracellular diplococci. In women, may be asymptomatic or associated with vaginitis or cervicitis. In men, urethral pain and creamy, purulent discharge may be present; may involve prostate or epididymis.
- *Herpes simplex virus (type 2):* Typically associated with tender grouped vesicles on an erythematous base. Virus lies latent in presacral ganglion, then reactivates. Viral shedding can by asymptomatic following initial infection or occur during a recurrence.

Prostatitis

- *Acute bacterial:* Signs and symptoms include sudden onset of fever and chills. Urinary symptoms may include dysuria, frequency, urgency, or perineal and low back pain. Prostate is tender, warm, and swollen on digital rectal exam. Most common organism is enteric gram-negative bacilli; enterococci and staphylococci also seen. Systemic bacteremia can result if an acutely inflamed prostate is massaged.
- *Chronic bacterial:* Signs and symptoms include relapsing UTIs and urinary symptoms of dysuria, frequency, and urgency. Dull perineal, suprapubic, or low back pain may be present. Prostate feels normal to indurated on exam.
- *Nonbacterial:* Most common form of prostatitis. Cause is unknown. Signs and symptoms are similar to chronic bacterial prostatitis. Cultures of urine and prostate secretions are sterile.

► **Clinical Therapeutics**

Acute cystitis and coliform urethritis

- *Single dose:* May result in higher recurrence rate; therefore, not current recommended treatment. Amoxicillin, 3 g PO; sulfasoxazole, 2 g PO; or trimethoprim-sulfamethoxazole (TMP-SMZ), 4 tablets of 80-mg trimethoprim and 400-mg sulfamethoxazole, are treatment options.
- *Three-day course of antibiotics:* Usual treatment for uncomplicated cystitis. TMP-SMZ, trimethoprim, or fluoroquinolones may be used.
- *Exceptions:* Pregnant women, those with multiple recent infections, symptoms more than 7 days, recurrent symptoms after initial 3-day antibiotic course, those with complicating factors (diabetes), and the elderly should receive a 7-day antibiotic regimen.

Recurrent cystitis: Single postcoital antibiotic dose or bedtime dose of antibiotic three times weekly can reduce number of cystitis episodes. Encourage postcoital voiding.

Urethritis associated with STDs

- *Chlamydial:* Sexual partners must be treated. Azithromycin, 1 g PO single dose; erythromycin or tetracycline, 500 mg qid; or doxycycline, 100 mg bid for 7 days are treatment options.
- *Gonococcal:* Sexual partners must be treated. Ceftriaxone, 250 mg intramuscularly (IM), is recommended; single dose of cefixime or fluoroquinolone orally can be used. Due to frequent concomitant chlamydial infection, erythromycin or doxycycline for 7 days should be given; single-dose azithromycin is also effective.
- *Herpes simplex virus:* Oral acyclovir, 200 mg five times daily × 7 to 10 days or until resolved, to reduce the frequency and severity of recurrent episodes. Topical acyclovir six times daily can be added and may help reduce both viral shedding and the interval to healing. Maintenance therapy with acyclovir 600 to 800 mg qd for recurrent genital infections. Famciclovir and valacyclovir can also be used for recurrent genital herpes episodes.

Prostatitis

- *Acute bacterial:* Often associated with cystitis. Antibiotic therapy dependent on organism cultured in urine or prostatic secretions. Initial treatment usually parenteral antibiotics. Once afebrile for 24 to 48 hours, oral TMP-SMZ or fluoroquinolone can be used. Treatment course is 4 to 6 weeks.
- *Chronic bacterial:* Usually caused by gram-negative enteric bacteria. Difficult to treat; can use TMP-SMZ or fluoroquinolone × 6 to 12 weeks.
- *Nonbacterial:* Treat with erythromycin for 14 days; continue 3 to 6 weeks if patient has good clinical response. Sitz baths and anti-inflammatory agents may provide symptomatic relief.

► **Clinical Intervention**

Sexually active young adults are at increased risk of STDs. Patient education is key to prevention. Treat to prevent complications of pelvic inflammatory disease and sterility.

2. Upper Urinary Tract Infections (Kidney)

▶ History & Physical

Presents as an acute illness; obtain history for evidence of recurrent infection, childhood infections, or stones. Signs and symptoms include flank, low back, or abdominal pain; fever and chills; tachycardia; headache; nausea and vomiting; malaise; costovertebral angle tenderness; dysuria, frequency, urgency may or may not be present. In children, symptoms may be absent or nonspecific. In chronic pyelonephritis, symptoms may be absent, nonspecific, or related to infection.

▶ Diagnostic Studies

Laboratory findings include leukocytosis in acute pyelonephritis. BUN/creatinine are normal or elevated. Microscopic exam of urine may reveal pyuria, WBC casts, and hematuria. Proteinuria usually less than 1 g/d. If acutely infected, Gram stain for bacteriuria. Urine culture for identification of causative organism, usually gram-negative bacteria. Blood culture is positive in 20% of patients with acute pyelonephritis. Radiodiagnostics are used to identify underlying pathology such as reflux, renal calculi, or other factors interfering with urine flow. Abdominal film to evaluate for radiopaque calculi and soft tissue evaluation. IVP reveals blunting of calyces and cortical scarring in chronic pyelonephritis. Voiding cystourethrogram in young children to evaluate for vesicoureteral reflux; retrograde cystogram may be helpful. Renal ultrasound and CT may identify obstruction or perinephric abscesses.

▶ Diagnosis

Acute pyelonephritis: Inflammation of the renal parenchyma. Spread of bacteria from bladder to kidneys; may result in sepsis. Responds to antibiotics in > 90% of cases; failure to respond should prompt further investigation. Generally not associated with long-term morbidity.

Chronic pyelonephritis: Result of recurrent or persistent infection. Associated with anatomic abnormalities of the urinary tract including vesicoureteral reflux, obstruction, and renal calculi. Most commonly seen in children with vesicoureteral reflux leading to renal scarring and damage (reflux nephropathy).

▶ Clinical Therapeutics

Acute pyelonephritis: Outpatient therapy for compliant, clinically stable (nontoxic) patient is 10- to 14-day course of antibiotic based on urine sensitivities. TMP-SMZ or a fluoroquinolone may be initial choice. Inpatient therapy for more acutely ill patient requires intravenous (IV) antibiotics pending urine and blood cultures. Once afebrile and stable, change to appropriate oral antibiotic and complete 10- to 14-day course. If fever or bacteriuria persist beyond 48 to 72 hours, need to evaluate for underlying urinary tract abnormality.

Chronic pyelonephritis: Difficult situation; may develop resistant organisms. Can progress to end stage renal failure. Goal is to prevent recurrent infection and glomerulosclerosis. If possible, eliminate any risk factors such as lesions obstructing urine flow, catheters, or calculi. Treat symptomatic episodes initially with 10 to 14 days of appropriate antibiotic. If patient fails 10- to 14-day course of antibiotics, may benefit from 6 weeks of antibiotics. Suppressive therapy with continuous prophylactic low-dose antibiotics in select patients over a 5- to 10-year time period may decrease renal scarring and reflux; choices include TMP-SMZ, nitrofurantoin, or methenamine mandelate. Surgical correction indicated for severe vesicoureteral reflux or when other complicating factors are present.

► Clinical Intervention

Prompt detection and treatment of UTIs in children and surgical repair of any underlying anatomic abnormalities to prevent further damage. Management of other complicating factors such as infected stones. Vesicoureteral reflux has familial tendency; may want to screen siblings.

► Health Maintenance Issues

Asymptomatic bacteriuria: All pregnant women should be treated with 2-week course of antibiotics due to increased risk of fetal prematurity and maternal pyelonephritis. May indicate vesicoureteral reflux in preschool and young girls; treatment and urological evaluation is indicated. In men and nonpregnant women (especially elderly) without evidence of obstructive uropathy or vesicoureteral reflux, no treatment indicated. Not usually seen in males until after age of 60 years.

Catheter-associated bacteriuria: Associated with asymptomatic and symptomatic UTIs; asymptomatic bacteriuria in patient with a catheter is not usually treated. Responsible for 40% of all nosocomial infections. In the hospital setting, urosepsis related to catheter bacteriuria is the most common source of gram-negative bacteremia. Recurrent episodes of infections are common if catheter not removed. Increased risk of *Candida albicans* infection. No indication for antibiotic prophylaxis in patient with chronic catheter.

B. Epididymitis

► Scientific Concepts

Can be sexually transmitted or non–sexually transmitted. Sexually transmitted type usually seen in men under age of 40 and is associated with either gonococcal or chlamydial urethritis. Non–sexually transmitted type seen in older men and associated with gram-negative bacterial UTIs or prostatitis.

► History & Physical

Symptoms of urethritis or cystitis may be present, as well as fever and scrotal swelling. Epididymis may be tender, warm, or swollen. Scrotal pain may radiate along spermatic cord. Lower abdominal tenderness or flank pain on the involved side and prostate tenderness may be present.

▶ Diagnostic Studies

Leukocytosis and left shift on complete blood count (CBC), Gram stain of urethral discharge, urinalysis for pyuria or bacteriuria, urine culture, scrotal ultrasound.

▶ Differential Diagnosis

Testicular tumors, torsion of spermatic cord, testicular trauma, orchitis.

▶ Clinical Therapeutics

Antibiotic therapy based on offending organism. Sexually transmitted types are treated for 10 to 21 days and sexual partners must be treated. Non–sexually transmitted types are treated for 21 to 28 days.

▶ Clinical Intervention

Bedrest with scrotal elevation, oral analgesics. Once treated, non–sexually transmitted epididymitis requires urinary tract evaluation to rule out other pathology.

▶ Health Maintenance Issues

Delayed or inadequate therapy can lead to complications, including orchitis, abscesses, or impaired fertility.

III. URINARY TRACT OBSTRUCTION AND TUMORS

A. Urinary Tract Obstruction

▶ Scientific Concepts

Can occur at any site in urinary tract and may be congenital or acquired disorder with either structural or functional obstruction. Classified by degree, duration, and site of obstruction.

▶ History & Physical

Obtain patient history. Symptoms vary with degree of obstruction. In setting of obstruction, anuria implies complete bilateral obstruction or obstruction of a single functioning kidney. Pain is more likely associated with acute obstruction; can vary in intensity/location. Chronic obstruction may present with no or vague symptoms. Urinary symptoms may include polyuria, nocturia, frequency, hesitancy, and decreased urinary stream. Palpable mass or distended bladder may be present as well as prostatic enlargement on rectal exam.

▶ Diagnostic Studies

Laboratory tests may reveal acute or chronic renal failure; abnormal blood chemistry. Urinalysis may be normal or have few red cells, white cells, or minimal proteinuria. Bacteria suggestive of underlying infection. Urine cytology to evaluate for malignancy. Urine volume may be normal, increased, or decreased. Anuria suggests complete bilateral obstruction. Plain film of abdomen to identify radiopaque stones. Bladder catheterization to evaluate for urinary retention or neuropathic bladder. Ultrasound may reveal hydronephrosis or tumors. CT can further identify cause of obstruction. IVP to evaluate upper urinary tract obstruction. Useful in patients with cysts and staghorn calculi. In patients with renal insufficiency, limited due to risk of radiocontrast nephrotoxicity. Retrograde pyelography to evaluate and visualize ureter and collecting system. Used when other testing is inconclusive and in patients with contrast allergy. Urodynamic studies; cystoscopy to evaluate and visualize urethra and bladder.

▶ Diagnosis

Congenital anomalies of urinary tract: Ureterovesical junction stenosis is more common in boys than girls and can be detected by ultrasonography in utero. Treatment is surgical. Ureteropelvic junction stenosis is most common in infants; more common in boys than girls and can be detected by ultrasonography in utero. Treatment is surgery or close monitoring in select patients. Urethral stricture; meatal stenosis.

Obstructing calculi: Must have bilateral obstruction or obstruction of single functioning kidney to cause renal failure.

Urethral stricture: Seen with trauma (urethral instrumentation) or infections (gonococcal, infections secondary to indwelling catheters). Treatment includes dilation, urethrotomy with endoscope, or surgical repair.

Renal tumors

- *Renal cell carcinoma:* Most common neoplasm of kidney. More common in men, usually fifth to seventh decades of life. Often found incidentally by sonogram or CT scan. Classic presenting triad of gross hematuria, flank pain, and palpable mass present in only 10 to 15% of patients. Acquired cystic disease of the kidney, which can develop in patients with end-stage renal disease, is a risk factor. CT scan is best method to evaluate suspected renal lesion. Treatment is radical nephrectomy. Radiation therapy may be used for metastatic disease. Chemotherapy of limited value as tumor is very resistant; immunotherapy is promising. Survival rate poor for those with positive lymph nodes and metastases.
- *Sarcoma:* Less than 5% of all malignant renal tumors. Treatment is radical nephrectomy.
- *Wilms' tumor (nephroblastoma):* Most common urologic tumor in children. Usually presents around age of 3 years. Familial and nonfamilial forms seen. Associated with congenital anomalies, including genitourinary malformations and aniridia. Asymptomatic abdominal mass is usual presentation; abdominal pain, hematuria, nausea and vomiting, anorexia, hypertension, and anemia may be present. Diagnosis made by ultrasound, CT scan, or IVP. Treatment includes surgery, radiation, and chemotherapy, depending on staging of tumor pathology. Metastasize early; 80% of patients have metastases by direct extension. Prognosis based on tumor type and staging.
- *Metastatic tumors:* Primary tumors including lung, breast, and lymphoma can metastasize to kidney. Prognosis usually poor.

Renal pelvis and ureteral tumors: Uncommon tumors with male predominance. Transitional cell carcinoma most common. Increased risk in smokers, analgesic abuse, and those with occupational exposure to certain chemicals. Painless gross hematuria is often the presenting symptom. Diagnosis by IVP or retrograde studies. Treatment is surgical excision; chemotherapy and radiation of limited value.

Bladder carcinoma

- *Transitional cell carcinoma:* Greater than 90% of all bladder cancers with male:female ratio of 3:1. Peak incidence is seventh decade of life. Most present with painless gross hematuria. Diagnosis made by cystoscopy and biopsy. Associated with the following environmental factors: occupational exposure (aniline dyes, rubber, leather, dry cleaning), analgesic abuse, radiation therapy, and cyclophosphamide therapy. Smoking increases risk by fourfold. Treatment is transurethral resection of tumor, intravesical immunotherapy or chemotherapy (intravesical bacillus Calmette–Guérin [BCG]), radiation, chemotherapy (cisplatin or combination chemotherapy), or partial or radical cystectomy.
- *Squamous cell carcinoma:* Associated more with bladder irritation from chronic catheters and chronic infections. More frequent in Egypt due to chronic infection with *Schistosoma haematobium.* Treatment is radical cystectomy.

B. Neuropathic Bladder

▶ Scientific Concepts

Normal bladder capacity 400 to 500 mL. Nerve supply from both autonomic and somatic nervous systems.

▶ History & Physical

Obtain history and physical with neurologic examination and palpation of bladder. Signs and symptoms may vary with cause; in spastic neuropathic bladder: involuntary urination, vague lower abdominal discomfort, autonomic dysreflexia, frequency, nocturia, urgency, double voiding; in flaccid neuropathic bladder: urine retention and overflow incontinence.

▶ Diagnostic Studies

BUN/creatinine; urinalysis; urodynamic studies: uroflowmetry, cystometic evaluation, urethral pressure measurement, electromyography; cystoscopy, retrograde cystogram; x-ray studies: VCUG, IVP, sonogram, CT scan.

▶ Diagnosis

Spastic neuropathic bladder: Associated with reduced bladder capacity, involuntary bladder contractions, high voiding pressures, detrusor hypertrophy, sphincter spasticity (ureteral reflux). Causes include dementia, cerebrovascular accident, multiple sclerosis, tumors, Parkinson's disease, and spinal cord injury. In spinal cord injury, autonomic dysreflexia may be present.

Flaccid neuropathic bladder: Associated with large bladder capacity and residual urine, lack of voluntary bladder contractions, low voiding pressures, mild hypertrophy of bladder wall, and decreased tone of external sphincter. Causes include injury to spinal cord at micturition center, radiation or surgical damage, and neuropathies (diabetes, pernicious anemia, posterior spinal cord injuries).

► Clinical Therapeutics

Spastic: Low-dose anticholinergic medications and parasympatholytic drugs (oxybutynin chloride, dicyclomine hydrochloride, methantheline bromide).

Flaccid: Parasympathomimetic drugs (bethanechol chloride).

► Clinical Intervention

Spastic: Bladder training, Foley catheter, condom catheter, sphincterotomy in males, sacral rhizotomy, neurostimulation of sacral nerve roots (bladder pacemaker), urinary diversion.

Flaccid: Bladder training, intermittent catheterization, surgery for BPH if bladder outlet obstruction present.

C. Enuresis

► Scientific Concepts

Involuntary passage of urine at night or while sleeping usually due to delayed maturation of central nervous system. Usually defined as bedwetting after age 3 years; 10% of children over 3 years may have enuresis.

► History & Physical

Urine stream is normal. Not associated with UTIs. Frequency and urgency may be present. Physical and urological exam normal.

► Diagnostic Studies

Daytime incontinence needs further investigation. Urological evaluation usually not indicated unless other organic disease (obstruction, urethral stenosis, ureteral reflux, neuropathic bladder) or infection is suspected.

► Differential Diagnosis

Obstruction, ureteral reflux, infection, neuropathic disease, urethral stenosis.

► Clinical Therapeutics

Imipramine drug of choice. Others include parasympatholytic drugs, sympathomimetic drugs, desmopressin nasal spray (antidiuretic hormone preparation), and psychotherapy.

► Clinical Intervention

Limit evening fluids, empty bladder at bedtime, awaken to void at night; mechanical devices such as alarm pads on bed may be helpful.

► Health Maintenance Issues

Bladder training should not start until after age 18 months. Anxiety of parents may be transferred to child. Psychological fear may cause enuresis.

D. Testicular and Prostate Disease

1. Testicular Carcinoma

▶ Scientific Concepts

Most common neoplasm in men between 20 and 35 years of age. Two to three cases per 100,000 males in the United States per year. Ninety to 95% are germ cell tumors (seminoma, nonseminoma), others are nongerminal tumors (Leydig cell, Sertoli cell, gonadoblastoma). Most common germ cell tumor in bilateral primary testicular carcinoma is seminoma. In the United States, more frequent in white males and those of higher socioeconomic classes. More common on right side than left due to higher incidence of cryptorchidism on right. Risk is higher in those with history of cryptorchidism (especially intra-abdominal testis), and the tumor is usually a seminoma. Surgery to relocate the testis into scrotum does not decrease risk of malignancy but aids in future examinations for tumors. Other risk factors include maternal exogenous estrogen during pregnancy, possibly trauma, and testicular atrophy due to infection.

▶ History & Physical

Signs and symptoms include painless enlargement of testis, testicular mass (usually firm and nontender), and testicular heaviness. Occasionally, pain from testicular hemorrhage, abdominal masses, lymphadenopathy, or gynecomastia present. Ten percent of tumors are asymptomatic on presentation; found after trauma, by partner, or on routine exam. Metastatic symptoms of back pain, dyspnea, cough, nausea, vomiting, anorexia, bone pain, and leg swelling due to venous obstruction may be present.

▶ Diagnostic Studies

Increased alpha fetoprotein (AFP) in nonseminomatous germ cell tumors but not in seminomas, increased human chorionic gonadotropin (hCG), increased total lactic dehydrogenase (LDH) and LDH isoenzyme-1, anemia, increased liver function tests, scrotal ultrasound, metastatic evaluation (chest x-ray, CT abdomen/pelvis, possibly CT of chest), 24-hour urine for CrCl if chemotherapy needed.

▶ Differential Diagnosis

Epididymitis, epididymoorchitis, hydrocele (transillumination of scrotum helpful), spermatocele, varicocele, epidermoid cyst.

▶ Clinical Therapeutics

Dependent on tumor type and staging. Radiation therapy or chemotherapy; seminomas are very radiosensitive.

▶ Clinical Intervention

Inguinal exploration with radical orchiectomy. Retroperitoneal lymph node dissection (nonseminomatous germ cell tumor); if no dissection, then surveillance with monthly follow-up for first 2 years, then bimonthly in third year with repeat tumor markers at each visit and chest x-ray and CT scan every 3 to 4 months; those with retroperitoneal lymph node dissection or radiation also require regular follow-up with physical exam, repeat AFP, hCG, LDH, and chest x-ray. Survival rate dependent on tumor type and stage; rates improving with advances in combination chemotherapy.

2. Prostate Carcinoma

▶ Scientific Concepts

Most common cancer in American males. Over 300,000 new cases diagnosed in 1996 and many more occult prostate cancers that are not clinically recognized. Incidence increases with age; rare under the age of 40 years, however, autopsy incidence of prostate cancer approaches 67% in men aged 80 to 89 years. Most tumors are adenocarcinomas. Environmental, dietary, genetic, and hormonal factors may all play a role in etiology.

▶ History & Physical

Most patients are asymptomatic and are found to have abnormal prostate by digital rectal exam. Urinary obstructive symptoms can occur but are more likely due to BPH. Symptoms of metastatic disease (cord compression, pathologic fractures) may be present.

▶ Diagnostic Studies

Digital rectal exam and prostate-specific antigen (PSA) with age-specific reference ranges. PSA useful for detecting, staging, and monitoring response to therapy, as well as evaluating for recurrence of tumor. Serum acid phosphastase used before PSA available and is more predictive of metastases. BUN/creatinine are elevated if obstruction present. Alkaline phosphatase and serum calcium elevated with bone metastases. Obtain prostate biopsy by transrectal ultrasound guidance. Transrectal ultrasound to image prostate can be used in staging of prostate cancer. Radionuclide bone scan to evaluate bone metastases.

▶ Differential Diagnosis

Benign prostatic hyperplasia, prostatitis, prostatic fibrosis, prostatic calculi or cysts.

▶ Clinical Therapeutics

Locally extensive cancers are at increased risk for local and distant relapse with radiation or surgery alone; other therapies under investigation include surgery or radiation with androgen deprivation (luteinizing hormone-releasing hormone [LHRH] agonists, estrogens, antiandrogens, orchiectomy), cryosurgery, advanced radiation, and hormonal therapy alone. Metastatic prostate cancer can be treated with testicular androgen deprivation (LHRH agonists, estrogens, orchiectomy) and adrenal androgen blockage with an antiandrogen (flutamide, bicalutamide). Hormone refractory disease is treated with palliative care. Chemotherapeutic agents of limited value; ongoing studies with use of suramin.

► Clinical Intervention

Based on TNM staging system (primary tumor, regional lymph nodes, distant metastases), age, and health of patient. Watchful waiting may be alternative in those with other medical illnesses or in older men (generally if life expectancy < 10 years) and those with small-volume or well-differentiated cancers. Localized disease and minimal extracapsular disease may respond to radiation therapy or prostatectomy.

► Health Maintenance Issues

Increased risk in blacks, those with positive family history of prostate cancer, and possibly in those with prior vasectomy.

3. Benign Prostatic Hyperplasia

► Scientific Concepts

Primary etiology unclear; hormonal and age-related factors possible. Increased frequency in men over 50 years of age.

► History & Physical

Urinary symptoms may include frequency, nocturia, hesitancy, dribbling, urgency, decreased force and caliber of urinary stream, incomplete emptying, and urinary retention. Symptoms generally progressive over years. A symptom score system has been designed to help select therapy. Obtain a careful history to rule out other urinary tract problems. Physical examination should include digital rectal exam, palpation of bladder, and genital exam to exclude structural deformity.

► Diagnostic Studies

Digital rectal exam, urinalysis may help establish other diagnosis; serum BUN/creatinine, ultrasound, uroflowmetry and postvoid residual urine, serum PSA, and urethrocystoscopy. Urethrocystoscopy not recommended for routine evaluation; useful when hematuria is present to exclude other structural abnormalities or prior to surgical therapy.

► Clinical Therapeutics

Alpha-1-adrenergic blockers: Alpha-1 and alpha-2 receptors are present in prostate and base of bladder and are increased in prostatic hyperplasia; blocking these receptors can reduce bladder outlet resistance. Alpha-1-adrenergic blockers are approved for treatment of BPH, increase urinary flow, and improve prostate symptom scores. Monitor for hypotension, lightheadedness, and dizziness. Terazosin, doxazosin, prazosin, alfuzosin are all alpha-1 selective while tamsulosin is selective to alpha-1a receptors.

5-alpha-reductase inhibitors: Finasteride is only drug in this class approved in the United States for treatment of BPH. Acts to decrease dihydrotestosterone, reduce obstructive symptoms, increase urinary flow rate, and lower PSA level. Only approved drug shown to reduce prostate volume.

Gonadotropin-releasing hormone (GnRH) agonists: Act to cause androgen deficiency, reduce obstructive symptoms, reduce prostate volume, and increase urinary flow rate. Side effects include hot flashes, loss of libido, and impotence. Drugs include leuprolide, nafarelin, and buserelin.

Antiandrogens: Block androgen receptor sites. High incidence of side effects, including gynecomastia and diarrhea, as well as lack of efficiency make these drugs poor choice for BPH. Drugs include flutamide and bicalutamide.

► Clinical Intervention

No therapy: Close monitoring may be reasonable when symptoms not severe.

Transurethral resection of prostate (TURP): Mainstay of therapy but invasive; for moderate to severe symptoms. Complications include postoperative failure to void, TUR syndrome (intraoperative fluid absorption), hemorrhage, UTI, bladder neck contracture, urethral stricture, incontinence, impotence, and obstruction necessitating second TURP.

Transurethral incision of prostate: Used in cases of bladder outlet obstructive symptoms when prostate is normal or small.

Open prostatectomy: Only 5 to 10% of operations in the United States for BPH. Reserved for cases in which prostate weight is more than 60 g or when other surgical procedures are required at the same time.

Urethral stents: Used for BPH and urethral strictures; limited long-term experience.

Laser prostatectomy
Microwave therapy
Electrovaporization

► Clinical Intervention for Urinary Tract Obstruction and Tumors

Relieve obstruction with catheter, suprapubic cystostomy, ureteral catheter, or nephrostomy tube. Postobstructive diuresis may occur. Close monitoring, pharmacological management, surgery, chemotherapy, radiation.

IV. NEPHROLITHIASIS

► Scientific Concepts

Renal calculi are more common in men, occur more often in hot and dry climates, are often recurrent, and usually present in third to fifth decade of life. Metabolic, hereditary, and infectious etiologies play a role in stone formation. Ninety percent pass spontaneously, especially if < 5 mm in size.

► History & Physical

Obtain history including onset of symptoms, timing of first stone and subsequent stones, previous evaluations (radiodiagnostics, stone analysis, hospitalizations), and family history of renal calculi. Evaluate for other known diseases associated with stone formation including primary hyperparathyroidism, renal tubular acidosis, medullary sponge kidney, and sarcoidosis.

Signs and symptoms of dysuria, frequency, and urgency may or may not be present. Hematuria may be gross or microscopic. Nausea and vomiting are occasionally associated. Renal colic results from pressure and dilatation of urinary system. It is abrupt in onset, increases in intensity over a period of time, reaches a plateau, then remains constant and severe. May begin in flank and radiate downward to groin, testicle, or vulva. Stones lodged at ureterovesicle junction may present with irritant voiding symptoms rather than renal colic. Asymptomatic stones are often found on x-ray. Stones are radiopaque except for uric acid stones.

► Diagnosis

Calcium stones: Most stones are a mixture of calcium oxalate or calcium oxalate/calcium phosphate. Causes include:

- *Low urine volume:* Urine saturation by crystalloids increases as urine volume decreases. Preventive goal in stone formers is to excrete at least 2 L of urine per day.
- *Hypercalciuria:* Usually idiopathic but primary hyperparathyroidism, renal tubular acidosis, sarcoidosis, Cushing's syndrome, and vitamin D excess are some of other causes. Idiopathic hypercalciuria is most common cause of hypercalciuria. Familial tendency, usually seen in men. Serum calcium normal, parathyroid hormone (PTH) level normal or low. High intestinal calcium absorption leads to increased urinary calcium excretion. Primary hyperparathyroidism is seen more in middle-aged or older women. Associated with elevated serum calcium and PTH levels. Hypercalciuria is the result of increased production of 1,25-dihydroxyvitamin D by kidney in response to PTH. Parathyroid adenoma is cause in 85% of cases; others due to parathyroid hyperplasia.
- *Hyperuricosuria:* May result from excessive dietary purine intake. Increased uric acid crystals in urine act as a surface for calcium oxalate deposition.
- *Hyperoxaluria:* Increased urinary excretion of oxalate can cause calcium oxalate stone formation. Seen with increased production of oxalate (primary hyperoxaluria, excess vitamin C intake) or increased absorption of oxalate either dietary or intestinal (Crohn's disease, malabsorption, ileal surgery).

Uric acid stones: Nonopaque by radiologic study. Associated mainly with acid urine pH (as seen in gout, idiopathic uric acid stones, chronic diarrhea associated with ileostomy or colostomy) and, in 20% of patients, an increased urinary uric acid concentration.

Cystine stones: Reduced renal tubular reabsorption of cystine. Seen only with hereditary disorder of cystinuria.

Struvite stones: Form as a result of urease-positive bacterial urine infection (often *Proteus* or *Providencia*). Contain both struvite and calcium phosphate and are often seen as large staghorn calculi in renal collecting system. Urine pH high, usually > 8.0. Can lead to chronic renal failure (if bilateral), persistent infection, or abscess. Infection difficult to resolve due to bacteria in stones.

► Diagnostic Studies

Urinalysis: Hematuria is commonly seen; may be microscopic or gross. Bacteriuria and crystalluria may be present. Cystine and struvite crystals are specific; other crystals can be seen in normal urine but may be significant if found in a patient with suspected stones.

Metabolic investigation: Laboratory tests may include serum calcium, serum phosphorus, PTH level, uric acid, creatinine, BUN, and urinalysis. Twenty-four-hour urine collection for measurement of urinary excretion of calcium, phosphate, uric acid, oxalate, citrate, cystine, creatinine, pH, sodium, and urine volume. Must collect all urine in 24-hour period. Three collections are recommended. Should be done in the patient's normal outpatient setting (not while hospitalized), with patient eating and drinking usual amount of food and beverages (not on any unusual diets), and with the patient participating in usual activities. Stone analysis.

Abdominal film

Renal sonogram

IVP

► Clinical Therapeutics

Treatment of calcium stones

- *Hypercalciuria state:* Idiopathic—restrict dietary sodium; high sodium intake in diet will increase renal calcium excretion and decrease the effect of thiazide diuretics. Dietary protein restriction may decrease calciuria. Dietary calcium restriction is not advised; should maintain moderate calcium intake of at least two to three servings daily as a low-calcium diet can lead to bone loss and also increases oxalate excretion. Thiazide diuretics used to decrease urine calcium excretion. Primary hyperparathyroidism—parathyroid surgery for adenoma or hyperplasia.

- *Hyperuricosuria state:* Reduce purine intake in diet. Pharmacological management with allopurinol.

- *Hyperoxaluria state:* Reduce excess oxalate in diet (colas, teas) and reduce vitamin C supplements. In cases of intestinal disease, treatment includes calcium supplements to bind intestinal oxalate, low-fat diet, and cholestyramine.

Treatment of uric acid stones: Alkalization of urine with bicarbonate; uric acid is more soluble in alkaline urine. Goal is urine pH 6.5 to 7.0. Reduce purine intake in diet. Allopurinol if hyperuricosuria is > 1,000 mg/24 hr. Acetazolamide can raise urine pH by causing bicarbonaturia.

Treatment of cystine stones: Goal is to increase urine volume to help dissolve excess cystine in urine. Need urine volume of ≥ 3 L daily and increased urine volumes at night. Penicillamine can help prevent cystine precipitation. Alkalization of urine is beneficial.

Treatment of struvite stones: Treat any associated metabolic stone disease. Suppress infection with chronic antibiotics. Choices include methenamine mandelate or TMP-SMZ. Acute infections should be treated with a 3-week course of antibiotic based on organism sensitivity. Achieving sterile urine is not generally successful. Surgery is a last resort measure for struvite stones causing obstruction, severe pain, serious infections, or substantial bleeding; stones can recur after surgical removal.

▶ Clinical Intervention

Increase fluid intake to at least 2 L/d. During acute episodes, strain all urine and provide analgesics. Urological management options include cystoscopy with retrieval by stone basket, extracorporeal shock wave lithotripsy, and percutaneous nephrolithotomy. Asymptomatic stones less than 5 mm may be followed without therapy.

▶ Health Maintenance Issues

Without intervention, 50% of patients will have recurrent stones in 5 years. Identify associated risk factors, including diet (increased dietary intake of animal protein, purines, oxalate, sodium), climate (increased frequency in hot and dry areas), family history, medication use (triamterene, acetazolamide), and conditions associated with stone formation (medullary sponge kidney, horseshoe kidney, polycystic kidney disease, etc.). Patient education on preventive measures can decrease stone recurrence rate.

V. RENAL FAILURE

A. Acute Renal Failure

▶ Scientific Concepts

Acute decline in renal function, which can be arbitrarily defined as an increase in creatinine of 0.5 mg/dL if baseline creatinine < 3.0 mg/dL or increase in creatinine of 1 mg/dL if creatinine > 3.0 mg/dL. A doubling of serum creatinine represents 50% loss of GFR. Prerenal azotemia and acute tubular necrosis (ATN) account for 70 to 75% of cases of acute renal failure.

▶ History & Physical

Identify onset of renal dysfunction—in hospital versus outpatient, acute illness versus chronic systemic process. Previous labs or history of elevated creatinine helpful in establishing timing of renal disease. Evaluate for history of trauma, drugs, drug overdose, or recent illness. Physical examination findings can vary. Decreased skin turgor, postural hypotension and tachycardia, and dry mucous membranes may indicate volume depletion. Edema, rales, elevated jugular venous pressure, ascites, and gallop rhythm may indicate cardiac failure, cirrhosis, or nephrotic syndrome. Fever and rash may indicate acute interstitial nephritis. Livedo reticularis, cyanotic toes or digital ulcers may indicate atheroembolic disease. Distended bladder or enlarged prostate may indicate obstruction.

▶ Diagnostic Studies

Elevated BUN/creatinine, urine volume (anuric, oliguric, normal), urinalysis (casts, protein, hematuria, cells), urine sodium and osmolality, serum tests for specific illness (antineutrophil cytoplasmic antibody [ANCA], antinuclear antibody [ANA], etc.). Radiodiagnostics include: abdominal plain film, renal ultrasound, IVP, renal angiogram, CT scan, renal scan, cystoscopy, retrograde pyelogram. Renal biopsy.

▶ Differential Diagnosis

Prerenal vs. ATN: Prerenal disease is a result of decreased renal perfusion. ATN is a result of intrinsic insult to the renal tubules from either ischemia or nephrotoxins. Urine and laboratory diagnostic indices:

Prerenal: BUN/creatinine ratio > 20:1, normal urinalysis, urine sodium < 20 mEq/L, urine osmolality > 500 mOsm/kg, fractional excretion of sodium < 1%.

ATN: BUN/creatinine ratio 10 to 15:1, urinalysis reveals granular casts and renal tubular epithelial cells and casts, urine sodium > 40 mEq/L, urine osmolality < 350 mOsm/kg, fractional excretion of sodium > 2%.

▶ Diagnostic Categories

Prerenal: Result of decreased renal perfusion.

- *Volume depletion:* Presents with signs of hypovolemia on examination. Causes may include GI losses (vomiting, diarrhea, bleeding), renal losses (diuretics, osmotic diuresis), and third-space losses (burns, tissue trauma from crush injury, pancreatitis). Treatment is fluid replacement.

- *Heart failure:* Associated with severe cardiac dysfunction (systolic or diastolic). Goal is to improve cardiac function (reduce ischemia or improve cardiac output with digitalis, vasodilators, ACE inhibitors, dopamine, dobutamine).

- *Cirrhosis:* Associated with a decrease in effective tissue perfusion. Increased renal vasoconstriction leads to acute renal failure in hepatorenal syndrome.

- *Hypotension:* Associated with shock or treatment of severe hypertension.

- *Bilateral renal artery stenosis:* Decreased renal perfusion due to renal artery disease. Use of ACE inhibitors in a patient with bilateral renal artery stenosis or renal artery stenosis in a patient with one functioning kidney can cause renal failure. ACE inhibitors lower systemic and intrarenal blood pressure. Because GFR is maintained by angiotensin II–mediated efferent arteriolar constriction, blocking angiotensin II formation with ACE inhibitors decreases GFR and may cause renal failure. Diuretics can enhance this effect.

- *NSAIDs:* Reduced renal vasodilator prostaglandin synthesis by NSAIDs in prerenal states such as volume depletion, heart failure, nephrotic syndrome, or cirrhosis can cause acute renal failure. In states of volume depletion, vasoconstrictors are activated and renal prostaglandins are needed to help compensate for the decreased perfusion to the kidneys. Blocking prostaglandin synthesis with NSAIDs can result in renal failure. Reversible with removal of offending agent.

- *Nephrotic syndrome:* Urinary protein losses cause hypoalbuminemia and plasma volume depletion. Characterized by proteinuria (3.5 g/d or greater), hypoalbuminemia, edema, hyperlipidemia, and a hypercoagulable state.

Intrinsic renal disease: Disorders within the kidney involving the blood vessels, glomeruli, tubules, or interstitium causing impaired renal function.

- ◆ *Tubular disease*
  - *Acute tubular necrosis (ATN):* Associated with a sudden decline in renal function lasting 7 to 21 days, followed by gradual improvement back to baseline. Tubular injury related to renal insult, usually ischemia or a nephrotoxin. Postischemic ATN is seen with severe prerenal disease such as hypotension and shock. Nephrotoxic ATN is seen with drugs, radiocontrast, and heme pigments.
    - *Aminoglycoside nephrotoxicity:* Most common cause of antiobiotic associated renal damage. Drug accumulates in the renal cortex. Seen in 7 to 36% of patients on aminoglycosides, and is related to dose and duration of therapy. Findings include an increase in the BUN and creatinine occurring 5 to 7 days into course of therapy. Toxicity risk minimized by maintaining drug levels in therapeutic range and monitoring serum creatinine. Usually reversible if drug discontinued.
    - *Radiocontrast nephrotoxicity:* Associated with an increase in the creatinine within 24 hours after the radiocontrast study. Creatinine peaks at 3 to 7 days, then quickly returns to baseline in most cases. Preexisting renal insufficiency, diabetes, volume depletion, and severe congestive heart failure are risk factors. Risk of renal failure low if creatinine < 1.5 mg/dL but increases with more advanced renal insufficiency and also with amount of contrast used, number of studies, and concomitant disease. Prevention in high-risk patients includes IV hydration before, during, and after the study as well as avoiding other nephrotoxic agents and limiting amount of contrast. Nonionic agents may offer small benefit in those with creatinine > 2.0 mg/dL, especially diabetics.
    - *Cisplatin:* Direct tubular toxin. Toxicity can be limited with IV hydration.
    - *Heme pigments associated with ATN:* Seen with rhabdomyolysis (myoglobinuria) or intravascular hemolysis (hemoglobinuria). Rhabdomyolysis is caused by trauma (tissue ischemia), intense exercise, seizures, and drugs (cocaine, heroin). Lab findings include myoglobinuria, urine dipstick positive for heme but no red blood cells (RBCs) seen on microscopy, urine red to brown with pigmented granular casts, plasma normal in color, markedly elevated serum creatine phosphokinase (CK) especially creatine kinase MM band (CK-MM), elevated serum creatinine out of proportion to BUN, elevated uric acid, potassium, and phosphorus levels, and decreased serum calcium. Treatment includes IV fluids, mannitol, furosemide, and sodium bicarbonate (alkalinizes urine and

increases solubility of heme proteins). Treat hyperkalemia and hyperphosphatemia. Intravascular hemolysis is caused by a transfusion reaction with mismatched blood and infections. Lab findings include hemoglobinuria, urine red to brown with pigmented casts, plasma red in color, low haptoglobin and hematocrit, and elevated levels of LDH, bilirubin, potassium, and plasma hemoglobin.

- *Multiple myeloma:* Characterized by overproduction of monoclonal immunoglobulin proteins by malignant plasma cells. Renal failure is due to tubular obstruction from casts and tubular cell toxicity. Presentation may include acute or chronic renal failure, proteinuria, anemia, weakness, bone pain, pathologic fractures, lytic lesions on x-ray, and hypercalcemia. Diagnosis confirmed by abnormal paraprotein found in serum or urine protein electrophoresis, immunoelectrophoresis of blood or urine for monoclonal light chains (Bence Jones proteins), bone marrow biopsy, or renal biopsy. Treatment includes hydration, alkalinization of urine, correction of hypercalcemia, decrease production of immunoglobulins (chemotherapy and steroids), plasmapheresis, or dialysis.

◆ *Interstitial disease*
- *Interstitial nephritis:* Characterized by interstitial inflammation, edema, and renal tubular cell damage; glomeruli and blood vessels not usually involved. Usually results from hypersensitivity to a drug (penicillin, methicillin, NSAIDs, sulfonamides, rifampin, cimetidine, diuretics) or related to infection. Presentation may include rash, arthralgias, or fever. Lab findings include eosinophiluria, mild proteinuria, hematuria, pyuria, WBC casts, and peripheral eosinophilia. Renal dysfunction can be mild or severe. Treatment is supportive; stop suspected drugs. Steroid therapy may offer some benefit. Recovery over weeks to months, although renal function may not return to baseline.

  Other causes of acute interstitial disease include infections (acute pyelonephritis, systemic infections), immunologic diseases (systemic lupus erythematosus, cryoglobulinemia), or idiopathic.

◆ *Glomerular disease*
- *Glomerulonephritis:* Term for inflammation of the glomerulus. Nephritic syndrome is associated with hypertension, edema, active urine sediment with hematuria, RBC casts, and proteinuria. Nephrotic syndrome associated with > 3.5 g/d proteinuria, hypoalbuminemia, hyperlipidemia, and edema. Lab tests include urinalysis (hematuria, proteinuria, cells, casts), BUN/creatinine, 24-hour protein and CrCl, urine and protein electrophoresis, complement levels, antistreptolysin-O (ASO) titer and other disease specific tests, renal sonogram, and renal biopsy.
  - *Poststreptococcal glomerulonephritis:* Caused by a nephritogenic strain of group A beta-hemolytic streptococci and may occur after pharyngeal or skin infection. Most common in children

5 to 15 years of age. Has latent period of 7 to 21 days from infection to onset of nephritis. Presenting signs and symptoms may include abrupt onset of hematuria (tea-colored urine), edema (usually periorbital), hypertension, oliguria, nonnephrotic range proteinuria, and RBC and other cellular casts. Lab tests include throat or skin culture positive for group A streptococci, decreased serum complements, and elevated titers for ASO, antistreptokinase, and antihyaluronidase. In children, disease course is self-limiting. Ninety-five percent of patients have normal renal function within 2 months. Antihypertensives, sodium restriction, and diuretics may be indicated.

- *Rapidly progressive glomerulonephritis (RPGN):* Associated with loss of renal function over days to weeks. Diagnosis confirmed by renal biopsy, which shows crescents in glomeruli; immunofluorescence and electron microscopy to determine specific type of disease (Wegener's granulomatosis, Goodpasture's disease, immune complex glomerulonephritis, idiopathic). Treatment includes antihypertensives, steroids, and cytotoxic agents depending on diagnosis; dialysis if needed.
- *Goodpasture's disease:* Form of glomerulonephritis associated with pulmonary hemorrhage and iron deficiency anemia. Lab tests include positive circulating anti-glomerular basement membrane antibodies. Renal biopsy identifies deposition of immunoglobulin G (IgG) along glomerular basement membrane (GBM). Treatment includes steroids, cyclophosphamide, and plasma exchange (remove circulating anti-GBM antibodies).

◆ *Vascular disease*
  - *Vasculitis:* Systemic condition associated with inflammatory changes in vessel walls thought related to immune response mechanisms. Causes include include temporal arteritis, polyarteritis nodosa, Kawasaki disease, Wegener's granulomatosis, and Henoch–Schönlein purpura. Presenting symptoms vary and are related to vessels and organs involved; may include fever, arthralgias, myalgias, headache, abdominal pain, and weight loss. Treatment is dependent on disease and severity; antiinflammatory drugs, corticosteroids, and cytoxic agents are choices.
  - *Malignant hypertension:* Presents with headache, blurred vision, dizziness, and confusion. Diagnostic findings are diastolic blood pressure > 130 mm Hg, retinopathy (hemorrhages and exudates), papilledema, increased creatinine, hematuria, proteinuria, and RBC casts. Initial treatment goal is to reduce diastolic blood pressure gradually to range of 100 to 110 mm Hg; initial drug choices may include IV sodium nitroprusside, nitroglycerine, labetalol, and diazoxide.
  - *Atheroembolic disease:* Atheromatous plaque causing obstruction of medium or small renal arteries. Presentation may include livedo reticularis, cyanotic toes, painful ulcerations of digits, fever, abdominal pain, anorexia, and GI bleeding due to bowel infarction. Usually associated with disruption of plaque during

angiography or surgical procedure. Renal dysfunction can be mild to acute renal failure; onset of renal failure is typically slow and progressive over 30 to 60 days; may or may not recover some renal function. Diagnosis based on history and suspicion as well as physical exam. Eosinophilia and mild proteinuria may be present. Differential diagnosis includes contrast-induced renal failure, vasculitis, ATN, interstial nephritis, and renal artery stenosis. Treatment is supportive; pain control, management of digital ischemic areas, amputation, avoid anticoagulant therapy, avoid further angiography procedures, and dialysis if needed. Those at increased risk for thromboembolic disease are elderly patients with extensive atherosclerotic and hypertensive disease, smokers, male gender, and those over the age of 70 years.

Postrenal: Obstruction of the urinary tract leading to reduced GFR. Causes are obstructive uropathy due to prostate (hyperplasia, tumor), tumors (bladder, pelvic malignancy, retroperitoneal fibrosis), bilateral ureteral obstruction (calculi), and urethral obstruction. Symptoms depend on location and cause of the obstruction. Urine volumes may vary. Ureteral obstruction must be bilateral or occur in setting of one functioning kidney to cause renal failure. Laboratory findings include elevated BUN/creatinine. Renal sonogram to evaluate for hydronephrosis. Bladder catheterization for postvoid residual urine can help establish a diagnosis. Treatment guided by the underlying cause.

B. Chronic Renal Failure

▶ Scientific Concepts

Progressive decline in renal function, generally over months to years. Loss of nephrons may lead to end-stage renal disease (ESRD). Diabetes mellitus and hypertension most common causes of ESRD.

▶ History & Physical

History of medication or other drug use, obstructive symptoms, past renal disease, hypertension, diabetes mellitus, proteinuria, hematuria, family history of renal disease or other illnesses. Symptoms may include fatigue, weakness, feeling cold, anorexia, nausea, vomiting, metallic taste, hiccup, sleep disturbance, irritability, restless legs, twitching, pruritus, decreased concentration, dyspnea, edema, or chest pain (pericarditis). Uremia indicative of severe renal insufficiency. Physical examination findings: may appear chronically ill, sallow complexion, skin excoriations, ecchymoses, retinopathy, uremic odor to breath, hypertension, rales, cardiomyopathy, pericardial rub, edema, drowsy, lethargic, confused, asterixis, myoclonus, rash, arthritis, palpable kidneys, prostate exam.

▶ Diagnostic Studies

Laboratory data: BUN/creatinine, anemia (normocytic, normochromic), metabolic acidosis, hypocalcemia, hyperphosphatemia, serum albumin, proteinuria, hematuria, urine casts, 24-hour urine for protein and creatinine clearance, other markers of specific disease (ANA, serum protein electrophoresis, ANCA, etc.).

Radiodiagnostics: Renal ultrasound (small kidneys, polycystic kidneys, chronic obstruction), abdominal x-ray, IVP, renal scan, CT/magnetic resonance imaging (MRI), renal angiogram, renal osteodystrophy on x-ray.
Renal biopsy

► Diagnostic Categories
Prerenal: Conditions leading to prolonged decreased tissue perfusion (heart failure, severe; cirrhosis).
Intrinsic renal
- ◆ *Tubular disease*
  - • *Polycystic kidney disease (PCKD):* Autosomal dominant inherited disorder which occurs 1 in every 400 to 1,000 live births. Fourth most common cause of end-stage renal failure. Characterized by enlargement of the kidneys with multiple cysts and slow deterioration in renal function over years, with 50% of patients progressing to end-stage renal failure by middle age or later. Cysts also found in liver, pancreas, and spleen but not associated with liver failure. Cerebral aneurysms may be associated with this disease in 5 to 10% of patients.

    Diagnosis based on positive family history, genetic testing, abdominal or flank pain, hematuria or urinary tract infections, finding of hypertension (70% of patients), renal insufficiency (mild or advanced), and minimal proteinuria. Renal sonogram (test of choice) or CT scan to confirm cysts. Screening for PCKD with renal ultrasound may be done in those with positive family history; more likely to diagnose in those over age 30. CT brain indicated if family history of cerebral aneurysm is present.

    Treatment is supportive; blood pressure control (ACE inhibitors), low-protein diet, and cyst drainage for severe pain. Dialysis or renal transplant for those with ESRD. Risk factors for disease progression include a younger age at diagnosis, hypertension, race (increased progression of disease in blacks), and kidney size. Complicating factors may include bleeding from cysts, UTIs, infected cysts, pain, renal calculi, cerebral hemorrhage, and renal cell carcinoma.
  - • *Medullary sponge kidney:* Characterized by development of cysts in terminal collecting ducts. Most patients are asymptomatic at presentation. Associated with increased incidence of renal calculi. Not associated with renal failure. Diagnosis made by IVP which reveals brush-like appearance to calyces. No specific treatment except for UTIs and stone complications.
- ◆ *Interstitial disease*
  - • *Analgesic abuse:* One to two percent of cases of ESRD in the United States. Increased risk with analgesics containing *both* aspirin and phenacetin (no longer available), acetaminophen, NSAIDs, combination analgesics, and possibly aspirin. Risk related to dose and duration of drug use. Clinical presentation is typically middle-aged women with chronic pain and analgesic use. May have hematuria or flank pain secondary to papillary necrosis, elevated BUN/creatinine, hypertension, or mild proteinuria. An increased risk of transitional cell carcinoma (especially bladder) is associated with phenacetin.

Diagnosis based on suspicion or history of analgesic use; IVP may detect papillary necrosis and sonogram or CT scan may show an irregular renal contour. Treatment is to discontinue analgesics (if continued, may progress to end stage renal disease) and control hypertension.

Other causes of interstitial disease: Chronic pyelonephritis, multiple myeloma.

◆ *Glomerular disease*

• *Diabetic nephropathy:* The major cause of ESRD, accounting for approximately 35% of dialysis patients. Marked glomerular sclerosis leads to renal failure. Glomerular disease usually not detected until diabetes present for 10 years. Lab findings of elevated BUN/creatinine; obtain 24-hour urine for protein and creatinine clearance. Microalbuminuria can be detected by radioimmunoassay prior to positive dipstick protein and is predictive of gross proteinuria and eventual renal insufficiency. Dipstick proteinuria indicates glomerulopathy and is usually seen between 17 ± 6 years after onset of type I diabetes, followed by progressive decline in renal function over years with ESRD occurring within 10 years of onset of proteinuria. Type II diabetics may present with proteinuria due to prolonged length of time from onset of disease to diagnosis. Type I diabetics with diabetes more than 5 years should have microalbuminuria screening yearly. Type II diabetics should have initial screening for microalbuminuria at diagnosis and yearly thereafter.

Diagnosis: In those patients with type I diabetes, if diabetes present at least 10 years and accompanied by proteinuria and retinopathy, a renal biopsy generally is not indicated unless other disease is suspected by history or exam. For type II diabetes, if no retinopathy is present, may need to evaluate for and rule out other forms of renal disease.

Treatment involves strict glucose control, especially early on in disease as well as blood pressure control. ACE inhibitors beneficial in reducing intraglomerular pressure and microalbuminuria; nondihydropyridine calcium channel blockers are also useful but with less effect on decreasing urine protein excretion. Dietary restriction may be helpful. Dialysis (hemodialysis or peritoneal) and renal transplant for those with ESRD.

• *Membranous nephropathy:* Most common cause of nephrotic syndrome in adults presenting with proteinuria and no other obvious systemic illness. Males > females, usually over 30 years of age. Can be associated with malignancy in those patients presenting over age 60. Associated with an increased risk of arterial and venous thrombosis, especially renal vein thrombosis. Disease is an immune-mediated process with immune complexes found in glomerular capillary walls. Course is variable and depends on serum creatinine, biopsy findings, age, sex, and amount of proteinuria; only 20 to 25% progress to ESRD over 20- to 30-year period, remainder have remission, stable, or very slow progression of renal disease. May be associated with other systemic illness or medication up to 30% of the time.

Diagnosis: Proteinuria (often nephrotic), microscopic hematuria, hypertension, edema, anasarca, anorexia, hyperlipidemia, hypoalbuminemia, lipiduria, normal or elevated BUN/creatinine. Treatment in those with normal renal function involves controlling edema with salt restriction and diuretics; NSAIDs and ACE inhibitors may help decrease proteinuria. Dietary protein restriction may be beneficial. Treat hyperlipidemia. Anticoagulants for those who have had a thrombotic event. Immunosuppressive therapy with corticosteroids and cytotoxic agents for those with progressive renal disease or severe nephrotic syndrome.

- *Focal glomerulosclerosis:* Characterized by segmental sclerosing lesions in glomeruli. Primary idiopathic and secondary forms (reflux nephropathy, human immunodeficiency virus [HIV]-associated nephropathy, morbid obesity) have been identified. Seen in children and adults. May progress to ESRD, usually 5 to 10 years from presentation.

  Diagnosis: Proteinuria, microscopic hematuria, and hypertension may be seen. Diagnosis confirmed by renal biopsy.

  Treatment is controversial. ACE inhibitors may be used to decrease proteinuria. Corticosteroids or other immunosuppressive drugs in patients with nephrotic syndrome, elevated creatinine, or significant findings on biopsy.

- *Lupus nephritis:* Disease associated with deposition of immune complex in tissues. Renal involvement varies from mild to ESRD. Physical examination findings include a malar rash, photosensitivity, oral ulcers, arthritis, serositis, and hypertension.

  Diagnosis: BUN/creatinine, proteinuria, hematuria, cellular casts in urine, lupus erythematosus prep, anti-DNA antibody, anti-Sm antibody, positive ANA, antiphospholipid antibody. Obtain renal biopsy to define renal pathology (class I–VI) and guide treatment.

  Treatment is corticosteroids for active lupus nephritis to promote remission of renal disease. Steroids and cyclophosphamide are used for more aggressive renal disease.

- *IgA nephropathy (Berger's disease):* Most common form of primary glomerulonephritis worldwide. Characterized by IgA deposition in mesangium of glomeruli. It is most common in children and young adults; male:female ratio 2 to 3:1. May present with hematuria 1 to 2 days following recent URI symptoms; hematuria may recur months to years later associated with pharyngitis, febrile state, or vigorous exercise. Other presentations include asymptomatic microscopic hematuria and proteinuria (< 1 g/d) or Henoch–Schönlein purpura.

  Diagnosis: Increased serum IgA levels (not specific), increased circulating IgA-containing immune complexes, elevated BUN/creatinine, proteinuria, renal biopsy.

  Treatment for acute disease may include steroids, cytoxic agents, anticoagulants, and plasmapheresis. Chronic disease treatment involves control of hypertension (ACE inhibitors), sodium and protein restriction, and steroids. Immunosuppressives are of unclear benefit. Dialysis and renal transplantation for those with ESRD. IgA nephropathy is a chronic disease with progressive worsening of renal function in 40% of patients, with half of those developing ESRD within 20 years from presentation; one-third of patients have persistent hematuria but no renal failure.

- *Amyloidosis:* Two forms of amyloidosis. Primary form is due to overproduction of monoclonal immunoglobulin light chains. Secondary form involves deposition of nonimmunoglobulin serum amyloid A protein. Amyloid deposits are found mainly in glomeruli and stain positively with Congo red. Other organ involvement (cardiac, GI, pulmonary) may be seen. May present with proteinuria, renal insufficiency, or monoclonal light chains in blood or urine.

  Diagnosis: renal biopsy, rectal, gingival, or fat pad biopsy.

  Treatment of primary amyloid includes melphalan, prednisone, and colchicine. Dialysis or renal transplantation for those with ESRD.

- *Minimal change nephropathy (Nil disease):* Presents as nephrotic syndrome. May occur in children or adults. In children, peak age of onset 24 to 36 months and males > females. Usually not associated with hypertension, hematuria, or renal dysfunction.

  Diagnostic findings include: nephrotic range proteinuria, hypoalbuminemia, edema, hypercholesterolemia, and oval fat bodies in urine. Renal biopsy confirms diagnosis. In children, initiate treatment with a trial of steroids before renal biopsy.

  Treatment is corticosteroids. For steroid-resistant or frequent relapsing cases, may use chronic low-dose steroids, cyclophosphamide, chlorambucil, or cyclosporine. In those patients who are unresponsive to therapy, management of edema with salt restriction and diuretics. ACE inhibitors or NSAIDs can be used to decrease proteinuria. Prognosis is good with complete remission or partial remission; relapses occur in 75 to 85% of patients. Relapses in most children disappear 10 years after onset of disease. Chronic renal failure rare in patients responsive to steroids. Complications are related to use of steroid drugs and cytoxic agents.

◆ *Vascular disease*
- *Hypertensive nephrosclerosis:* Cause of renal failure in 30% of patients with ESRD. Vascular and glomerular damage usually occurs over years. Risk of chronic renal failure secondary to hypertension is six times more likely in blacks, especially black males. Most patients are asymptomatic on presentation.

  Diagnosis: Elevated BUN/creatinine, urinalysis benign or with minimal protein.

  Treatment focused on management of hypertension. Must rule out other possible causes of renal disease. Dialysis or renal transplantation for those with ESRD.

- *Renovascular hypertension (renal artery stenosis):* Renal artery disease can cause hypertension. This form of hypertension accounts for less than 5% of all cases of hypertension and is the result of increased renin release. Causes of renovascular hypertension are fibromuscular hyperplasia (young patients) or atherosclerotic disease. Those at increased risk include patients with sudden-onset hypertension below age 20 or over age 50, accelerated hypertension, presence of abdominal bruits, other atherosclerotic disease, acute decline in renal function after use of ACE inhibitor, or difficult-to-control hypertension.

Diagnosis: Renal artery Dopplers, captopril renal scan, renal angiography (gold standard of diagnosis), renal vein renin levels, or magnetic resonance (MRA). Asymmetric kidneys on renal sonogram may be clue to diagnosis.

Treatment includes hypertension control (ACE inhibitor may cause acute renal failure in those with bilateral renal artery disease), renal artery angioplasty, renal artery stenting, or surgical revascularization.

Postrenal: Obstructive uropathy represents approximately 2% of causes of ESRD. Congenital anomalies and neuropathic bladder are other causes of postrenal failure. Prolonged time before diagnosis is made contributes to chronic renal failure.

▶ Clinical Therapeutics

Slow progression with efforts to control hypertension, control blood glucose, and reduce urinary protein excretion with ACE inhibitor. Drug dosing in chronic renal failure:

- Dose medications on estimation of creatinine clearance by Cockcroft and Gault equation:

$$\text{CrCl} = \frac{(140 - \text{age}) \times \text{weight (in kg)}}{72 \times \text{serum creatinine}}$$

Multiply result by 0.85 in females

- Caution with use of NSAIDs and ACE inhibitors (can decrease GFR) in those with known renal disease.

▶ Clinical Intervention

Slow progression with dietary protein restriction. Avoid radiocontrast material and other nephrotoxins. Monitor labs for metabolic acidosis, hyperphosphatemia, hyperuricemia, hyperkalemia, hypocalcemia, and anemia. Dialysis and renal transplantation for those with ESRD.

ESRD: Preparation includes early nephrology referral to begin teaching, counseling, dialysis preparation information, management of abnormal blood chemistries and uremic symptoms. Spare nondominant arm from venipunctures in anticipation of future dialysis access. Permanent dialysis access should be placed at least 1 to 2 months prior to start of dialysis. For acute hemodialysis access, temporary cuffed or noncuffed catheters are placed. These should preferably be inserted in the internal jugular vein as use of subclavian vein can lead to stenosis and prevent future placement of permanent access in affected arm (femoral vein may also be used). For chronic dialysis access, choices include a primary arteriovenous fistula (preferred), synthetic arteriovenous graft, or peritoneal dialysis catheter. Indications for dialysis include fluid overload, congestive heart failure, pericarditis, progressive uremic symptoms (especially neurologic or GI), encephalopathy, uremic coagulopathy, and in cases of severe hypertension, hyperkalemia, or metabolic acidosis resistant to management. In general, CrCl < 10 mL/min in a patient with other symptoms, earlier in diabetics.

Dialysis

- *Hemodialysis:* Most common form of dialysis. Requires creation of permanent access (primary arteriovenous fistula or synthetic arteriovenous graft); noncuffed temporary or tunneled cuffed dialysis catheters are not recommended for long-term dialysis. Hemodialysis involves diffusion of solutes across a semipermeable dialyzer membrane and fluid removal by the hydrostatic pressure gradient. Usual treatment 3 to 4 hours, three times weekly on fixed schedule at an outpatient dialysis unit.

  Key management goals include blood pressure control with fluid removal and antihypertensives, erythropoietin for anemia, nutritional support to maintain serum albumin (low serum albumin associated with increased mortality), dietary restriction (potassium, phosphorus, fluids), measurement of dialysis adequacy by urea reduction ratio or urea kinetic modeling, and monitoring of psychological status (decreased employment rates, increased disability and depression).

  Complications include vascular access difficulties (clotting, stenosis, malfunction, infected catheters), hypotension on dialysis, muscle cramps, allergic reactions, renal osteodystrophy from secondary hyperparathyroidism, and disequilibrium syndrome (neurologic symptoms or seizures related to rapid removal of urea). In United States, gross annual mortality is 20 to 22% for all dialysis patients. Risk is higher for diabetics and elderly; nutrition and compliance are key factors.

- *Peritoneal dialysis:* Requires insertion of a peritoneal catheter into the abdomen. Involves diffusion of solute across peritoneal membrane and fluid removal due to hyperosmotic dialysate fluid. Technique involves instillation of an electrolyte and dextrose solution (dialysate) into peritoneum over a period of time then removal of fluid on a continuous cycle. Done by patient at home, either intermittently (chronic ambulatory peritoneal dialysis [CAPD]) or with a continuous cycler machine (continuous cycle peritoneal dialysis [CCPD]) nightly.

  Key management goals include regulation of blood pressure with volume removal or antihypertensives, anemia control with erythropoietin, increased protein requirements due to protein loss in dialysate, psychosocial factors (more independent with care, responsible for own dialysis), and measurement of dialysis adequacy (peritoneal membrane kinetics). Complications include peritonitis, exit site or catheter tunnel infection, peritoneal membrane failure, and renal osteodystrophy.

Renal transplantation

- *Pretransplant evaluation:* May be done before patient is on dialysis. Involves general health assessment, including active illnesses and infectious diseases as well as systemic examinations including dental, ophthalomologic, urologic, cardiac, pulmonary, GI, immunologic, and psychosocial evaluations. Blood work including blood ABO group type, human lymphocyte antigen (HLA) histocompatibility tissue typing, HIV and hepatitis screening, panel-reactive antibodies, and recipient–donor cross-match are obtained. Once a patient is deemed a candidate for renal transplant, he or she is placed on the United Network for Organ Sharing (UNOS) waiting list; average length of wait for cadaveric kidney is 24 months.

Contraindications include serious infections, active malignancies (those treated and free of disease for 2 years may be a candidate), ongoing substance abuse, other end-organ disease (i.e., severe cardiac disease), and noncompliant patient. Age alone is not a contraindication unless significantly advanced or other illnesses present.

- *Donor:* Donor kidney source may be cadaveric, living related donor, or living unrelated donor.
- *Post-transplant:* Immunosuppressives are the key to successful renal transplantation and are evolving constantly. Three phases of immunosuppressive therapy are induction (initial), maintenance, and rejection treatment. Generally given in combination as cyclosporine or tacrolimus (FK506), azathioprine, and corticosteroids. Rejection is decreased by attempts to match major histocompatibility antigens. Can be hyperacute (within 24 hours), acute (within first 3 months) or chronic. Acute rejection often reversible with corticosteroids or anti-T cell antibody therapy. Chronic is usually irreversible and progressive and is the most common cause of late graft loss. Occasionally, recurrent disease in graft may cause loss of transplant kidney.

Management post-transplant involves careful measure of renal function and immunosuppressive drug levels (avoid toxicity and side effects), monitor for rejection (oliguria, fever, tenderness over graft, declining renal function, hypertension) and monitor for consequences of immunosuppression. Survival rates are improving. One-year graft survival 91% for living related and 81% for cadaveric donor transplants. Patient survival rate at 5 years is dependent on age; ranges from 82% in those aged 60 to 64 years with living donor transplants (63% cadaveric donor) to 94% in those aged 30 to 34 years with living donor transplants (81% cadaveric donor). Renal transplantation improves quality of life, increases life expectancy in diabetics and the young, and is the most cost-effective method of care for those with ESRD.

VI. ELECTROLYTE IMBALANCES

A. Hyponatremia

▶ Scientific Concepts

Serum sodium concentration < 135 mEq/L. Frequently seen in hospitalized patients.

▶ History & Physical

Signs and symptoms vary depending on the severity and rate of decline of serum sodium as well as age of patient. Sudden development of severe hyponatremia may cause serious central nervous system symptoms. Nausea, anorexia, malaise, headache, altered sensorium, lethargy, seizures, brain edema and herniation, and Cheyne–Stokes respirations may be present.

► Diagnostic Studies

Serum sodium, electrolytes, plasma osmolality (low in true hyponatremia, normal or high in pseudohyponatremia), urine osmolality (true hyponatremia suppresses antidiuretic hormone [ADH] release resulting in urine osmolality < 100 mOsm/kg), urine sodium (< 10 mEq/L in volume depletion, > 20 mEq/L in syndrome of inappropriate antidiuretic hormone [SIADH]).

► Diagnosis

Hyponatremia with hypovolemia: Renal volume loss (urine sodium > 20 mEq/L) may be due to excessive diuretics—especially thiazides (clue is hypokalemic metabolic alkalosis); salt-losing nephropathy—usually associated with advanced renal disease; mineralocorticoid deficiency (Addison's disease)—hyponatremia and hyperkalemia present; osmotic diuresis (glucose, urea, mannitol)—both water and electrolyte loss. Extrarenal losses (urine sodium < 10 mEq/L) may be due to GI losses (vomiting, diarrhea) or third-space losses (pancreatitis, peritonitis, burns, severe muscle injury).

Hyponatremia with volume overload: Seen in edematous states including cardiac failure, cirrhosis, nephrotic syndrome, and renal failure. Urine sodium < 10 mEq/L (if not on diuretic therapy). In renal failure, urine sodium may be > 20 mEq/L due to renal tubular dysfunction and inability to conserve sodium.

Hyponatremia with euvolemia: SIADH is associated with low plasma osmolality, high urine osmolality, and high urine sodium. May be seen with carcinoma (especially oat cell carcinoma of lung), pulmonary infection or acute disease, central nervous system disorders (stroke, infections, tumors, acute psychosis), or drugs (chlorpropramide, carbamazepine, several tricyclic antidepressants and serotonin reuptake inhibitors, and others). Postoperative hyponatremia results from administration of excess hypotonic fluids in setting of increased ADH levels due to surgery or postoperative pain. Primary polydipsia is a condition in which there is increased water intake beyond ability of the kidney to excrete (usually > 10 L/d). Associated with normal plasma osmolality and urine osmolality < 100 mOsm/kg. May be seen in patients with psychiatric disease. Severe hypothyroidism; glucocorticoid deficiency (secondary adrenal insufficiency).

Hyponatremia with increased extracellular fluid osmolality: Hyperglycemia is associated with an increased plasma osmolality. For each 100 mg/dL rise in blood glucose, serum sodium decreases by 1.6 mEq/L. Mannitol administration is associated with an increased plasma osmolality. Water is pulled into extracellular space diluting the serum sodium.

Pseudohyponatremia: Plasma osmolality normal in pseudohyponatremia. Hyperlipidemia and hyperproteinemia cause pseudohyponatremia. High levels of lipids and proteins occupy larger portion of plasma volume, therefore less water and sodium per liter of plasma (this effect is not seen if direct-reading potentiometry technique is used). Plasma sodium concentration in relation to plasma water is normal. Glycine irrigation during urologic surgery is another cause of pseudohyponatremia. A dilutional fall in serum sodium occurs due to absorption of fluid.

► Clinical Therapeutics

Demeclocycline antagonizes effect of ADH on kidney. Used to treat SIADH when it is not responsive to fluid restriction. Hypertonic saline is indicated for severe hyponatremia with central nervous system symptoms. Usually given with furosemide.

► Clinical Intervention

Correct extracellular volume depletion, remove offending drug, and treat underlying condition. Restrict fluid intake to less than urine output plus insensible losses.

► Health Maintenance Issues

Rate of correction for hyponatremia is dependent on duration and severity of hyponatremia and patient symptoms. Rapid correction of hyponatremia can cause central pontine myelinolysis. The increase in serum sodium concentration should be 0.5 mEq/L/hr, not to exceed 12 mEq/L over first 24 hours or more than 25 mEq/L over the first 48 hours of treatment. For symptomatic hyponatremia, rate of correction is 1.5 to 2.0 mEq/L/hr over first 3 to 4 hours. Aim for serum sodium concentration of 130 to 135 mEq/L over the first 48 hours of treatment to avoid overcorrection.

B. Hypernatremia

► Scientific Concepts

Serum sodium concentration > 150 mEq/L. Represents a disorder of water balance. Protective mechanism against hypernatremia is thirst and ADH secretion. Most commonly the result of impaired thirst or inability to get fluids in the setting of water loss (especially infants, elderly).

► History & Physical

Signs and symptoms are primarily neurologic. Lethargy, weakness, coma, twitching, seizures, and irritability may be present. The severity of symptoms is more dependent on the rate of developing hypernatremia (acute versus chronic) than to the serum sodium level.

► Diagnostic Studies

Serum sodium, electrolytes, urine sodium, increased plasma osmolality, urine osmolality (inappropriately low in central and nephrogenic diabetes insipidus; high or maximally concentrated in sodium overload, insensible water loss, and hypodipsia).

► Diagnosis

Hypernatremia with hypovolemia: Extrarenal losses from GI tract (diarrhea) or excessive sweating can cause hypernatremia. With GI losses, the urine is hypertonic and urine sodium < 10 mEq/L due to renal sodium and water conservation. Renal losses from osmotic diuresis (glucose, urea, mannitol).

Hypernatremia with euvolemia: Extrarenal losses from insensible water losses (fever, respiratory, burns). Renal losses from central diabetes insipidus or nephrogenic diabetes insipidus can cause hypernatremia. In central diabetes insipidus, there is inadequate vasopressin release and hypotonic urine with increased plasma osmolality. In nephrogenic diabetes insipidus, there is impaired kidney response to vasopressin. This can be secondary to renal or other diseases and drugs (lithium, demeclocycline). Hypothalamic disorders including reset osmostat (higher plasma sodium level seen as normal) or hypodipsia.

Hypernatremia with volume overload: Hypertonic salts (hypertonic saline, large amounts of sodium bicarbonate) and ingestion of sodium (high-sodium enteral feedings).

► Clinical Therapeutics

Goal is to correct cause. Volume-expanded states without advanced renal disease respond to diuretics. Diuretics cause renal loss of sodium and water; must replace urine water loss with free water. Central diabetes insipidus (DI) responds to ADH.

► Clinical Intervention

Fluid replacement based on calculation of water deficit. In volume-depleted states, isotonic saline should be administered to the hypotensive patient until extracellular fluid volume is restored, then hypotonic saline may be given to correct plasma osmolality.

► Health Maintenance Issues

Avoid overly rapid correction to prevent brain edema. Chronic hypernatremia should be corrected over 48 hours or longer with goal to lower serum sodium concentration by 0.5 to 1.0 mEq/L/hr.

C. Hypokalemia

► Scientific Concepts

Serum potassium concentration < 3.5 mEq/L. Potassium is the major intracellular cation.

► History & Physical

Signs and symptoms depend on level of serum potassium and include the following systems: cardiac (arrhythmias, electrocardiogram changes—flat T waves and prominent U waves, increased sensitivity to digitalis), neuromuscular (muscle weakness, cramps, paresthesias, rhabdomyolysis, ileus), and renal (polyuria, polydipsia).

► Diagnostic Studies

Serum potassium, urine potassium, serum electrolytes, glucose, urine sodium and chloride, evaluate for acid–base disorders, plasma renin and aldosterone levels, and blood pressure.

► Diagnosis

Extracellular to intracellular redistribution of potassium: Insulin administration/excess, metabolic alkalosis, respiratory alkalosis, beta-adrenergic agonists, toluene poisoning (glue or spray paint sniffing), and hypokalemic periodic paralysis (hereditary disorder).

Potassium losses: Extrarenal losses including GI (diarrhea, laxative abuse), extreme sweating, and extensive burns. Renal losses including diuretics, vomiting (release of aldosterone in response to volume depletion causing renal potassium loss), excess mineralocorticoid (Cushing's syndrome, licorice), renal tubular acidosis, hypomagnesemia, and primary hyperaldosteronism.

Decreased potassium intake: Uncommon cause of hypokalemia because of potassium content in various foods and ability of kidney to conserve potassium efficiently.

► Clinical Therapeutics

Correct underlying cause. If hypomagnesemia present, this must be corrected for potassium balance to be restored. Various types of potassium salts are available for replacement therapy. In cases of hypokalemia with metabolic alkalosis or unclear cause, use only potassium chloride. For hypokalemia with metabolic acidosis, use a bicarbonate salt. Potassium-sparing diuretics can be used in those with primary hyperaldosteronism. Caution when used in those with renal insufficiency.

► Clinical Intervention

Route of potassium replacement may be oral or intravenous. Oral is preferred route of replacement. Usual rate of intravenous replacement is no greater than 10 mEq/hr; in urgent cases, no greater than 20 to 40 mEq/hr with close cardiac monitoring. Potassium concentration of IV fluids should be no greater than 40 mEq/L due to risk of phlebitis unless infused into a large vein. Avoid glucose solutions and alkali as these can further decrease serum potassium by causing intracellular shift of potassium.

► Health Maintenance Issues

Monitor serum potassium levels in those on diuretics, especially those on cardiac glycosides or with cardiovascular disease; mild hypokalemia may predispose to arrhythmias.

D. Hyperkalemia

► Scientific Concepts

Serum potassium concentration > 5.0 mEq/L. Potassium is the major intracellular cation. Hyperkalemia is often iatrogenic.

► History & Physical

Signs and symptoms depend on level of serum potassium. Often asymptomatic until level 6.5 mEq/L or greater. May include cardiac (electrocardiogram changes—peaked T waves, prolonged PR interval, widening of QRS, arrhythmias), and neuromuscular (paresthesias, weakness, tingling) systems.

► **Diagnostic Studies**

Serum potassium, serum electrolytes, BUN/creatinine, evaluate for acid–base disorders, urine pH, plasma aldosterone and cortisol levels, rule out pseudohyperkalemia; history and physical examination.

► **Diagnosis**

Increased intake: Transient hyperkalemia unless renal potassium excretion is impaired.

Transcellular redistribution: Insulin deficiency, acidosis (especially hyperchloremic metabolic acidosis), cell breakdown (rhabdomyolysis, tumor cell lysis), digoxin toxicity, nonselective beta-adrenergic blocker, and hyperkalemic periodic paralysis (rare hereditary disorder).

Impaired renal excretion: Renal failure with oliguria, mineralocorticoid deficiency (Addison's disease, hyporeninemic hypoaldosteronism, drugs including NSAIDs and ACE inhibitors), and renal tubular dysfunction (hyperkalemic type I distal renal tubular acidosis, drugs including potassium sparing diuretics and trimethoprim).

Pseudohyperkalemia: Traumatic blood draw with hemolysis, excessive fist clenching or tourniquet pressure with blood draw, thrombocytosis, and marked leukocytosis.

► **Clinical Therapeutics**

Reserved for potassium > 6.0 mEq/L or if electrocardiographic changes present. Evaluate and correct causes such as pseudohyperkalemia and transcellular redistribution of potassium. Antagonize cell membrane effects with IV calcium gluconate. Shift potassium intracellularly with sodium bicarbonate, glucose/insulin, and beta-2-adrenergic agonists. Remove excess potassium with cation exchange resin (Kayexalate, oral or enema) or loop diuretics.

► **Clinical Intervention**

Remove excess potassium by dialysis, either hemodialysis or peritoneal dialysis (slower method of potassium removal); dietary potassium restriction.

► **Health Maintenance Issues**

Identify those patients at risk for hyperkalemia (renal insufficiency, mineralocorticoid deficiency). Use caution with certain drugs (NSAIDs, ACE inhibitors, trimethoprim, potassium-sparing diuretics) in this population.

VII. ACID–BASE DISORDERS

A. Respiratory Acidosis

► **Scientific Concepts**

Hypercapnia as result of decreased alveolar ventilation.

► History & Physical

Signs and symptoms associated with acute-onset respiratory acidosis include somnolence, confusion, myoclonus, asterixis, coma, papilledema, bradypnea, and hypopnea.

► Diagnostic Studies

Decreased pH, increased partial pressure of carbon dioxide (PCO_2), increased bicarbonate.

► Differential Diagnosis

Respiratory center depression (sleep apnea, brain stem infarct, sedative overdose), neuromuscular disorders (multiple sclerosis, amyotrophic lateral sclerosis, Guillain–Barré syndrome, poliomyelitis), restrictive disorders (pneumo/hemothorax, kyphoscoliosis, acute respiratory distress syndrome), and acute or chronic pulmonary disease (interstitial fibrosis, chronic obstructive pulmonary disease [COPD], bronchospasm).

► Clinical Therapeutics/Interventions

Treat underlying cause and improve ventilation. Consider naloxone if sedative overdose suspected.

B. Respiratory Alkalosis

► Scientific Concepts

Hypocapnia as a result of increased rate of pulmonary carbon dioxide excretion. Hyperventilation is most common cause.

► History & Physical

Signs and symptoms include lightheadedness, anxiety, paresthesias, tachypnea, and hyperpnea.

► Diagnostic Studies

Increased pH, decreased carbon dioxide, decreased bicarbonate.

► Differential Diagnosis

Hyperventilation and other causes of hypoxia (high altitude, severe anemia), central nervous system events (infarction, trauma, tumor, infection), sespis with endotoxin, drugs (salicylates, progesterone), pulmonary disease (pneumonia, pulmonary edema or embolism), and excessive mechanical ventilation.

► Clinical Therapeutics/Interventions

Treat underlying cause and maintain oxygenation.

C. Metabolic Acidosis

► Scientific Concepts

Anion gap helpful in determining cause. Anion gap = (Na) − (HCO_3 + Cl), normal anion gap is 9 ± 3 mEq/L.

► History & Physical

Signs and symptoms are related to underlying disorder and may include diarrhea, oliguria, anuria, Kussmaul respirations, hypotension, arrhythmias, and lethargy.

▶ Diagnostic Studies

Decreased pH, decreased PCO_2, decreased bicarbonate; anion gap, electrolytes, urine or serum ketones, and serum lactate.

▶ Differential Diagnosis

Metabolic acidosis with increased anion gap seen in ketoacidosis, lactic acidosis, drug intoxications (ethylene glycol, methanol, salicylates), and advanced renal failure. Metabolic acidosis with normal anion gap seen with GI bicarbonate loss (diarrhea and drainage of small bowel or pancreatic secretions), renal bicarbonate loss (acetazolamide, renal tubular acidosis), and inorganic acids (ammonium chloride, sulfur).

▶ Clinical Therapeutics/Interventions

Treat underlying disorder; sodium bicarbonate administration for moderate to severe metabolic acidosis. For ketoacidosis, treat with fluids, correct electrolytes and glucose; insulin for diabetic ketoacidosis; thiamine for alcoholic ketoacidosis. For lactic acidosis, goal is to restore tissue perfusion and oxygenation. Treatment for drug intoxication is based on specific drug ingested. Ethylene glycol and methanol poisoning are treated with ethanol infusion and hemodialysis. Salicylate overdose is treated by alkalinization of urine and may require hemodialysis.

D. Metabolic Alkalosis

▶ Scientific Concepts

Elevated plasma bicarbonate. Generated by loss of hydrogen ion or chloride and maintained by decreased renal bicarbonate loss.

▶ History & Physical

Signs and symptoms include weakness, neuromuscular irritability, and symptoms of volume depletion.

▶ Diagnostic Studies

Increased pH, increased PCO_2, increased bicarbonate; decreased potassium and chloride; anion gap may be increased; urine chloride.

▶ Differential Diagnosis

In volume-depleted states (low urine chloride), consider gastric acid loss (vomiting, nasogastric suction) or renal loss from diuretics (urine chloride low after diuretic stopped). In volume-repleted states (high urine chloride), consider mineralocorticoid excess (hyperaldosteronism, Bartter's syndrome, Cushing's syndrome, licorice excess) or severe hypokalemia.

▶ Clinical Therapeutics/Interventions

If present, correct extracellular volume deficit with chloride containing solutions or treat other underlying disorders. Acetazolamide can be used in volume-expanded patients. Rarely, acid infusion required (sodium chloride, ammonium chloride, dilute hydrochloric acid).

BIBLIOGRAPHY

Black RM. *Rose & Black's Clinical Problems in Nephrology,* 1st ed. Boston: Little, Brown and Company; 1996.

Greenberg A, ed. *Primer on Kidney Diseases,* 2nd ed. San Diego: Academic Press; 1998.

Rose BD, ed. *Pathophysiology of Renal Disease,* 2nd ed. New York: McGraw-Hill; 1987.

Schrier RW, ed. *Manual of Nephrology,* 4th ed. Boston: Little, Brown and Company; 1995.

Tanagho EA, McAninch JW, eds. *Smith's General Urology,* 15th ed. New York: McGraw-Hill; 2000.

Tierney LM Jr et al., eds. *Current Medical Diagnosis and Treatment 1998,* 37th ed. Stamford, CT: Appleton & Lange; 1998.

Male Genitourinary Disorders 8

Stephen M. Thomas, BHS, PA-C, John W. Rafalko, MS, PA-C

I. BLADDER TUMORS

► Scientific Concepts

The second most common site for tumors of urinary tract. Types include transitional cell carcinomas (most common), epidermoid tumors, adenocarcinoma, and sarcoma with systemic disease. Highest occurrence in males over 50.

► History & Physical

Include symptoms of hematuria, urinary frequency, reduced urinary stream, dysuria, suprapubic pain, and palpable bladder mass.

► Diagnostic Studies

Urinalysis, urine culture, intravenous pyelogram (IVP), ultrasound, computed tomographic (CT) scan, cystoscopy/biopsy.

► Diagnosis

Rule out renal calculus, cystitis, nephritis. Specific diagnosis by tissue biopsy. Metastasis from other locations is rarely seen.

► Clinical Therapeutics/Preventions

Specific cause is unknown. Risk factors include alcoholism, smoking, teratogens (pesticides, etc.), and radiation exposure.

► Clinical Intervention

Tumor staging, surgery, radiation/immuno/hormonal and chemotherapies.

► Health Maintenance Issues

Genetic link may be present. Also increased incidence noted in rural and farm populations. There are no good screening tests. Presenting symptoms are often vague (back or abdominal pain). Gross hematuria often presenting symptom, but the use of urinalysis as a screener is nonspecific. Issues of smoking cessation and alcohol consumption should be discussed.

II. EJACULATORY DISORDERS

► Scientific Concepts

Inability to consistently control ejaculatory reflex. Includes ejaculation before wanted to delayed or absent reflex in spite of normal erection. Also includes retrograde ejaculation in which semen is forced back into the bladder during ejaculation. Causes include peripheral neuropathy, prior urogenital surgery, multiple sclerosis, diabetes mellitus, psychogenic factors, and drugs.

► History & Physical

Historical responses range from ejaculation before wished to absent ejaculation, including intercourse and masturbation. Premature tends to be more common in adolescent and younger age groups. Retrograde and delayed/retarded are more common in older males with concurrent systemic disease (i.e., heart disease, diabetes mellitus), or prescription drug use (i.e., nasal decongestants).

► **Diagnostic Studies**

Detailed sexual history. Appropriate management/diagnosis of other metabolic and neurologic disorders. Laboratory studies are usually normal. Postejaculate urinalysis may confirm retrograde ejaculation.

► **Diagnosis**

Generally made by detailed history, but consultation with endocrinology, neurology, urology may be in order.

► **Clinical Therapeutics**

Identification and treatment of any medical causes. Prescriptions may be altered or discontinued if appropriate. Voiding prior to intercourse may help retrograde ejaculation. Interpersonal therapies (i.e., counseling for communication and sexual disorders).

► **Clinical Intervention**

Appropriate management of systemic disease and referral/treatment for psychogenic factors.

► **Health Maintenance Issues**

Office screenings and good sexual history important. Mental health services if appropriate nonorganic source. Proper management of cardiovascular and endocrine disorders (i.e., vascular and lipid disorders, hypertension, diabetes). Lifestyle modifications such as diet, smoking cessation, exercise should be discussed.

III. ENURESIS

► **Scientific Concepts**

Involuntary urination. Nocturnal (determined by nighttime frequency of > 1/mo in females older than 5 years old and males older than 6 years old). Daytime (during waking hours). Primary (child never completely toilet trained), secondary (the return of involuntary loss after toilet training). Occurs in males > females, incidence 10% of children.

► **History & Physical**

Important information includes age, primary or secondary, nocturnal or daytime, other developmental milestones, and toilet training history. Familial history of diabetes mellitus. Associated genitourinary symptoms (dysuria, frequency, etc.). Thorough examination of lower back for spinal dysrhaphia and neurological examination of genitalia and lower extremities (i.e., spina bifida, tethered cord syndrome). Also consider emotional problems as a trigger for secondary enuresis.

► Diagnostic Studies

Urinalysis, urine culture. Renal ultrasound, IVP, voiding cystourethrogram helpful if urinary tract infections (UTIs) are associated with the enuresis. Spinal cord/column imaging if physical abnormalities noted on examination.

► Diagnosis

Generally a disorder that can be diagnosed by history and limited diagnostic studies. Differential diagnosis includes diabetes mellitus, diabetes insipidus, renal tubular disorders, and spinal cord tumors or malformations.

► Clinical Therapeutics

Tricyclic antidepressants (imipramine, desipramine), desmopressin acetate can be used with high early success rates. Both medication regimens have a high relapse rate following withdrawal. Overall success rate around 40%.

► Clinical Intervention

Measures including fluid restrictions prior to bedtime, behavioral training, and bed alarms are utilized with good success rates. The use of alarms actually has the best success and lowest recurrence rate.

► Health Maintenance Issues

Reassurance according to age-related statistics is important in the early age groups. Medical workup more important in cases of advanced age, recurrent infections, etc. Supportive approach important in children, and reassurance of decreased incidence with advancing age.

IV. EPIDIDYMITIS

► Scientific Concepts

Unilateral inflammation of the epididymis resulting in scrotal pain. Inflammation usually unilateral but may spread to both testicles and the scrotal wall. Hydrocele formation occurs in some situations. Caused by urinary pathogens, sexually transmitted diseases (STDs), and sterile inflammation.

► History & Physical

Highest incidence in young, sexually active men. Older age groups next with UTIs. Rarely occurs in prepubertal boys. Scrotal elevation and support improves pain. Physical findings include urethral discharge, UTI symptoms, pain and inflammation extending from the posterior epididymis to the scrotal wall. Fever and chills can occur with severe infection and abscess formation.

► Diagnostic Studies

Urinalysis, Gram stain of urethral discharge, urethral culture. Cultures should be for gonorrhea and chlamydia. Ultrasound of scrotum, radionuclide scan.

► Diagnosis

Differential diagnosis includes testicular torsion, mumps orchitis, tumor, hydrocele, varicocele, spermatocele, trauma, postvasectomy congestion.

► Clinical Therapeutics

STDs should be treated for gonococcal/nongonococcal organisms (doxycycline, ceftriaxone, ciprofloxin, norfloxin). With bacteriuria, should treat for urinary pathogens (trimethoprim-sulfamethoxazole [TMP-SMZ], tetracycline, ciprofloxacin, norfloxacin).

► Clinical Intervention

Appropriate analgesia (nonsteroidal anti-inflammatories [NSAIDs] for mild to moderate pain, (opiates for severe pain). Additionally, scrotal elevation and cold packs may help with pain. Pain improves within 1 to 3 days, but swelling may take several weeks to resolve. Sterility sometimes a complication.

► Health Maintenance Issues

Screening in patients with high-risk behaviors (i.e., multiple partners, no barrier methods practiced, change in sexual partner in last 6 to 12 months). Counsel, educate, and encourage the use of condoms. Discuss issues of promiscuity, abstinence, and risk behavior management.

V. PRIAPISM

► Scientific Concepts

Penile erection, often painful. Not related to sexual stimulation. Incidence/prevalence in the United States is unknown.

► History & Physical

Penile erection that is painful and prolonged. Accompanying painful urination, eventual loss of sexual function.

► Diagnostic Studies

There are no primary diagnostics for priapism. However, appropriate diagnostics for disease processes involved are indicated. A good history and physical examination are principal diagnostics.

► Diagnosis

Causes for priapism are numerous. Blood dyscrasias (leukemia, sickle cell), vascular thrombosis, pelvic masses (hematoma, neoplasm), spinal cord tumors, urinary calculi and infections, and drugs (trazodone, chlorpromazine, some antihypertensives).

► Clinical Therapeutics

Generally pharmaceutical management involves pain management and observation.

► Clinical Intervention

In sickle cell, hydration and exchange transfusion is appropriate. If a neurogenic cause is determined, caudal or spinal anesthesia is appropriate. Urologic referral for surgery. Placement of shunts or invasive release of congestion in cavernosum/spongiosum. Treat other underlying causes.

► Health Maintenance Issues

Proper screening and management of blood disorders. Familial history is vital in the screening of these blood disorders. Atherosclerotic disease should be noted in the differential diagnosis (i.e., lipid disorders, smoking, hypertension, diabetes).

VI. TESTICULAR TORSION

► Scientific Concepts

Acute ischemia of testis caused by twisting of cord and vascular supply. Torsions involving the entire testicular structure as well as within the tunica vaginalis can occur.

► History & Physical

History of trauma (20%), prior history of testicular pain. Exercise, cold temperature, and sexual stimulation may play a role. Peak occurrence at age 14, but occurs in all age groups. Two-thirds of cases occur in second decade. Scrotal enlargement, pain, redness, and edema are common. Accompanying nausea, vomiting, and fever may occur.

► Diagnostic Studies

Urinalysis, CT or ultrasound, Doppler ultrasound, and radionuclide testicular scintigraphy with technetium.

► Diagnosis

Differential diagnosis includes epididymitis, orchitis, hernia, hematoma, hydrocele, varicocele, tumor, infiltrate, and abscess.

► Clinical Therapeutics

Pain management and rapid diagnosis is essential. Testicular salvage is related to length of time torsion persists. Manual reduction of torsion may be successful; this can be facilitated by 1% lidocaine injection.

► Clinical Intervention

Rapid surgical exploration of scrotal contents is essential for testicular salvage. Removal of necrosed testis may be indicated. Fixation of testis recommended.

► Health Maintenance Issues

High level of suspicion in young age groups. No screening measures are available to determine risk. Open communication with young male patients about testicular exam should take place. This is to facilitate better communications with parents and providers. Reporting of testicular problems is often delayed to a point of poor outcome.

VII. URETHRITIS

▶ Scientific Concepts

Urethral inflammation, discharge, and painful urination are hallmarks of the urethral syndrome. Predominantly an STD seen in sexually active postpubertal males. Can also be seen in other UTIs such as cystitis, prostatitis, and epididymitis. Causative organisms, in order of incidence, include *Neisseria gonorrhoeae, Chlamydia trachomatis, Ureaplasma, Trichomonas,* cytomegalovirus, herpes simplex virus, human papillomavirus, other bacteria.

▶ History & Physical

Higher incidence seen in males < 35 years old, multiple sexual partners, and prior history of STDs. Avoidance of condoms considered high risk. Contact with a known carrier is best actively treated, even if asymptomatic. Symptoms include dysuria, urethral discharge, and suprapubic tenderness. Associated symptoms of proctitis, pharyngitis, and conjunctivitis are sometimes seen. Inguinal lymphadenopathy can be seen.

▶ Diagnostic Studies

Culture or rapid reagins of urethral discharge, Gram stain, urinalysis, urine culture, and wet prep. Viral cultures are indicated if physical examination indicates.

▶ Diagnosis

Differential diagnosis includes STDs, UTIs, trauma, foreign bodies (i.e., venereal warts, polyps), Reiter's syndrome.

▶ Clinical Therapeutics

Current recommended drug treatment is ceftriaxone, 250 mg intramuscularly (IM), plus doxycycline, 100 mg bid. Alternate regimens include macrolides and fluoroquinolones. Metronidazole is used in cases of trichomoniasis. Increasing incidence of drug resistance should be noted. Treat sexual partners, and consider post-treatment repeat of positive cultures.

▶ Clinical Intervention

None, except surgical treatment of underlying causes (i.e., polyps, condyloma). Medical management of associated conditions (i.e., Reiter's syndrome).

▶ Health Maintenance Issues

Counseling regarding sexual abstinence, condom use, and risks related to multiple sexual partners is essential. Stress importance of compliance to treatment regimens, avoidance of intercourse until treatment completed, and communication to partners.

VIII. PROSTATE DISORDERS

A. Prostatic Hypertrophy

▶ Scientific Concepts

Benign prostatic hypertrophy (BPH) has unknown etiology but appears to be hormonally influenced. The resulting obstructive uropathy is responsible for characteristic signs and symptoms. The transition zone, next to the urethra, is first affected. Risk factors include previous family history and any male > 50 years old.

▶ History & Physical

Increased frequency, urgency, nocturia, weak stream, hesitancy, and dribbling are characteristics. An enlarged prostate is palpable on rectal examination. A distended bladder, secondary to urinary retention, may be identified when the lower abdomen is examined. The International Prostate Symptom Score (I-PSS) is recommended to grade BPH and monitor treatment. Total score ranges from 0 to 35; the greater the BPH symptoms, the higher the score.

▶ Diagnostic Studies

Urinalysis may reveal hematuria and infection characteristic of UTIs. Elevated blood urea nitrogen (BUN) and creatinine may reflect urinary retention.

▶ Diagnosis

Diagnosis based on the history and clinical examination of the patient, while excluding other causes of obstructive uropathy. These include prostate cancer, acute prostatitis, urethral stricture, or neurogenic bladder. Prostate-specific antigen (PSA) may be elevated in BPH (> 4 ng/mL but < 10 ng/mL). Intravenous urography, uroflowmetry, and cystourethroscopy can narrow the diagnosis. Consider postvoid residual volumes.

▶ Clinical Therapeutics

Conservative treatment with pharmacologic trial is the first line of therapy due to slow natural progression of disease. Alpha-sympatholytic agents (terazosin), which relax prostate smooth muscle, or 5-alpha-reductase inhibitors (finasteride), which block testosterone conversion, are utilized in treatment of BPH.

▶ Clinical Intervention

Surgical treatment for complications or recurrent symptoms. Transurethral resection of the prostate (TURP) most common operation. Other therapies include laser, ultrasound, microwave, and stents.

▶ Health Maintenance Issues

BPH is a natural process of aging in men; their health care provider should inform them about anticipated signs and symptoms. Medications should be checked. BPH symptoms can result from probanthine or phenylephrine use.

B. Prostate Cancer

▶ Scientific Concepts

The second most common cause of cancer death in males. Increased incidence with age. Majority of prostate cancer localized to peripheral zone. Etiology is unknown; however, genetic, endocrine, diet, and environmental factors are suspected. Most are adenocarcinomas.

▶ History & Physical

Risk factors include family history, African-American males, and age > 50 years old. Most men with prostate cancer are asymptomatic. Weight loss or bone pain suggests late stage with metastases. Rectal examination reveals a firm, indurated, rock hard, nontender, localized area.

▶ Diagnostic Studies

PSA, although not solely specific to prostate cancer, is useful in narrowing the diagnosis and monitoring treatment. Transrectal ultrasound (TRUS) with needle biopsy confirms the diagnosis. Magnetic resonance imaging (MRI) and radionuclide bone scan verify metastases.

▶ Diagnosis

Once a definitive diagnosis is made, the Gleason pathology grading and tumor, node, metastases (TNM) staging system are applied for prognosis and determining treatment.

▶ Clinical Therapeutics

Treatment is based on the above classification system identifying localized disease or metastases. Radiation therapy by external beam or internal implants are a mainstay for treatment. Hormone treatment offers androgen deprivation to sensitive tumors.

▶ Clinical Intervention

Bilateral orchiectomy provides radical antiandrogen effects. The main surgical therapy is radical prostatectomy.

▶ Health Maintenance Issues

The role of prostate screening poses a serious dilemma. PSA was not designed to be a screening tool. Prostate screening remains controversial because PSA is not specific to prostate cancer. Annual digital rectal examination is recommended in males at 50 years of age.

C. Prostatitis

▶ Scientific Concepts

Classified as acute or chronic. Usually caused by gram-negative rods (*Escherichia coli*) or gram-positive organisms (*Enterococcus*). Bacteria ascend up the male urethra. Nonbacterial prostatitis is relatively common. Viruses and atypical microorganisms (mycoplasma) should be considered if bacterial organisms are eliminated.

▶ History & Physical

History of UTI. Perineal, suprapubic, and lower back pain. Dysuria, frequency, urgency, and obstructive symptoms. Fever may be present. Digital rectal examination reveals a boggy, tender, indurated prostate that is warm to palpation. Aggressive massage of prostate is cautioned with acute prostatitis because of the risk of sepsis.

▶ Diagnostic Studies

Digital rectal examination. Urine is collected in series of initial void, midstream, and postprostatic massage. Prostate secretions are collected, as is the urine. Analysis reveals hematuria, many bacteriuria (> 100,000 colony-forming units [CFU]/mL), or pyuria (> 10 white blood cells per high-power field [WBC/HPF]). Cultures and sensitivity to identify offending organism. Complete blood count (CBC) shows elevated WBC.

▶ Diagnosis

History, physical, and urinalysis should establish the diagnosis. Consider urethritis, cystitis, pyelonephritis, and epididymitis in the differential diagnosis.

▶ Clinical Therapeutics

Treat with systemic antibiotics until sensitivities are known. TMP-SMZ is often the antibiotic of choice. Several weeks of antibiotic therapy are essential. Follow-up urinalysis and culture are needed after antibiotic treatment to test for cure. Consider NSAIDs for pain.

▶ Clinical Intervention

Chronic prostatitis may require 6 weeks to 3 months of antibiotic therapy to suppress recurrent UTIs.

▶ Health Maintenance Issues

Age > 50 years old, frequent catheterization, and most males with urethritis age 15 to 30 years old are at risk of prostatitis.

IX. URINARY TRACT INFECTIONS

▶ Scientific Concepts

Any UTI in an adult male mandates a thorough workup. Anatomy is thought to prevent infection. Rare in young men. Female to male ratio, 30:1. Males who are homosexual, are noncircumcised, or have a partner with vaginal colonization have a greater incidence. In men > 50 years of age, UTIs are often associated with diseases of the prostate or instrumentation. Above age 50 years, incidence in men equals women.

▶ History & Physical

Age > 50 years. Dysuria, frequency, urgency, hematuria, and nocturia. Flank pain and costovertebral angle tenderness if upper UTI.

► Diagnostic Studies

Dipstick with positive nitrate and leukocyte esterase tests. Urinalysis and culture. Use midstream catch for culture and sensitivity. Standard is > 100,000 CFU/mL. Microscopic spun urinalysis under HPF prior to culture, look for bacteria or WBCs.

► Diagnosis

UTI is a simple diagnosis. The workup for a UTI is often complex, focused on obstructive uropathy. Cystourethroscopy, intravenous urography, and uroflowmetry are indicated in male UTI. Treat the cause.

► Clinical Therapeutics

Gram-negative rods (*E. coli*) most common pathogen. TMP-SMZ for simple UTI. Broad-based antibiotic selection initially, then focused on sensitivities to urine culture growth. Follow-up culture indicated if complicated UTI.

► Clinical Intervention

Nosocomial infections are related to indwelling catheter. Straight catheterization recommended. Recurrent infections are often due to urological abnormalities or chronic bacterial prostatitis.

► Health Maintenance Issues

Frequent hydration. Eight glasses of water per day. Cranberry juice to acidify the urine. Avoid alcohol. Regular bathroom trips and try not to hold urine.

X. TRAUMA

A. Ureteral Trauma

► Scientific Concepts

Uncommon urologic injury. Associated with blunt multisystem or penetrating trauma. Iatrogenic injury seen with instrumentation.

► History & Physical

High index of suspicion required based on mechanism of injury. Flank pain, oliguria, anuria, fever, with or without hematuria. Lower abdominal pain on physical examination.

► Diagnostic Studies

Diagnosis identified with IVP or an incidental finding on exploratory laparotomy.

► Diagnosis

Consider with any associated injury to the genitourinary area. Missed diagnosis can result in urine leak, ileus, fever, sepsis, or ureterocutaneous fistula.

▶ **Clinical Therapeutics**

Minor injury may divert urine by ureteral stenting. Foley catheter to decompress bladder and monitor urine output. Broad-spectrum antibiotics to prevent infection.

▶ **Clinical Intervention**

Major injury demands early diagnosis and repair. Ureteroureterostomy most common operative repair. Prompt urological consult.

▶ **Health Maintenance Issues**

Anticipatory guidance. The best treatment is prevention of trauma. Avoid alcohol, drugs, and conflict. Mostly due to penetrating trauma and iatrogenic injury. Inform patients at risk.

B. Urethral Trauma

▶ **Scientific Concepts**

Blunt injury occurs greater than penetrating. High index of suspicion with deceleration mechanism of injury. Associated pelvic fractures. Disruption may be complete or partial.

▶ **History & Physical**

Motor vehicle accident, fall from horse or bicycle with resulting pelvic fracture is often mechanism of injury. Blood at the tip of the urethral meatus is the classic presentation. Hematuria, anuria, perineal edema, or tender and distended lower abdomen and "high-riding" prostate on digital rectal examination.

▶ **Diagnostic Studies**

Retrograde urethrogram is mandated for the evaluation of a urethral injury.

▶ **Diagnosis**

Differential diagnosis includes both lower and upper urinary tract injuries.

▶ **Clinical Therapeutics**

Do not insert Foley or straight catheter until retrograde urethrogram is performed. If extravasation of contrast is noted, a suprapubic catheter is then placed to decompress the bladder. Prompt urological consult.

▶ **Clinical Intervention**

Primary repair with stenting for small lacerations or delayed primary repair with suprapubic cystostomy for complex injury. Complications include stricture, impotence, and incontinence.

▶ **Health Maintenance Issues**

Most commonly seen with blunt injury associated with automobile accidents.

C. Bladder Trauma

▶ Scientific Concepts

Intraperitoneal and/or extraperitoneal rupture. Both associated with pelvic fractures. Distended bladder is susceptible to contusion, laceration, or perforation. All common with associated multisystem trauma. Blunt to penetrating ratio, 5:1. Iatrogenic injuries common.

▶ History & Physical

History of lower abdominal trauma. Anuria, oliguria, and gross or microscopic hematuria. Localized suprapubic or diffuse abdominal pain. Tenderness to percussion or palpation. Intraperitoneal rupture will result in acute abdomen secondary to peritonitis.

▶ Diagnostic Studies

Hemorrhagic shock may result from associated injuries. Follow serial hemoglobin/hematocrit. Retrograde urethrogram to rule out suspected urethral injury if indicated by blood at tip of meatus. If negative, Foley catheter insertion to decompress bladder. Urinalysis dipstick to identify microhematuria if gross hematuria is not noted. Pelvic x-ray may show associated pelvic fracture. Cystography to note extravasation. Cystogram is radiologic study of choice. IVP to rule out kidney or ureteral injury often will miss bladder injury.

▶ Diagnosis

Bladder trauma is a diagnosis of exclusion, eliminating other genitourinary tract injuries. A missed diagnosis can have increased mortality and morbidity.

▶ Clinical Therapeutics

Conservative management is indicated for bladder contusions with Foley catheter decompression and irrigation of clots. Intravenous fluid resuscitation as needed. Broad-spectrum antibiotics. *Caution:* bladder decompression > 1,000 cc should never be allowed without adequate intravenous fluid replacement. Historically, gradual bladder decompression has been emphasized.

▶ Clinical Intervention

Extraperitoneal ruptures may be managed conservatively with catheter decompression or require surgery for repair and drainage. Intraperitoneal ruptures mandate exploration, repair with absorbable sutures, and drainage.

▶ Health Maintenance Issues

See previous trauma topics about prevention and anticipatory guidance.

BIBLIOGRAPHY

Ashcraft KW. *Pediatric Urology.* Philadelphia: WB Saunders; 1990.

Berkow R, Fletcher AJ. *The Merck Manual of Diagnosis & Therapy,* 16th ed. Rahway, NJ: Merck & Company; 1992.

Currey R. Epididymitis: Recognition & management. *PA Today* 6(12):10–13; 1998.

Goldberg JS. *The Instant Review for the USMLE Step 3,* 2nd ed. Stamford, CT: Appleton & Lange; 1997.

Ho MT, Saunders CE. *Current Emergency Diagnosis & Treatment,* 4th ed. Norwalk, CT: Appleton & Lange; 1992.

Way LW. *Current Surgical Diagnosis & Treatment,* 10th ed. Norwalk, CT: Appleton & Lange; 1994.

Moore KL. *Clinically Oriented Anatomy,* 3rd ed. Philadelphia: Williams & Wilkins; 1992.

Rutherford A. Enuresis: Its diagnosis and management, a general practice perspective. *Aust Fam Phys* 17(9):749–754; 1988.

Tanagho EA, McAninch JW. *Smith's General Urology,* 15th ed. New York: McGraw-Hill; 2000.

Tierney LM. *Current Medical Diagnosis and Treatment,* 38th ed. Stamford, CT: Appleton & Lange; 1999.

Walsh PC, Gittes RF, Perlmutter AD. *Campbell's Urology.* Philadelphia: WB Saunders; 1989.

Obstetrics and Gynecology 9

Dawn Morton-Rias, RPA-C

I. VAGINA/VULVA

A. Vaginal Infections and Sexually Transmitted Diseases

Vaginal infections are probably the most common gynecological complaint of women. Complaints range from mild itching of the vagina or vulva with or without discharge to severe swelling of the labia and vulva, profuse discharge, itching, and pain. Many vaginal infections are sexually transmitted and may be chronic and/or recurrent. Asymptomatic infection is common.

1. *Trichomonas vaginalis*

▶ Scientific Concepts

Caused by protozoa, may be carried symptomatically or asymptomatically by men and women; transmitted sexually.

▶ History & Physical

Profuse, frothy, gray-greenish, malodorous leukorrhea worse after menstruation, with or without secondary vulvar pruritus. Dysuria and urinary frequency are common. Vulvar and/or labial swelling or inflammation, cervical petechiae (strawberry spots).

▶ Diagnostic Studies

Trichomonads visualized on saline wet mount, potassium hydroxide (KOH) prep under darkfield, phase contrast, ordinary microscope or identified on Pap smear. Vaginal pH is usually > 5.0.

▶ Diagnosis

Rule out other etiologic agents.

▶ Clinical Therapeutics

Metronidazole, 2 g PO one dose or 500 mg bid × 7 days for both partners or a single dose of 2 g orally.

▶ Health Maintenance Issues

Patient education, use of condoms, avoid high-risk sexual behaviors. Patient and partner should be advised to avoid alcohol or vinegar during treatment as they may interact with metronidazole, causing severe nausea, vomiting, sweating, weakness, and other complications.

2. Condyloma Acuminata (Human Papillomavirus)

▶ Scientific Concepts

Many types, transmitted via direct contact with human papillomavirus (HPV) through mucous membranes or skin abrasions. Incubation period may be 1 to 6 months. Infection with HPV is associated with cervical cancer.

▶ History & Physical

May be symptomatic or subclinical, may include pruritus, burning, pain, bleeding, and dyspareunia. Single or multiple exophytic warts from a few millimeters to large fleshy lesions covering the entire genitalia or flat grey lesions.

► Diagnostic Studies
May be identified on appearance, Pap smear, colposcopy, or biopsy. Application of 3 to 5% acetic acid causes warts to turn white; may aid in diagnosis.

► Diagnosis
Rule out other genital ulcer disease including chancroid, condyloma lata of secondary syphilis, and genital herpes.

► Clinical Therapeutics
Trichloroacetic acid (TCA), podophyllum resin (Podophyllin), applied by health professional. Podifilox or Imiquimod may be applied by patient. Podophyllum resin is not approved for use during pregnancy; TCA is approved for use in pregnancy. Larger warts may require laser treatment, cryotherapy with liquid nitrogen, electrocautery, or surgical excision.

► Clinical Intervention
HPV highly contagious and is implicated in cervical cancer; warts may grow rapidly during pregnancy, may predispose infant to genital warts or laryngeal papillomatosis.

► Health Maintenance Issues
Patient education, use of condoms, avoid high-risk sexual behaviors. Consider screening for human immunodeficiency virus (HIV) infection. If topical therapy is instituted, patient must follow directions carefully to avoid inflammation.

3. Herpes Simplex Virus

► Scientific Concepts
Two primary types, type 2 (80 to 90%), type 1 (10 to 20%), mucosal contact with herpes simplex virus (HSV)-infected secretions/lesions, asymptomatic shedding, or perinatal transmission. This virus is frequently found in association with other sexually transmitted diseases (STDs).

► History & Physical
May be symptomatic or subclinical. Prodromal symptoms include tingling, irritation, pruritus, or vaginal discharge. Primary episode associated with pain, dysuria, and dyspareunia with lesions; inguinal lymphadenopathy; fever and multiple tender, vesicular lesions at site of infection. Recurrent outbreaks tend to be slightly less severe.

► Diagnostic Studies
Identification of multinucleated giant cells in Wright–Giemsa stain, viral culture, serological assay, enzyme-linked immunosorbent assay (ELISA)/Western blot.

► Diagnosis

Rule out other genital ulcer disease, chancroid, HPV, and syphilis.

► Clinical Therapeutics

Currently no cure; acyclovir, famciclovir, and valacyclovir PO for up to 5 days offers symptomatic relief, may diminish severity of recurrences. Current treatment of primary episode: acyclovir, 400 mg PO tid × 7 to 10 days; famciclovir, 250 mg PO × 7 to 10 days; or valacyclovir, 1 g PO × 7 to 10 days. Current prophylaxis for severe recurrent disease: acyclovir, 200 mg PO bid, tid, or qid or 400 mg PO bid.

► Clinical Intervention

Clinical picture may be exacerbated by other serious illness, immunocompromise, or stress. Epidemiologic link to cervical cancer; high mortality rate in neonatal disease.

► Health Maintenance Issues

Patient education, use of condoms, avoid high-risk sexual behaviors. Consider screening for HIV infection.

4. *Chlamydia*

► Scientific Concepts

Currently the most common STD in the United States, causing nongonococcal cervicitis in women and urethritis in men. Causative agent *Chlamydia trachomatis*. Sequelae of infection include infertility, pelvic inflammatory disease (PID), and ectopic pregnancy. Perinatal transmission associated with neonatal chlamydial conjunctivitis and pneumonia.

► History & Physical

The majority of lower genital tract chlamydial infections are asymptomatic, detected by routine screening. Patients may present with no signs or symptoms, mild to severe vaginal discharge, dysuria, pelvic pain, urethritis, and infection of Bartholin glands to cervicitis with mucopurulent cervix.

► Diagnostic Studies

Urinalysis positive for greater than 500 polymorphonuclear neutrophils (PMNs)/1,000 and Gram stain positive for polymorphonuclear lymphocytes (PMLs) without gonococci are nonspecific tests for *Chlamydia trachomatis*. Cell culture that detects organisms from the endocervical swab demonstrates specificity close to 100% and has been the "gold standard" but delays diagnosis 3 to 7 days. Direct immunofluorescence techniques (MicroTrak): amplified chlamydia test (AMP-CT, Gen Probe), which detects chlamydia in the urine; enzyme immunoassay (Chlamydiazyme) and chlamydia polymerase chain reaction (PCR) and ligase chain reaction (LCR), which amplify deoxyribonucleic acid (DNA), are newer, more sensitive and specific approaches for detection of chlamydia.

► Diagnosis

Rule out infection of other etiologic origin. Untreated infection associated with multiple complications.

► Clinical Therapeutics

Azithromycin (Zithromax), 1 mg PO; doxycycline, 100 mg PO bid × 7 days; or ofloxacin, 300 mg PO bid × 7 days. If pregnant: erythromycin, 500 mg PO qid × 7 days. If PID develops, treat with ceftriaxone, 250 mg intramuscularly (IM) × 1 dose, and doxycycline, 100 mg PO bid × 7 days, or ofloxacin, 400 mg PO bid, and metronidazole, 500 mg PO bid.

► Health Maintenance Issues

Patient education, use of loose-fitting clothing, use of condoms, avoid high-risk sexual behaviors, concurrent treatment of all partners, and delay sexual relations until treatment is complete.

5. Lymphogranuloma Venereum

► Scientific Concepts

Caused by one of the aggressive L serotypes of *Chlamydia trachomatis*. More common in the tropical and subtropical nations. More common in women than men; incubation period 7 to 21 days.

► History & Physical

In early phase, vesicopustular eruption progressing to inguinal and vulvar ulceration, pronounced inguinal lymphadenopathy, positive "groove sign" (line between lymph nodes), fever, joint pain, and body aches. Strictures and narrowing of the vagina or rectum common complication of ulcerations.

► Diagnostic Studies

Isolation of *Chlamydia trachomatis* via culture or microimmunofluorescent and complement fixation tests, if available.

► Diagnosis

Rule out other ulcerative infectious disease. Diagnosis correlates well with degree of suspicion.

► Clinical Therapeutics

Treatment includes doxycycline, 100 mg PO bid × 21 days (preferred); tetracycline, 500 mg PO qid × 21 days; or erythromycin, 500 mg PO bid × 21 days.

► Clinical Intervention

Concurrent abscesses may require incision and drainage. If untreated, long-term complications include perianal scaring, vaginal, anal, rectal, and sigmoid strictures, requiring surgical intervention including colostomy. Consider screening for HIV infection.

► Health Maintenance Issues

Risk increases with unprotected sexual activity. Prevention achieved with use of condoms and avoidance of high-risk behaviors.

6. Bacterial Vaginosis

Previously referred to as *Gardnerella vaginalis,* the most common cause of bacterial vaginitis and vaginal discharge in sexually active patients.

► **Scientific Concepts**

Polymicrobial condition involving interactions between several components of the vaginal flora, especially anaerobes, elevation of vaginal pH, and production of amines.

► **History & Physical**

Grey/white, malodorous, creamy, noninflammatory vaginal discharge, little to no vulvar irritation or pruritus, most pronounced symptom is odor; discharge and signs of inflammation may or may not be evident.

► **Diagnostic Studies**

Wet mount and Gram stain reveal "clue cells" (unstained exfoliated epithelial cells with a large number of gram-negative bacteria); cultures seldom necessary.

► **Diagnosis**

Presence of 3 to 4 of the following: clue cells on microscopic examination; white, noninflammatory, adherent discharge; vaginal fluid pH > 4.5; positive "whiff test" (fishy odor worse with addition of 10% KOH).

► **Clinical Therapeutics**

Metronidazole, 500 mg PO bid × 7 days or single dose of 2 g PO; metronidazole vaginal gel, 0.075% per vagina qd or bid × 5 days; or clindamycin, 300 mg bid × 7 days. In pregnancy, treatment of choice is metronidazole, 250 mg PO tid × 7 days (second and third trimester). Clindamycin is not recommended during pregnancy.

► **Clinical Intervention**

Obstetric and gynecologic complications associated with untreated bacterial vaginosis in pregnancy include premature rupture of membranes (PROM), chorioamnionitis and PID in the nonpregnant female.

► **Health Maintenance Issues**

Patient education, treat both partners, use of condoms, avoid high-risk sexual behaviors.

7. Gonorrhea

► **Scientific Concepts**

STD caused by direct contact with *Neisseria gonorrhoeae,* asymptomatic in 85% of infected female patients. Incubation period is 3 to 5 days following infection.

► **History & Physical**

No symptoms to mild to severe purulent vaginal discharge, pelvic pain, urethritis, dysuria, urinary frequency, infection of Bartholin glands, fever, signs of nonspecific vaginitis to cervicitis with mucopurulent cervix, pain on pelvic examination, and adnexal tenderness. Other symptoms may include anorectal inflammation, pharyngitis, tonsillitis, conjunctivitis, and disseminated infections such as septic arthritis, endocarditis, meningitis, polyarthralgias, tenosynovitis, and dermatitis.

▶ Diagnostic Studies

Routine cervical, urethra, pharynx, and rectum sampling for culture using Thayer–Martin medium; Gram-stained smear will identify gram-negative intracellular diplococci with PMLs.

▶ Clinical Therapeutics

With the emergence of resistant strains, treatment of choice is a single dose of ceftriaxone, 125 mg IM, plus doxycycline, 100 mg PO bid × 7 days; doxycycline or tetracycline, 500 mg qid × 7 days, should be given routinely because of high risk of coexisting chlamydial infections. Many clinicians still rely on the old standard treatment, penicillin G (Procaine PCN), 2.4 million units IM, with probenecid, 1 g PO.

▶ Clinical Intervention

Evaluate for extragenital infection.

▶ Health Maintenance Issues

All partners should be treated; patient education and follow-up including safe sex practices should be provided. Sexual activity should not be resumed until a follow-up culture is negative. Consider screening for HIV infection.

8. Chancroid

▶ Scientific Concepts

STD more common in the tropics and Southeast Asia. Caused by *Haemophilus ducreyi*, chancroid is a cofactor for HIV transmission and has been found in coexistent syphilis and herpes infections. Incubation period is short, with lesions appearing 3 to 5 days following exposure.

▶ History & Physical

Symptoms include the presence of painful, vesicopustular lesions, progressing to nonindurated, saucer-shaped weal that produces a profuse, foul-smelling discharge, found on the external genitalia, perineum, thigh, or cervix. Lymphadenopathy, buboes in the lymph nodes, and abscess formation are common.

▶ Diagnostic Studies

The diagnosis is clinical, with cultures and smears less reliable, and *H. ducreyi* is difficult to isolate.

▶ Diagnosis

Rule out other ulcerative disorders including lymphogranuloma venereum, herpes, and syphilis.

► Clinical Therapeutics

Azithromycin, 1 g PO in one dose, or ceftriaxone, 250 mg IM in one dose.

► Health Maintenance Issues

Sitz baths and meticulous hygiene are beneficial, use of condoms and avoidance of high-risk behaviors encouraged. Consider screening for HIV infection.

9. Syphilis

► Scientific Concepts

STD caused by direct sexual contact with the spirochete, *Treponema pallidum*. Infection in utero, via needle sticks and blood transfusion uncommon. A diagnosis of another STD is considered a risk factor for syphilis, and previous treatment does not confer immunity against future infections.

► History & Physical

Primary lesion (chancre, painless indurated ulcer) at site of inoculation approximately 10 to 90 days after contact. Heals spontaneously. *Secondary* stage heralded by a maculopapular rash approximately 6 weeks post healing of primary lesion. Associated with malaise, fever, generalized lymphadenopathy, condyloma lata (moist papules), and alopecia. *Latent* phase occurs approximately 2 to 6 weeks post resolution of the rash, considered infectious for first 1 to 2 years in latency. One-third of all untreated patients develop *tertiary* syphilis, which is associated with serious cardiovascular and central nervous system (CNS) sequelae.

► Diagnostic Studies

Serologic tests *nontreponemal tests* (rapid plasma reagin [RPR], Veneral Disease Research Laboratory [VDRL], automated reagin test [ART]) *treponemal tests* used in follow-up to positive nontreponemal tests (microhemagglutination test for *T. pallidum* [MHATP], fluorescent treponemal antibody-absorption test for syphilis [FTA-ABS]). Darkfield microscopy may be used in evaluating chancres, condyloma lata, and mucous patches; useful in diagnosing primary and secondary syphilis. PCR is specific for detection of *T. pallidum* in amniotic fluid, neonatal serum, and spinal fluid.

► Diagnosis

Positive RPR/VDRL and follow-up FTA. Rule out other ulcerative disorder.

► Clinical Therapeutics

Primary, secondary, and early latent (< 1 year) are treated with Penicillin G benzathine (Bicillin), 2.4 million units IM in single dose. Alternative for penicillin-allergic, nonpregnant patient is doxycycline, 100 mg PO bid × 2 weeks. Tertiary or late syphilis is treated with penicillin G benzathine (Bicillin), 2.4 million units IM 1/wk × 3 consecutive weeks, or tetracycline hydrochloride, 500 mg PO qid × 14 days, or doxycycline, 100 mg PO bid × 2 weeks.

► Clinical Intervention

Pregnancy does not alter the course of the infection. Risk of fetal infection correlates with degree of exposure to spirochetemia and gestational age. The earlier the fetus is exposed, the greater the risk of premature delivery or stillbirth. Infected neonates may not develop symptoms until weeks or months later and may include lymphadenitis, hepatosplenomegaly, osteochondritis, and irregular epiphyseal juncture on x-ray. Treatment in pregnancy as above, except if penicillin allergic, then desensitize patient with gradually increasing doses of oral penicillin and then proceed with treatment as above.

► Health Maintenance Issues

Partners should be treated; patient education and follow-up. Consider screening for HIV infection.

10. Atrophic Vaginitis

► Scientific Concepts

Most common cause of vaginal discharge in the postmenopausal woman. Estrogen deficiency precipitates thinning of vaginal mucosa.

► History & Physical

Symptoms include dysuria, pruritus, burning, soreness, bleeding, and dyspareunia. Thin, erythematous mucous membranes; loss of rugae; and watery discharge are common. Vaginal pH 7.0.

► Diagnostic Studies

Serum follicle-stimulating hormone (FSH), luteinizing hormone (LH), wet mount, and Pap smear.

► Diagnosis

Rule out other cause of vaginal discharge, STD, urinary tract infection (UTI), foreign body, allergen.

► Clinical Therapeutics

Exogenous estrogen (topical or systemic) and lubricants.

► Health Maintenance Issues

Avoid irritants, encourage lubrication with sexual activity. Increased sexual activity may improve condition.

11. Candidiasis

► Scientific Concepts

Mycotic vaginitis is the second most common cause of symptomatic vaginal discharge. Infections typically caused by yeasts (*Candida albicans,* most commonly), which may be precipitated by cyclic hormones including oral contraceptives, diabetes mellitus, chemical irritation, immunocompromise, pregnancy, or recent antibiotic therapy.

► History & Physical

Thick, white vaginal discharge; mild to severe vulvar pruritus and burning; red, swollen vulva and vaginal mucosa; white exudate on cervix or vaginal mucosa.

► Diagnostic Studies

Wet mount or KOH prep slide with visualization of budding yeast or hyphae, or culture on Nickerson's medium.

► Diagnosis

Classic clinical presentation is common.

► Clinical Therapeutics

Topical application of antifungal cream or vaginal suppositories such as miconazole, terconazole, clotrimazole, butoconazole, or nystatin at bedtime × 3 days or at bedtime × 7 days; systemic treatment with fluconazole or ketoconazole.

► Clinical Intervention

Treat underlying condition. Further evaluation is necessary for recurrent or recalcitrant infections. Similarly, treatment may be prolonged.

► Health Maintenance Issues

Provide health education and referral for evaluation of recurrences.

B. Prolapse of Vaginal Walls

► Scientific Concepts

Defects in pelvic support structures may result in prolapse of urethra (urethrocele), bladder (cystocele), rectum (enterocele), or uterus (uterine prolapse). Loss of muscle tone may be attributed to advancing age, pregnancy, multiple or difficult childbirth, or increased intra-abdominal pressure. May progress postmenopause.

► History & Physical

Symptoms related to degree of prolapse and structures involved. When descent is limited to the upper two-thirds of the vagina, it is said to be first degree; second degree is present when the structure approaches the vaginal introitus, and third degree involves descent outside of the vaginal opening. Symptoms include fullness, pressure, urinary symptoms including incontinence, frequency, urgency, incomplete voiding; relaxed vaginal outlet.

► Diagnostic Studies

Diagnosis is by physical and pelvic exam. Q-tip test (assessment of degree of upward motion of a Q-tip placed in the urethra when the patient strains), urodynamic testing, and evaluation of urinary function are diagnostic studies employed to assess pelvic relation including cystocele.

► Diagnosis

Rule out urethral obstruction. Herniation of other structures may be simultaneously diagnosed.

► Clinical Therapeutics

Medical measures include vaginal pessaries, Kegel isometric exercise, and estrogen replacement therapy. Treatment with anticholinergic drugs (propantheline bromide), beta-sympathomimetic agonists (metaproterenol sulfate), musculotropic drugs (flavoxate hydrochloride), diazepam, and bromocriptine mesylate have been effective in providing improvement, depending on the problem. Surgical interventions may be employed depending on anatomical defect. Vaginal hysterectomy or Moschowitz procedures may be offered if the defect causes secondary urinary retention, obstruction, or other significant complication.

► Clinical Intervention

Kegel exercises may be recommended. If pessary is placed, regular removal and replacement are recommended.

► Health Maintenance Issues

Patient education plays an important role in treatment and management. Nonmedical treatment interventions include biofeedback and bladder training.

C. Vulvar and Vaginal Neoplasms

1. Vulvar Carcinoma

► Scientific Concepts

A disease of postmenopausal women, now seen in younger women. Associated with lower socioeconomic status and infection with HPV and HSV. Other risk factors include obesity, hypertension, diabetes with vulvar irritation, vulvar dystrophy, and history of granulomatous STD.

► History & Physical

Patients may be asymptomatic or present with a long history of pruritus, pain, bloody discharge, vulvar mass, or rash, which may range from leukoplakia, as in Paget's disease, to hyperpigmentation, as in Bowen's disease. Vulvar pruritus is the most common presenting complaint.

► Diagnostic Studies

The visibility of the region lends itself to early detection and treatment. Toluidine blue staining of the vulva and incisional biopsy of any lesion or suspicious areas as well as computed tomographic (CT) scan to rule out metastatic disease are most helpful.

► Diagnosis

Suspicious lesions should be biopsied; prognosis is worse with pelvic lymph node involvement. Early vulvar intraepithelial neoplasia

(VIN) may be classified as VIN I (mild dysplasia), II (moderate dysplasia), or III (severe dysplasia or carcinoma in situ).

► Clinical Intervention

Assess tumor size, node involvement, and metastasis (TNM staging). Good surgical outcome with radical vulvectomy; less extensive surgery for early disease. Radiation therapy prior to surgery for more advanced disease. Chemotherapy not useful.

► Health Maintenance Issues

Careful and regular pelvic exams and early detection and treatment provide best opportunity for recovery.

2. Vaginal Carcinoma

► Scientific Concepts

Relatively rare disease. Etiology unknown, yet chronic irritation from pessary use, prior existence of preinvasive carcinoma in situ (CIS) and HPV have been implicated. Squamous cell carcinoma accounts for the majority of invasive vaginal cancer. Clear cell adenocarcinoma, usually related to diethylstilbestrol (DES) exposure before 18 weeks' gestation in utero, and vaginal melanoma account for a small percentage of vaginal carcinomas.

► History & Physical

Early stages (preinvasive carcinoma of the vagina) generally asymptomatic. Abnormal painless vaginal bleeding or ulcerated lesions as noted on routine exam, illustrating need for continued regular Pap smears in the postmenopausal female and those who have undergone hysterectomy. Vaginal bleeding or discharge are the most common symptoms of invasive vaginal cancer.

► Diagnostic Studies

Abnormal Pap smear, incisional biopsy of gross lesion, colposcopy to identify smaller lesions.

► Diagnosis

Biopsy to rule out other causes of red ulcerated or white hyperplastic lesions of the vagina.

► Clinical Intervention

Staging based on extent and structural involvement. Primary treatment radiotherapy, then surgical or vaporization with carbon dioxide laser or 5-fluorouracil cream.

► Health Maintenance Issues

Must rule out other gynecologic cancer as vaginal cancer may represent metastasis of cervical cancer. The larger the mass, the worse the prognosis. Lymph node involvement and tumor location are important factors.

II. FALLOPIAN TUBES

▶ Scientific Concepts

PID is a general term for acute, subacute, recurrent, or chronic infection of the oviducts and ovaries often with involvement of adjacent tissues. PID has become increasingly recognized and may frequently be due to a coexisting infection with either *N. gonorrhoeae* or *Chlamydia trachomatis* or both. Pathways of dissemination include lymphatic (i.e., postpartum and postabortal), endosalpingo, and peritoneal spread of microorganisms as in intrauterine device (IUD)-related infections, and in rare cases hematogenous routes such as tuberculosis.

▶ History & Physical

Insidious or acute onset of lower abdominal cramps and pelvic pain, mild to severe purulent vaginal discharge, urethritis, dysuria, urinary frequency, fever > 38°C (100.4°F), leukocytosis, erythema of the vaginal mucosa, purulent cervicitis, with rebound tenderness, inguinal lymphadenopathy, adnexal tenderness and pain on motion of cervix (chandelier sign), palpable tubo-ovarian abscess (~ 15% of cases), pelvic abscess (may include infection), and unilateral tenderness of Bartholin glands.

▶ Diagnostic Studies

Beta-human chorionic gonadotropin (hCG) and cultures obtained from the from cervix, urethra, anus, and pharynx when appropriate. Cervical cultures, including for *N. gonorrhoeae*, grown on a Thayer–Martin agar plate and kept in a carbon dioxide–rich environment are diagnostic for *N. gonorrhoeae*. Gram-stained smear may identify gram-negative intracellular diplococci with leukocytes or endocervical culture or antigen test for *Chlamydia* may be positive. Culdocentesis is generally productive of a cloudy fluid, which should also be cultured with sensitivity. Blood work may reveal increased white blood cells (WBCs) with a shift and an increased sedimentation rate. Laparoscopy and pelvic sonogram may reveal a tubo-ovarian mass.

▶ Diagnosis

Rule out ectopic pregnancy, acute abdomen, ovarian torsion, and ovarian mass. Concomitant signs of infection suggest PID.

▶ Clinical Therapeutics

Hospitalization may be necessary, if a surgical emergency (i.e., appendicitis and ectopic pregnancy), if a pelvic abscess is present, if patient is pregnant, if patient is an adolescent, if severe illness precludes outpatient management, or if the patient fails to respond to outpatient therapy with 72 hours of initial treatment. Inpatient regimens include cefoxitin, 2 g intravenously (IV) q6h, plus doxycycline, 100 mg PO bid or IV q12h. Post hospital discharge, treatment is doxycycline, 100 mg PO bid for a total of 10 to 14 days. Outpatient regimens include ofloxacin, 400 mg PO bid × 14 days, and metronidazole, 500 mg PO bid × 14 days, or ceftriaxone, 250 mg IM in one dose, plus doxycycline, 100 mg PO bid × 14 days, or cefoxitin, 2 g IM, with probenecid, 1 g PO. Surgical intervention such as colpotomy (drainage of cul de sac) or salpingo-oophorectomy may be necessary.

► Clinical Intervention
Patients with suspected pelvic abscess who fail to respond to antibiotic therapy may require surgical intervention, CT-guided percutaneous drainage, colpotomy drainage, and perhaps exploratory laparotomy.

► Health Maintenance Issues
Acute or chronic PID may result in infertility, chronic pelvic pain, and increased incidence of ectopic pregnancy.

III. CERVIX

A. Abnormal Pap Smear

► Scientific Concepts
Widespread use of the Pap smear and early cytologic detection of abnormal preinvasive cervical lesions have resulted in early intervention and management of dysplastic cervical lesions. Rule out fungal, bacterial, viral, or other infection and benign inflammatory changes. Sexually transmitted viruses may induce malignant transformation of lesions.

► History & Physical
Risk factors include cervical mucosa previously altered by HPV, repeated STDs, cervicitis, cigarette smoking, multiple sexual partners, early age at first intercourse, and DES exposure. May be asymptomatic, cervix appearing normal; cervical discharge and/or postcoital bleeding possible. HPV infection is a major risk factor.

► Diagnostic Studies
Pap smear findings as reported in common descriptive conventions (Table 9-1). Cultures, colposcopy, colposcopic biopsy, and cone biopsy are essential for further evaluation and treatment.

► Diagnosis
Abnormal findings on Pap smear warrant further evaluation.

► Clinical Therapeutics
Depends on etiology and extent; treat underlying infection; electrocautery, cryotherapy, laser vaporization, loop electrosurgical excision, cone biopsy, chemotherapy agents.

► Clinical Intervention
Close follow-up, repeat Pap smear in 3 months, then 6 months; annual colposcopy for 2 years.

► table 9-1

COMMON DESCRIPTIVE CONVENTIONS

Class System	CIN System	Bethesda II System
Class I	Negative	Negative
Class II	Atypia or inflammatory changes	Atypical squamous cells of undetermined origin (ASCUS) cellular changes with or without atypia
Class III, mild to moderate dysplasia	Mild to moderate cervical intraepithelial neoplasia (CIN I or II)	Low-grade squamous intraepithelial lesion (LGSIL) and high-grade (HGSIL)
Class IV, severe dysplasia	Severe cervical intraepithelial neoplasia (CIN III)	HGSIL
Class V	Suggestive of cancer or carcinoma in situ (CIS)	Squamous cell cancer

► Health Maintenance Issues

Cervical screening with annual Pap smear is recommended at the onset of sexual activity or age 18. Patient education and counseling on importance of regular Pap testing and prompt and appropriate treatment of any cervical lesion.

B. Cervicitis/Endocervicitis

► Scientific Concepts

Nonspecific term to describe infectious process; may be localized to the cervix; may be caused by same etiologic agents as vaginal infections, HPV, STDs, and PID. Risk factors include early coitus and multiple partners.

► History & Physical

May be asymptomatic to complaints of yellow vaginal discharge, postcoital bleeding, and dyspareunia. Infective agent may be identified on abnormal Pap smear.

► Diagnostic Studies

Pap smear, cervical culture, enzyme assays, colposcopy, and serology to rule out syphilis.

► Diagnosis

Identify causative or infective agent.

► Clinical Therapeutics

Depends on etiology and extent; treat underlying infection. Treatment may include electrocautery, cryotherapy, laser vaporization, loop electrosurgical excision, cone biopsy, or topical chemotherapeutic agents.

► Clinical Intervention

Close follow-up, with repeat Pap smear following treatment, in 3 to 4 months for the next year, then every 4 to 6 months during the second year; annual colposcopy for 2 years.

▶ Health Maintenance Issues

Patient education and counseling on importance of regular Pap testing and prompt and appropriate treatment of any cervical lesion. Screen pregnant women for infectious cervicitis because of risk to fetus.

C. Cervical Polyps

▶ Scientific Concepts

Benign, pedunculated multiple or single growths, which vary in size. More common in multiparous women. Most originate from the endocervix, composed of vascular connective tissue stroma and covered by epithelium.

▶ History & Physical

Usually symptomatic, may include leukorrhea, postcoital bleeding, menorrhagia, postmenopausal bleeding, or bloody discharge. Soft, red, pedunculated growths may be visible extending from cervical os or endocervix.

▶ Diagnostic Studies

Pap smear and biopsy; rule out endometrial polyp. Some may be visible via hysterography or identified via dilatation and curettage (D&C).

▶ Diagnosis

Microscopic examination and biopsy of polyp confirms diagnosis. Rule out cervical neoplasia, chronic cervicitis, or prolapsed submucosal myoma.

▶ Clinical Therapeutics

Treat accompanying vaginal infection, if any.

▶ Clinical Intervention

Most polyps are removed surgically with concurrent antibiotic therapy if infection occurs. Close follow-up and repeat Pap smear regularly.

▶ Health Maintenance Issues

Prevention of vaginal and cervical infections that can precede cervical polyps. Patient education and counseling on importance of regular Pap testing.

D. Cervical Cancer

▶ Scientific Concepts

Common but treatable cancer in women, which begins as cervical dysplasia and progresses over time into malignancy in the exo/endocervix; hematogenous spread or locally via the lymphatics. Regional pelvic lymph nodes are generally affected and metastasis is to the lungs, brain, bone, and liver.

► History & Physical
Risk factors include early coitus, multiple sexual partners, cervical mucosa previously altered by HPV, repeated STDs or cervicitis, cigarette smoking, and DES exposure. May be asymptomatic; intermenstrual or postcoital bleeding most common early symptoms. Later-stage symptoms include change in urinary or bowel habits or function, bone pain, weakness, weight loss, and anemia. Cervix may appear normal to ulcerative with friable lesion(s).

► Diagnostic Studies
Abnormal Pap smear findings (see Abnormal Pap Smear), cultures, colposcopy, colposcopic biopsy, cone biopsy, magnetic resonance imaging (MRI), abdominal CT scan, lymphangiography, intravenous pyelogram (IVP), and sigmoidoscopy with biopsy aid in diagnosis and staging.

► Diagnosis
Rule out other ulcerative cervical disorders including cervicitis, condyloma acuminata, syphilis, and chancroid.

► Clinical Therapeutics
Proper technique in performing the Pap smear is essential for early diagnosis and treatment. Treatment may include surgical intervention such as partial, extended, or radical hysterectomy; radiation (most effective and widely used) or chemotherapy (least effective). Pelvic exenteration (radical hysterectomy with surgical removal of rectum, bladder, and/or vulva) may be necessary.

► Clinical Intervention
Excellent prognosis with early identification and treatment.

► Health Maintenance Issues
Preventive measures include avoidance of high-risk behaviors and known risk factors. Patient education and counseling on importance of regular Pap testing and prompt and appropriate treatment of any cervical lesion.

IV. UTERUS

A. Leiomyoma of the Uterus

► Scientific Concepts
Commonly known as uterine fibroids, leiomyomas are smooth muscle, estrogen-dependent tumors of the uterus that rarely progress to malignancy. Common to women over age 30 and more common in African-American and Asian women, uterine fibroids may be subserosal (outside of the uterine wall), intramural (within the myometrium), or submucosal (within the endometrium).

► History & Physical

Depending on size and location, the patient may be asymptomatic to experiencing abdominal pressure, dyspareunia, dysmenorrhea, menorrhagia, rectal pressure, complications in pregnancy (e.g., infertility, habitual abortion, premature labor), and anemia. Uterine fibroids may be multiple, and the uterus is generally irregularly enlarged.

► Diagnostic Studies

Uterine size may be assessed with bimanual pelvic exam and pelvic ultrasound. Leiomyoma may also be identified during cesarean section.

► Diagnosis

Pregnancy, endometrial carcinoma, ovarian neoplasia, tubo-ovarian mass, and diverticula are included in the differential of a woman with an enlarged uterus.

► Clinical Therapeutics

In the past, the primary treatment was surgical (hysterectomy). More recently, myomectomy has been performed for fertility considerations. Depending on severity of pain, anemia, urinary symptoms, or concomitant complications of leiomyoma, conservative therapy (observation) is recommended. Leiomyomas are estrogen dependent; hence, reduction of uterine size, fibroids, and complication associated with leiomyoma diminish in the postmenopausal period. Gonadotropin-releasing hormone (GnRH) agonists, 50 to 500 μg daily or 3- to 6-mg implant q3mo may retard growth. Common clinical effect of GnRH is short-lived regrowth following discontinuation of therapy.

► Clinical Intervention

Observation is the mainstay. Treatment is individualized depending on symptoms, complications, and interest in future conception.

► Health Maintenance Issues

Leiomyomas are time limited. Patient education and empowerment are important for patient management.

B. Endometrial Polyps

► Scientific Concepts

Mass of tissue that projects outward from cervical os. Rule out endometrial polyp versus submucosal myoma. Location fundal in origin. Can undergo neoplastic changes. Sensitive to estrogen (like leiomyoma).

► History & Physical

Patient generally complains of recurring menorrhagia, premenstrual and postmenstrual bleeding. On pelvic exam, uterus is normal size. Sudden bleeding in the postmenopausal female with crampy pain could be infarction of a polyp. If bleeding still after D&C, think polyp.

▶ Diagnostic Studies

Ultrasound not useful; MRI is helpful, but hysteroscopy is the most useful test.

▶ Diagnosis

Rule out endometrial and cervical carcinoma with biopsy.

▶ Clinical Therapeutics

Surgical excision is the treatment of choice. Endometrial polyps may be cut during D&C; one must look specifically for endometrial polyps (often overlooked).

▶ Clinical Intervention

Polyps may recur and should be excised.

▶ Health Maintenance Issues

Patient education and routine follow-up indicated.

C. Endometrial Hyperplasia and Cancer

▶ Scientific Concepts

Endometrial hyperplasia and endometrial adenocarcinoma are common. Endometrial hyperplasia may be considered a precancerous state. Endometrial carcinoma is the most common gynecologic malignancy. Histologic grade and depth of myometrium invasion are the most important prognostic factors. Adenosquamous, clear cell squamous, and papillary serous carcinoma have worse prognoses than the more common adenocarcinoma. Incidence increases with age, 45 to 65 most common age group.

▶ History & Physical

Postmenopausal bleeding is the most common sign. Most commonly associated with obesity, hypertension, diabetes mellitus, early menarche, and late menopause. Related to prolonged exposure to unopposed estrogen.

▶ Diagnostic Studies

Pap smear is rarely positive. D&C and endometrial biopsy are most useful. CA-125 may be elevated. Other diagnostic studies including chest x-ray, CT scan, bone scan, mammography, and barium enema to rule out metastasis. Test for occult blood because of association with colorectal cancer.

▶ Diagnosis

Rule out atypical hyperplasia, endometriosis, or other gynecologic cancer.

▶ Clinical Therapeutics

Chemotherapeutic agents such as cisplatin and adriamycin may be used. Surgical staging, hysterectomy, and regional radiation are the mainstay. Best outcome associated with early detection and minimal invasion.

► Clinical Intervention

Surgical treatment related to degree of invasion and node involvement. Obese, hypertensive, or anovulatory females may reduce risk with weight loss or by taking oral contraceptives.

► Health Maintenance Issues

Estrogen replacement therapy should also include progestational agents. Recurrence most common within the first 2 years following treatment. Pap smear q3mo for 2 years and endometrial biopsy recommended.

D. Dysfunctional Uterine Bleeding

► Scientific Concepts

Dysfunctional uterine bleeding (DUB) includes abnormal menstrual bleeding, amenorrhea, and/or anovulatory cycles not due to other causes such as pregnancy, systemic disease, or cancer. DUB represents abnormal hormonal regulation rather than the cyclical fluctuating gonadotropins and hormones.

Amenorrhea: Primary—absence of menarche by the age of 18 generally due to congenital abnormalities or genetic disorders (i.e., absent uterus or vagina, imperforate hymen, testicular feminization). Secondary—absence of menses for 3 to 6 successive cycles in a woman who has previously experienced menarche, most commonly due to pregnancy. An occasional cause is continued hypothalamic suppression after discontinuing oral contraceptives, hormonal imbalance, or excessive weight loss.

Menorrhagia: Heavy, prolonged menstrual flow that may be due to submucosal myomas, endometrial hyperplasia, malignant tumors.

Metrorrhagia (intermenstrual bleeding): Bleeding that occurrs at any time between menstrual periods. Endometrial polyps, hyperplasia, endometrial and cervical carcinomas are pathologic causes. In recent years, exogenous estrogen administration has become a common cause of this type of bleeding.

Oligomenorrhea: Menstrual periods that occur more than 35 days apart. Estrogen-secreting tumors will produce oligomenorrhea prior to other patterns of abnormal bleeding.

► History & Physical

Uterine bleeding unrelated to menses, absence of menses, or irregular bleeding in the absence of other systemic symptoms or disorders. Examination may be unremarkable; note evidence of hirsutism or virilization. Abdominal mass and irregular uterus suggests myoma; symmetrically enlarged uterus is more typical of adenomyosis or endometrial cancer.

► Diagnostic Studies

Obtain Pap smear and consider endometrial biopsy, complete blood count (CBC) with platelet, prothrombin time (PT), partial thromboplastin time (PTT), pregnancy, and thyroxine/thyroid-stimulating hormone (TSH). Consider FSH/LH and androgens as indicated. D&C in those who have higher risk for endometrial hyperplasia. D&C is diagnostic and therapeutic.

▶ Diagnosis
Rule out other medical condition.

▶ Clinical Therapeutics
Treat underlying cause. Investigate hormonal status, correct anovulatory cycles with hormones or oral contraceptives; surgical measures to correct endometriosis, myoma, and other surgical disorders. After exclusion of organic disease and pregnancy, treat with any combined progestin–estrogen oral contraceptives. In acute unstable situations, treat with estrogen, 25 mg IV q4h. When bleeding stops, and thereafter, induce shedding with 10 mg medroxyprogesterone qd × 10 to 13 days. Long-term management is achieved with low-dose oral contraceptives.

▶ Clinical Intervention
D&C, hysteroscopy, and endometrial ablation may be therapeutic as well as evaluative of organic lesions. Hysterectomy may be recommended in severe cases and if preservation of fertility is not desired. Estrogens should not be administered to perimenopausal women or those at risk for endometrial cancer.

▶ Health Maintenance Issues
Most anovulatory cycles in young women can be successfully managed. Uterine bleeding in the perimenopausal female requires full evaluation.

V. OVARY

A. Ovarian Cysts

▶ Scientific Concepts
The growth and regression of intraovarian structures appear to predispose the ovary to multiple abnormalities of structure and function. They may be solid, cystic, or mixed. Etiology unknown. Risk of ovarian malignancy increases with age.

Functional tumors (producing sex hormones) include follicular cysts, lutein cysts, theca-lutein cysts, and polycystic ovary. Follicular cysts are caused by the failure of the ovarian follicle to rupture in the course of follicular development and ovulation. The cyst is formed by one or more layers of granulosa cells. Lutein cysts form when the corpus luteum becomes cystic or hemorrhagic or fails to degenerate after 14 days. Development of theca-lutein cyst is accompanied by increase in beta-hCG. Examples include hydatidiform mole, choriocarcinoma, or ovulation induction with gonadatropins. Polycystic ovary (Stein–Leventhal syndrome) is characterized by multiple inactive follicle cysts of the ovary, androgen excess, and chronic anovulation. Inflammatory ovarian tumors include salpingo-oophoritis and tubo-ovarian abscess and result from inflammation of tube or ovary or tubo-ovarian cysts. Neoplastic epithelial tumors include stromal or germ cell tumors. Epithelial tumors, serous tumors, mucinous tumors, and endometroid tumors possess the highest potential for malignancy. Stomal tumors are derived from sex cords, fibromas, and Sertoli–Leydig cell tumors (germ cell tumors), and dermoid cysts are derived from embryonic germ cells. Calcifications are common. Benign cystic or germ cell tumors are the most common ovarian neoplasms. Epithelial neoplasia are the most common malignant ovarian tumors. Stromal neoplasia is uncommon. During the reproductive years, 70% of all noninflammatory tumors are functional, 20% are neoplastic, and 10% are endometriomas. After menopause, one-half of all ovarian tumors are malignant.

▶ History & Physical

Ovarian tumors and cysts are often clinically silent except for nonspecific pressure, low pelvic pain, dyspareunia. Functional cysts may cause menstrual abnormalities. Ruptured cysts are more painful. Adnexal mass and uterine enlargement may be noted (4- to 8-cm tumor on bimanual exam). Regression following menses. Benign tumors are characteristically unilateral, cystic, and mobile. Malignancies are usually solid, fixed, and nodular. May cause ascites.

▶ Diagnostic Studies

Pelvic exam, CBC, beta-hCG, and transabdominal or transvaginal ultrasound most important. Abdominal CT, barium enema, colonoscopy, or IVP may be indicated.

▶ Diagnosis

Rule out ovarian malignancies, uterine myoma diverticulitis, ectopic pregnancy.

▶ Clinical Therapeutics

Observation or monophasic oral contraceptives for 4 to 6 weeks.

▶ Clinical Intervention

If cyst is < 6 cm, observation; regression likely. If > 6 cm or cyst persists more than 6 to 8 weeks, cystectomy or wedge resection recommended.

▶ Health Maintenance Issues

Risk of ovarian cancer increases with age; annual pelvic exam is recommended.

B. Ovarian Malignancy

▶ Scientific Concepts

A variety of malignancies arise from ovarian epithelium, stromal or germ cells. Ovarian cancer accounts for over 50% of gynecologic cancer deaths. Risk increases with age, positive first-degree family history, low parity, infertility, and high-fat diet.

▶ **History & Physical**

Often asymptomatic, pelvic pressure, vague gastrointestinal (GI) symptoms, fullness or abdominal distention may be the only signs or symptoms.

▶ **Diagnostic Studies**

Pelvic ultrasound, serum CA-125, CT scan, carcinoembryonic antigen (CEA), liver function studies, and barium enema as warranted.

▶ **Diagnosis**

GI or other malignancy or tubo-ovarian abscess.

▶ **Clinical Therapeutics**

Surgical staging, excision, and debulking are critical.

▶ **Clinical Intervention**

Concurrent use of chemotherapy (cisplatin, carboplatin, paclitaxel, or cyclophosphamide) may be indicated. Alternative drugs include etoposide, 5-fluorouracil, adriamycin, or other alkylating agents.

▶ **Health Maintenance Issues**

Follow-up with routine monitoring of CA-125 is recommended. Attention to potential protective factors is encouraged, and annual pelvic exams are recommended.

VI. MENSTRUAL DISORDERS

A. Dysmenorrhea

▶ **Scientific Concepts**

Dysmenorrhea (pain associated with menses), categorized as primary or secondary. Dysmenorrhea represents a source of disability for many.

Primary: No identifiable cause of pain, normal pelvic organs. Etiologic theory, excess prostaglandin produced in the endometrium. Smooth muscle stimulant causes increased uterine contractions resulting in increased intrauterine pressure. Usual onset late teens to early 20s, declines with age.

Secondary: Clinically identifiable cause (endometriosis, leiomyomas, or other structural abnormalities), becomes worse with age. Neither affected by childbearing.

▶ **History & Physical**

Primary: History is more characteristic, recurrent month after month, first 1 to 3 days of menstruation, lower abdomen and suprapubic area, radiation to back and thighs. Other symptoms include nausea, vomiting, diarrhea, fatigue, low backache, and headache.

Secondary: Symptoms less severe and more general in nature. Complaints of menorrhagia with pain suggests myomas or polyps.

In primary, physical and pelvic examinations are usually normal. In secondary, history and physical findings suggest underlying disorder (abdominal fullness, rectal pain, etc.).

▶ Diagnostic Studies

None specific; cultures for evaluation of infection; consider pelvic ultrasound to rule out structural abnormalities.

▶ Diagnosis

Secondary dysmenorrhea, evaluate underlying condition.

▶ Clinical Therapeutics

Primary: Nonsteroidal anti-inflammatory agents (NSAIDs), mefenamic acid (Ponstel), diet, exercise, patient education, or oral contraceptives.
Secondary: Treat underlying condition.

▶ Clinical Intervention

Primary: Dietary supplementation with vitamin B_1, 100 mg PO qd × 3 months, and fish oil may also be beneficial.

▶ Health Maintenance Issues

Primary: Reassurance, exercise, and diet low in animal fat, dairy products.
Secondary: Routine follow-up and management of underlying cause.

B. Premenstrual Syndrome

▶ Scientific Concepts

Premenstrual syndrome (PMS) is a group of physical, mood, and behavioral changes that occur in a regular cyclic relationship to the late luteal phase of the menstrual cycle. Three-fourths of all menstruating women have premenstrual symptoms. Most prevalent in women in their 30s to 40s. Etiology unknown, yet many theories exist. Psychiatric basis: stress related; endocrinologic basis: abnormal luteal-phase steroid levels, higher estradiol levels relative to progesterone; diet basis: related to intake of salt and refined carbohydrates resulting in premenstrual hypoglycemic episodes; endorphin basis: alleviation of symptoms with increased endorphin production/release through exercise; serotonin basis: lower in patients with PMS and with depression; prostaglandin basis: excess production (late luteal phase) and prostaglandins are produced in breast, brain, GI tract, kidneys, and reproductive system; and fluid retention basis: alternations in renin–angiotensin–aldosterone axis.

▶ History & Physical

Mood changes (depression, hostility, irritability, etc.), somatic changes (appetite, bloating, fatigue, headache, hot flashes, mastalgia), cognitive changes (confusion, poor concentration), and behavioral changes (hyperphagia, social withdrawal).

► Diagnostic Studies

None specifically. Menstrual diary most useful. History and physical examination to rule out other disorders. *Diagnostic and Statistical Manual (DSM)* criteria: five or more symptoms, disturbance in the absence of other conditions, (timing) symptoms increase up to 14 days before menses, relieved within 4 days of the start of the menses and does not recur until at least the 12th day of the cycle.

► Diagnosis

Rule out psychiatric syndromes. The history and physical may suggest other entities.

► Clinical Therapeutics

Pharmacologic interventions such as trial of oral contraceptives, NSAIDs, diuretics, and more invasive therapy. Danazol, alprazolam, medroxyprogesterone as indicated.

► Clinical Intervention

Therapy should be comprehensive, including education, lifestyle modification (exercise; relaxation therapy; diet; decrease salt, caffeine, alcohol, etc.). Dietary supplementation (B_6, calcium, primrose oil, multivitamins, magnesium, vitamin E) is helpful.

► Health Maintenance Issues

Patient education and empowerment are important.

VII. MENOPAUSE

► Scientific Concepts

Characterized as the sequelae of symptoms related to cessation of menses. Climacteric is the period in which ovarian function declines and estrogen production diminishes. The estrogen receptors located throughout the body respond to diminishing circulating estrogens, hence the multisystemic impact of menopause experienced by most women. Mean age at menopause is 51; range, 40 to 58. Menopause may also be surgically induced.

► History & Physical

Gradual decrease and ultimate cessation of menses; atrophy of estrogen-dependent tissue (skin, breast, uterus, bladder, and vagina); vasomotor changes (hot flashes and sweating); psychological changes, including depression, nervousness, and anxiety; increased risk of arteriosclerosis and osteoporosis.

► Diagnostic Studies

Usually none are required. If diagnosis is questionable in a young patient, an elevated serum FSH suggests ovarian failure. Endometrial biopsy and/or D&C in patients who have intermenstrual or postmenopausal bleeding.

▶ **Diagnosis**

Rule out pregnancy.

▶ **Clinical Therapeutics**

General measures include adequate calcium intake (elemental calcium, 1,500 mg/d PO). Estrogen replacement therapy (ERT) for prophylaxis against osteoporosis and coronary artery disease is recommended unless otherwise contraindicated. Conjugated estrogen, .625 mg PO, micronized estradiol, 1 mg, for the first 25 days of each month, a 4-cm estrogen patch, or estrogen-containing vaginal creams alone or in combination may be indicated. Progesterone should be added for its protective effect against endometrial cancer if the uterus has not been removed.

▶ **Clinical Intervention**

Medroxyprogesterone acetate, 150 mg IM, may be used by those who cannot take estrogens. Other interventions include use of soy products, B complex vitamins; alternative therapies such as Dong Quai and Black Cohosh; exercise and cessation of cigarette smoking.

▶ **Health Maintenance Issues**

During the perimenopausal period, women should be reminded to use contraception as ovulation and subsequent pregnancy remain a possibility. Annual Pap smears; pelvic and breast exams; annual mammography and endometrial biopsy in patients with abnormal vaginal bleeding are recommended. Estrogen therapy is contraindicated if there is a preexisting malignant breast disease and should be discontinued if breast cancer develops.

VIII. BREAST

A. Inflammatory Breast Disease

▶ **Scientific Concepts**

Inflammatory changes and infection in the breast are more common in lactating women. Breast abscess can be associated with lactation, duct occlusion, or fistulous tracts secondary to squamous epithelial neoplasia. *Staphylococcus aureus* from the infant's nose or throat, abrasion of the nipple, and prolonged engorgement are common causes of breast infection or inflammation (mastitis). Without treatment, may lead to breast abscess.

▶ **History & Physical**

Unilateral tender breast mass, generalized breast tenderness, swelling, erythema, nipple drainage, and generalized malaise are common.

▶ **Diagnostic Studies**

Diagnosed by history. CBC, erythrocyte sedimentation rate (ESR), and culture with sensitivity of drainage to identify pathogen.

► Diagnosis

Rule out inflammatory carcinoma. History most significant in making diagnosis.

► Clinical Therapeutics

NSAIDs for inflammation. If infection is present, erythromycin, 250 to 500 mg PO qid; cephalexin, 500 mg bid; or amoxicillin-clavulanate, 250 mg PO tid.

► Clinical Intervention

Cold compresses and expression of milk provide symptomatic relief. Aspiration under ultrasound or incision and drainage may be indicated.

► Health Maintenance Issues

Routine health measures include reassurance, especially to exclude carcinoma; regular expression of milk; and early treatment of inflammation or infections.

B. Fibrocystic Breast Disease

► Scientific Concepts

Benign breast neoplasm characterized by painful, lumpy breasts. The lumps may be physiologic, vary with menstrual cycle, more common in younger women (21 to 25); ropy thickening, more common in the upper outer quadrant, or cystic, most common in the perimenopausal period.

► History & Physical

Etiology unknown; family history of cystic breast is common. Cyclic, bilateral or unilateral tenderness, engorgement, fluctuant masses, breast thickening, which improve following menses, are common.

► Diagnostic Studies

Patient history is most helpful. Ultrasound and mammography may be first diagnostic interventions. Serum prolactin and TSH as well as fine-needle aspiration and biopsy, or excisional biopsy may be indicated (rare).

► Diagnosis

Rule out breast cancer, inflammation of the chest wall.

► Clinical Therapeutics

Treatment is related to severity of symptoms. Spironolactone, 10 mg bid premenstrually; vitamin A, 150,000 IU qd × 3 months; vitamin E, 300 to 600 IU qd × 3 months; oral contraceptives and NSAIDs alone or in combination provide relief.

► Clinical Intervention

In severe cases, progestins, danazol, bromocriptine, and tamoxifen may be indicated. Dietary restriction of caffeine, primrose oil, cessation of cigarette smoking, and well-fitting supportive brassiere are recommended.

► **Health Maintenance Issues**
Reassurance and regular breast exams are encouraged.

C. Fibroadenoma

► **Scientific Concepts**
This solid, benign neoplasm is more common is young women but may occur at any age after menarche.

► **History & Physical**
Well-circumscribed, firm, mobile, rubbery nodule.

► **Diagnostic Studies**
Ultrasound, mammography, and aspiration cytology (fine-needle biopsy) are most useful in making diagnosis.

► **Diagnosis**
Rule out breast cancer.

► **Clinical Therapeutics**
Clinical examination, radiologic studies, and fine-needle biopsy to make diagnosis, observation, or excision.

► **Clinical Intervention**
As above.

► **Health Maintenance Issues**
This condition is generally benign. Reassurance and routine, age-appropriate mammography.

D. Nipple Discharge

► **Scientific Concepts**
Although considered one of the warning signs of breast cancer, 90% of women with nipple discharge have benign disease. Nipple discharge with nipple discomfort, burning, or itching is suggestive of duct ectasia. Bloody discharge is suggestive of intraductal papilloma.

► **History & Physical**
Unilateral, spontaneous nipple discharge of clear to milky fluid or sticky yellow-green, multicolored, or blood-tinged fluid requires further evaluation for endocrine or local disorder.

► **Diagnostic Studies**
Cytology and/or culture and sensitivity.

► **Diagnosis**
Rule out breast cancer.

▶ Clinical Therapeutics

Clinical examination, radiologic studies, and fine-needle biopsy to make diagnosis. Observation or excision based on finding.

▶ Clinical Intervention

As above.

▶ Health Maintenance Issues

This condition is generally benign. Reassurance and routine, age-appropriate mammography.

E. Breast Cancer

▶ Scientific Concepts

Malignant neoplasm in the breast. Classified as noninvasive (in situ) and invasive (infiltrating). Family history is the most important epidemiologic factor.

▶ History & Physical

Long history of unopposed estrogen, nulliparity, early menarche, and late menopause are considered risk factors for breast cancer. Inconclusive risks include high dietary fat and obesity. Signs include discrete breast mass, puckering of breast skin, dimpling, nipple retraction, lymphedema, and lymphadenopathy.

▶ Diagnostic Studies

Physical examination, ultrasound, mammography, fine-needle aspiration, and biopsy with cytologic confirmation are recommended.

▶ Diagnosis

Extensive, includes benign disorders such as abscesses, hematomas, or fibroadenomas; fibrocystic changes; hyperplasia; sarcomas and lymphomas.

▶ Clinical Therapeutics

Treatment includes hormonal therapy (most commonly tamoxifen), chemotherapy (cyclophosphamide, methotrexate, or fluorouracil); radiotherapy and/or surgery are employed depending on staging and patient preference.

▶ Clinical Intervention

Surveillance for recurrent disease is integral. The status of axillary lymph node involvement is an important indicator of disease relapse.

▶ Health Maintenance Issues

Starting in puberty, all women are encouraged to perform monthly self breast exams (SBEs) to become familiar with normal tissue and to detect changes. In addition, women over 18 are advised to have yearly clinical breast exams. Screening mammography and clinical breast exams are recommended at age 40 and every 1 to 2 years thereafter until the age of 50. Women over 50 are advised to have annual screening mammography and clinical breast exams.

IX. HEALTH MAINTENANCE

A. Screening

▶ Scientific Concepts

The primary care provider has the opportunity to impact on women's health maintenance. An evaluation of reproductive health status should address general health status, with emphasis on health promotion and disease prevention; patient psychological and emotional health as well as screening, early intervention, treatment, and management of the conditions common to the gynecological patient.

▶ History & Physical

Menstrual history, sexual history, obstetric history, fertility, contraception, and history of STDs should be considered. Routine physical examination includes pelvic, rectal, rectovaginal, and bimanual exams.

▶ Diagnostic Studies

Age specific, including Pap smear, cultures, breast exam, and instructions on SBE, lipid profile, rubella status, RPR, and perhaps HIV.

▶ Diagnosis
N/A.

▶ Clinical Therapeutics

The general gynecologic exam should be done annually along with counseling regarding tobacco, alcohol, caffeine, diet, exercise, adult immunizations, routine health screening, and safety.

▶ Clinical Intervention
N/A.

▶ Health Maintenance Issues
N/A.

B. Contraception

▶ Scientific Concepts

One of the most sensitive and intimate decision made by an individual or by a couple is that of fertility control. This decision is affected by religious/philosophical convictions, patient age, long- and short-term goals of childbearing (now, later, never), patient's lifestyle and sexual patterns, patient's comfort level with her own body, cost, and existent medical conditions.

Methods of Contraception
1. Barrier methods
  • **Latex condoms:** Cover penis during coitus and prevent deposition of semen in the vagina. *Advantages:* Highly effective when used properly and regularly, convenient, inexpensive, no prescription needed, provides major protection against STDs. *Dis-*

advantages: Both partners may experience some reduction of sensation; must be used properly, failure related to error in technique and/or timing of placement or removal. Cultural barriers to use of condoms and partner reluctance to use must be explored. Effectiveness is increased with concurrent use of spermicidal foam, jelly, or cream.

- **Vaginal diaphragm/cervical cap:** Provides a mechanical barrier between vagina and cervical canal, to be used with spermicidal agent. *Advantages:* Use of device is limited to episodes of sexual activity (no long-term contraception agents in circulation or indwelling uterine devices), relatively inexpensive, concurrent use of spermicidal agent increases effectiveness and offers protection against STDs. *Disadvantages:* Device must be "fit" by a health professional. Must be inserted properly, failure related to error in technique and/or timing of placement or removal. Patient must be able and willing to insert the device regularly and properly. Slight incidence of cervical dysplasia and toxic shock syndrome. Device must be kept in place at least 6 hours (24 to 48 hours for cervical cap). Slight incidence of reaction to spermicidal agent.

- **Spermicidal preparations (contraceptive sponge, foams, jellies, and creams used alone):** Function to kill sperm cells and act as a mechanical barrier to entry of sperm into cervical canal. *Advantages:* Convenient, inexpensive, no prescription needed. *Disadvantages:* Unreliable due to displacement and incomplete coverage of cervical os. Slight incidence of reaction to spermicidal agent.

2. **Intrauterine device (IUD):** Plastic or metal device introduced into the endometrial cavity through the cervical canal. Mode of action unknown; theory suggests that the placement of a foreign body creates a hostile environment to the ovum and prevents implantation. *Advantages:* Long-term protection, requires a single decision, is reversible. *Disadvantages:* Requires insertion by a trained health professional. *Side effects and complications:* Pain or discomfort during insertion, uterine perforation (rare), uterine cramping reaction to material used and size of device; pregnancy (rate is ~ 0.4 to 2.8/100 women in 12 months of use); spontaneous expulsion (rate varies with size, shape, and stiffness of device); increased menstrual flow and dysmenorrhea; increased incidence of extrauterine pregnancy; increased incidence of pelvic infections/PID and related sequelae. Currently, the Copper T Cu 380 can be retained for up to 8 years; Progestasert must be replaced annually. The IUD is not recommended for women who have had multiple sexual partners, who have STDs, or who have not been pregnant.

3. **Hormonal contraceptives:** Synthetic steroids similar to natural female hormones (estrogens and progestins) that, when used in combination, inhibit ovulation. Combined pills (estrogen and progestin) are started on the fifth day of the cycle, continued 20 to 21 days; withdrawal bleeding generally occurs 3 to 5 days after completion of cycle (menses like blood flow, slight shedding), cycle is then repeated. During a typical cycle, under combined oral contraceptive regimen, there is no rise in FSH and LH during the

first half of the cycle; thus, follicle growth is not initiated, ovulation does not occur. Hormonal implants consist of progestin capsules placed under the skin, slowly releasing hormones that block ovulation. Hormonal implants are effective for up to 5 years. Hormonal injections, most commonly medroxyprogesterone (Depo-Provera), also function to suppress ovulation but also function to alter the cervical mucous and inhibit implantation. *Advantages:* Highly effective; regular and less painful menses; possible decrease in the incidence of ectopic pregnancy, ovarian cancer, endometrial cancer, and benign breast disease; decreased menstrual fluid loss; decreased incidence of dysmenorrhea; increased protection against osteoporosis. *Disadvantages and side effects:* Increased incidence of thromboembolic disease, including pulmonary embolism, cerebral thrombosis, deep vein thrombosis, and coronary thrombosis; risk increases with age and with concurrent cigarette smoking; risk of endometrial and cervical cancers have been reduced with the introduction of triphasic oral contraceptives, which contain a lower dose of progestin and estrogen. None of the hormonal therapies offer protection against STDs, and all require administration or prescription from a health care provider.

4. **Rhythm or ovulation method:** Requires that coitus be avoided during the time of the cycle when a fertilized ovum and sperm could meet in the oviduct. Accurate prediction or indication of ovulation is essential to the success of the rhythm method. Means of predicting ovulation:

   • **Calendar method:** Based on a formula of menstrual pattern recorded over several months, coitus should be avoided on day 14 ± 3 days.

   • **Basal body temperature (BBT) method:** Temperature taken rectally or orally in morning before any physical activity is undertaken; slight drop in temperature 24 to 36 hours after ovulation, then rises abruptly 0.3 to 0.4°C or 0.5 to 0.7°F. The third day after rise in temperature is considered to be the end of the fertility period.

   • **Luteinizing hormone peak:** Most accurate method of determining ovulation time. Test is performed on serum and is costly and time consuming but very useful in the treatment of infertility when the timing of coitus or artificial insemination is of great importance. *Advantages:* Considered natural methods of contraception; nearly no cost except LH peak analysis. *Disadvantages:* Unreliable, increased margin of error, and variability of menstrual cycle.

5. **Induced abortion:** Deliberate termination of pregnancy in a manner that ensures that the embryo or fetus will not survive. Very controversial; subject to social, legal, and religious pressures. Indication for induced abortion may be categorized as maternal, paternal, fetal, social, etc. Some of the more common indications include obstetric (prior major uterine injury or damage, increased maternal age, multiparity, recurrent preeclampsia, eclampsia, etc.); medical complications (surgical, orthopedic, hematologic, cardiovascular pulmonary, urologic, immunologic, endocrine neu-

rologic, oncologic, infectious, psychiatric disorders, maternal inability to care for child, etc.). Whatever the reason, the decision and right to carry a child to term is the decision of the mother.

Method of induced abortion is determined primarily by the duration of pregnancy, patient's health, and physical facilities. *Suction curettage* is the most efficient, rapid method; used to terminate pregnancies less than 12 weeks, can be performed on an outpatient basis, with local or light anesthesia, limited blood loss and least likelihood of uterine perforation. Complications, although rare, include infection (< 2%), excessive bleeding (~2%), uterine perforation (under 1%). *Sharp curettage* must be performed during the first trimester and is performed as a standard D&C such as for the diagnosis and treatment of abnormal uterine bleeding. Blood loss, duration of surgery, and likelihood of damage to the cervix or uterus are greatly increased when surgical curettage is used. At least 5% of abortions in the United States are still performed by sharp curettage. *Induction of labor by intra-amniotic instillation of an oxytocic agent (saline abortion)* involves the aspiration of amniotic fluid and replacement with saline, urea, or most commonly, one of the prostaglandins, generally during the second trimester. The patient must be monitored until the fetus and placenta are delivered. Complication rate can be high (up to 20%) and can include disseminated intravascular clotting, sepsis, retained placenta, hemorrhage due to uterine inertia, hypernatremia, cervical laceration resulting form tumultuous labor in an "unripe" cervix, and delivery of a live fetus. *Abortifacients* such as prostaglandins have been used orally, parenterally, by intra-amniotic injection, or vaginally in the form of suppositories alone or in combination with a *Laminaria* tent to evoke labor (*Laminaria* tent placed in the cervix for a few hours to soften the "unripe" cervix). Side effects include severe nausea, vomiting, diarrhea, tachycardia, substernal pressure, and paralytic ileus.

6. **Sterilization:** A permanent method of contraception chosen increasingly by men and women. Sterilization is the most frequent indication for laparoscopy in the United States. Clear, comprehensive counseling is essential for women and men considering sterilization. Patients must be informed of the risks, effectiveness, and chances of reversibility with this procedure. There are several procedures that may be performed and vary according to the portion of oviduct in women and vas deferens in men, which are sutured or cut and the method employed. Complications are uncommon in men and women. Women may experience pain, menstrual disturbances, and psychological problems. Complications in men usually involve slight bleeding, skin infections, reactions to sutures or local anesthetics. Sterilization in men and women should be considered permanent.

▶ **History & Physical**
Complete history and physical examination are recommended prior to use of the vaginal diaphragm; cervical cap; hormonal contraceptives taken orally, implanted, or injected; IUDs; surgical steriliza-

tion. Condoms, sponges, and spermicide do not require complete history and physical prior to use.

► Diagnostic Studies

Pap smear, cultures recommended prior to use.

► Diagnosis

Rule out pregnancy prior to use of any contraceptive.

► Clinical Therapeutics

Patient education and counseling are integral to effective use of any contraceptive. Risk factors, convenience, instruction on proper use, and protection from STDs and HIV should be discussed with patient prior to use.

► Clinical Intervention

As above.

► Health Maintenance Issues

Monitoring as appropriate for each method.

X. OTHER DISEASES AND DISORDERS

A. Infertility

► Scientific Concepts

Fertility is considered to be compromised if a couple fails to conceive after 1 year of unprotected intercourse. Sterility refers to an intrinsic inability to conceive. *Primary infertility:* never having conceived. *Secondary infertility* refers to previous history of conception but current inability to conceive after 1 year. Fertility challenges plague 10 to 15% of all couples. The incidence increases with age. Several factors contribute to infertility, including genital or pelvic factor (endometriosis, tubal occlusion, or cervical anomalies); endocrine dysfunction (hypothyroidism or hypogonadism), or ovulatory dysfunction. Male and female factors are equally contributory to incidence of infertility, with etiology unknown in ~ 10% of cases.

► History & Physical

Evaluation includes menstrual, sexual, and obstetric history; history of pelvic surgery, exposure; medication; drug use; and history of pelvic infections. Endometriosis is often associated with cyclic premenstrual pain and dysmenorrhea.

► Diagnostic Studies

Evaluation should follow in a logical, stepwise fashion, including complete history and physical on both partners, semen analysis, postcoital test, cervical mucus assessment, BBT, serum progesterone, hysterosalpingogram, and endometrial sampling.

► Diagnosis

Identify underlying disorder, condition, or factor.

► Clinical Therapeutics

Therapeutics are related to cause of infertility. Clomiphene citrate, 50 mg PO qd × 5 days to induce ovulation; surgery (in vitro fertilization or intrauterine insemination for tubal or cervical factor).

► Clinical Intervention

Treatment may be prolonged. Patient education, exploration of options, and limits of intervention should be discussed.

► Health Maintenance Issues

Prevention of STDs and subsequent pelvic infection.

B. Endometriosis

► Scientific Concepts

Endometriosis typically occurs between the ages of 25 and 40 but may also affect those as young as 18. Over 2 million women in the United States are affected and incidence transcends all races. Endometrial tissue, normally found in the uterine epithelial lining, escapes the uterine cavity and grows outside the uterus. Exact etiology unknown, yet theory suggests that retrograde menstruation flows through the fallopian tubes and outside into the pelvic cavity and wayward endometrial cells implant on the ovaries, fallopian tubes, cul de sac, uterosacral ligament, bladder, and intestines. The presence of extrapelvic sites suggests lymphatic or vascular metastases. Risk factors include short menstrual cycles (< 27 days), menstrual flow duration of 8 days or more, women with uninterrupted menstruation for more than 15 to 20 years, nulliparity (by choice or otherwise), and positive family history.

► History & Physical

Low back pain, rectal pain, increase 1 to 2 days before menses begins and persist throughout flow; premenstrual spotting; midcycle bleeding; irregular bleeding; menorrhagia, dyspareunia, and dysmenorrhea; urinary and bowel dysfunction and pain. Physical examination should be done at midcycle and again before or during menses (if endometrial nodules or implants are present, they should be larger during perimenstrual exam); retrovaginal palpation is best means to examine (common site for implants). Pelvic fullness and tenderness may be noted on pelvic exam. Colored lesions may be present on umbilicus, vulva, vagina, or cervix.

► Diagnostic Studies

Imaging tests and serum immunoassay markers are noninvasive methods but are suboptimal due to limited sensitivity. Serum immunoassay CA-125 increases in ovarian cancer as well as endometriosis but may be useful if monitoring response to treatment. Laparoscopy may be diagnostic and therapeutic, with laser vaporization of implants, drainage and lysis of pelvic lesions.

▶ Diagnosis

Differential includes all causes of acute abdomen, intra- and extrauterine pregnancy, ruptured ovarian cysts, as well as urinary and GI disorders.

▶ Clinical Therapeutics

Treatment must be individualized and guided by the age of the patient, future childbearing plans, and severity of symptoms. GnRH agonists such as nafarelin, 400 μg/d intranasally, leuprolide acetate, and goserelin implants may be used. Alternative drugs include danazol, 400 to 800 mg/d × 9 months, medroxyprogesterone, and megestrol as well as continuous oral contraceptives.

▶ Clinical Intervention

Close patient monitoring and additional diagnostic interventions may be indicated.

▶ Health Maintenance Issues

While endometriosis cannot be prevented or cured, signs and symptoms generally regress with menopause.

XI. COMPLICATED PREGNANCY

A. Adolescent Pregnancy

▶ Scientific Concepts

Pregnancy before the age of 19 poses added risk for mother and child. Incidence of ectopic pregnancy, spontaneous abortion, prematurity, intrauterine growth retardation, and newborns with low birth weight is greater in teen pregnancy.

▶ History & Physical

Concurrent STDs; malnutrition; sexual, alcohol, and substance abuse complicate teen pregnancies.

▶ Diagnostic Studies

Complete history and physical examination, including Pap smear and cultures, beta-hCG, screening for STDs as per routine.

▶ Diagnosis

Early diagnosis of pregnancy and prompt initiation of prenatal care are recommended. Patients age 16 and younger have an increased risk of preeclampsia–eclampsia.

▶ Clinical Therapeutics

Prenatal vitamins that include iron and folate.

▶ Clinical Intervention

Routine prenatal care, screening, support services, and referral for interventions appropriate to pregnant teens.

► Health Maintenance Issues

Patient education and support as needed.

B. High-Risk Pregnancy

► Scientific Concepts

High-risk pregnancy is broadly defined as one in which the mother or fetus/newborn is or will be at risk for morbidity or mortality before or after birth. Maternal nutrition, prenatal care, preexisting medical condition, genetic abnormalities, or obstetric disorders may impose higher risks for mother and fetus.

► History & Physical

Initial screening to include maternal age (higher risk with adolescent and advanced maternal age), obstetric history (history of habitual abortion, previous stillbirth, neonatal death, premature or small- or large-for-gestational-age infant, grand multiparity, previous Rh isoimmunization, previous preeclampsia–eclampsia, previous or known genetic anomaly), history of reproductive disorders, medical complications of pregnancy, or history of exposure to teratogens. Complete physical examination, including Pap smear and pelvic exam with special attention to thyroid, breast, heart, lungs, abdomen, and vasculature.

► Diagnostic Studies

Diagnostic studies specific to condition. Beta-hCG (qualitative and quantitative), serum alpha-fetoprotein, ABO and Rh, sickle cell prep, and pelvic sonogram as per routine. Amniocentesis may be indicated.

► Diagnosis

Identify underlying condition or risk.

► Clinical Therapeutics

Specific to condition.

► Clinical Intervention

As above.

► Health Maintenance Issues

Reassurance, close monitoring, patient education and counseling depending on diagnosis.

C. First-Trimester Complications

1. Extrauterine Pregnancy

► Scientific Concepts

Extrauterine pregnancy, most commonly in the ampulla or other portion of the fallopian tube, less often in the pelvis, ovary, or abdomen. Risk increased with IUD for contraception, history of pelvic infection, adhesions, previous tubal pregnancy or surgery, history of endometriosis or endometritis.

► History & Physical

Early pregnancy symptoms, amenorrhea followed by irregular bleeding, pelvic pain, colicky abdominal pain and cramping. Shoulder pain, syncope, and peritoneal signs are associated with intraperitoneal bleeding.

► Diagnostic Studies

Urine pregnancy test, serial hCG (quantitative and qualitative), culdocentesis, laparoscopy, laparotomy.

► Diagnosis

Rule out spontaneous abortion, appendicitis, salpingitis, ruptured ovarian cyst.

► Clinical Therapeutics

Nonsurgical management for small, unruptured ectopic pregnancy may include methotrexate. More commonly laparoscopic surgery and segmental resection of the tube are indicated. Salpingectomy may be indicated in the treatment of a large ruptured ectopic pregnancy.

► Clinical Intervention

Early treatment (prior to rupture) is ideal. Complications include hemorrhage, hypovolemic shock, infection, infertility, and loss of reproductive organs.

► Health Maintenance Issues

Reliable contraception and reduction of risk factors recommended.

2. Abortion

► Scientific Concepts

Abortion refers to the separation of the products of conception from the uterine endometrium prior to potential for fetal survival outside of the uterus. A potentially viable fetus weighs at least 500 g or has a gestational age of 20 weeks or greater. *Stillbirth* commonly refers to death of preterm infants weighing ≥ 500 g and infants up to 28 days of age. *Spontaneous abortion* implies expulsion of the products of conception without notable provocation. *Complete abortion* refers to expulsion of all of the products of conception, whereas *incomplete abortion* refers to expulsion of part but not all of the products of conception. An *early abortion* occurs prior to 12 weeks' gestation, and a *late abortion* occurs between 12 and 20 weeks' gestation. A *threatened abortion* is characterized by vaginal bleeding with or without contractions and without cervical dilatation, rupture of membranes, and expulsion of the products of conception. *Inevitable abortion* refers to intrauterine bleeding prior to 20 weeks, with continuous and progressive cervical dilatation, rupture of membranes, and expulsion of the products of conception. *Induced abortion* refers to interruption of the pregnancy either by medical or surgical means. *Infected abortion* involves infection of the products of conception and maternal reproductive organs, as opposed to *septic abortion,* which refers to dissemination of a pathogen into the maternal circulation. *Habitual abortion* refers to three or more consecutive spontaneous abortions. Exact etiology of most spontaneous abortions is unknown, yet chromosomal abnormalities account for most. Exposure to toxins, drugs, alcohol, endocrine dysfunction, abnormalities of maternal reproductive structures, and infectious processes also contribute to the incidence. Spontaneous abortions are more common in the very young (< 16 years) and women of advanced years (> 35).

► History & Physical

Vaginal bleeding or spotting with a pink, brownish discharge is common. Uterine cramping, pelvic pain, cervical dilatation, rupture of membranes, and possible passage of clotted or other nonviable products. Uterine enlargement, softening of the cervix, and adnexal tenderness may be noted on bimanual exam.

► Diagnostic Studies

Sterile speculum exam to determine bleeding source, cultures, beta-hCG (qualitative and quantitative), and ultrasound examination for identification of gestational sac and to access fetal viability are most useful.

► Diagnosis

Rule out ectopic pregnancy, cervical polyp, molar pregnancy (hydatidiform mole), and membranous dysmenorrhea.

► Clinical Therapeutics

Observation, beta-agonists (isozuprine), bedrest, and nothing per vagina may effectively manage threatened abortion. D&C with suction is generally indicated for incomplete and inevitable abortions; IV or PO antibiotic therapy for infected and septic abortions and analgesia as needed.

► Clinical Intervention

Bleeding following D&C may be effectively treated with oxytocin, 3 to 10 units IM, or methylergonovine, 0.2 mg IM. Karyotyping of products of conception, genetic screening, and special care for subsequent pregnancies including surgical reinforcement of the cervix (cerclage stitch) may be warranted for habitual abortion.

► Health Maintenance Issues

Prognosis for future pregnancies after threatened abortion and D&C for incomplete or inevitable abortion is good. Guilt and sadness are common; counseling and support recommended.

D. Second-Trimester Complications

1. Premature Rupture of Membranes/Prematurity

► Scientific Concepts

Premature labor is defined as uterine contractions and cervical changes before the 37th week of gestation. Premature labor may or may not progress to mature rupture of membranes. Prematurity is a common sequela of premature rupture of membranes (PROM). Risk factors for preterm labor and PROM include incompetent cervix, uterine surgery, uterine anomalies, multiple gestation, intrauterine and urinary tract infections, abnormal placental placement, dehydration, stress, and cigarette smoking.

► History & Physical

The signs may be subtle, including increased uterine activity, contractions, intestinal cramping, vaginal discharge or bleeding, and pressure or pain in the pelvis, back, or thighs. Patient may report a sudden gush of fluid or continuous leakage.

► Diagnostic Studies

Sterile speculum exam, fern test (assessment of pooled fluid, air dried on a slide, noting arborization, fern pattern), nitrazine test (positive suggests presence of amniotic fluid), L/S ratio (assessment of fetal maturity), ultrasound, and, in some cases, amniocentesis. Cervical secretions should also be sent for culture and sensitivity.

► Diagnosis

Monitor patient, rule out rupture of membranes.

► Clinical Therapeutics

Depending on severity; if no rupture of the membranes, monitoring, hydration, bedrest, tocolytics (terbutaline, 0.25 mg subcutaneously × 6 doses), and outpatient use of beta-sympathomimetics (ritodrine) may be employed. Other clinical therapeutics include magnesium sulfate, indomethacin, or calcium channel blockers. The goal is to sustain pregnancy to as close to 35 weeks as possible. If membranes have been ruptured, delivery should be accomplished within 24 hours. Medical induction of labor with IV pitocin (Oxytocin) may be indicated if spontaneous labor does not occur within 12 to 24 hours of rupture.

► Clinical Intervention

Management is individualized according to status of membranes (intact vs. ruptured) and gestational age. Risk to fetus is greatest in pregnancy < 24 to 26 weeks' gestation. Risk of intrauterine, fetal, and maternal infection increases as rupture allows pathogens to access the fetus and maternal circulation.

► Health Maintenance Issues

Identification of etiology is most important in minimizing recurrence. Patient and family support recommended.

2. Incompetent Cervix

► Scientific Concepts

Incompetent cervical os is characterized by cervical effacement and dilatation between 18 and 22 weeks' gestation and may be a result of cervical instrumentation, surgery, laceration, or congenital anomaly. Increased incidence in multiple gestation, history of cervical conization, cervical amputation, and intrauterine exposure to DES.

▶ History & Physical
Symptoms include painless vaginal discharge of pink or bloody fluid, contractions, and pelvic pressure. Progressive thinning and dilatation of the cervix may be evident on pelvic exam.

▶ Diagnostic Studies
Diagnosis is made on history of repeated second-trimester spontaneous abortions and physical examination.

▶ Diagnosis
Measurement of cervical os > 1 cm or painless passage of a #8 Hegar dilator. Rule out other etiology of miscarriage.

▶ Clinical Therapeutics
No medical intervention.

▶ Clinical Intervention
Surgical intervention includes prophylactic placement of a transvaginal cerclage at 12 to 16 weeks' gestation or in a nonpregnant patient.

▶ Health Maintenance Issues
Education, counseling, bedrest, and restriction of coital activity are recommended. The cerclage is easily removed prior to delivery.

3. Infection of the Genitourinary Tract

▶ Scientific Concepts
Pregnant women have a greater risk of developing UTIs. Genitourinary tract infections as well as asymptomatic bacteriuria in pregnancy are associated with low birth weight and preterm labor and are the most common cause of miscarriage during the second trimester of pregnancy. Risk increases with history of recurrent UTI in nonpregnant state and diabetes mellitus. Approximately one-third of all pregnant women with asymptomatic bacteriuria progress to develop pyelonephritis.

▶ History & Physical
Patients may be asymptomatic or complain of urgency, frequency, dysuria without vaginal discharge. Back pain, fever, vomiting, and costovertebral angle tenderness may suggest pyelonephritis.

▶ Diagnostic Studies
Urine dipstick may be positive for leukocyte esterase, nitrite, and protein. Full culture and sensitivity of the urine are indicated, especially in cases of suspected pyelonephritis, even though the results are not likely to change the management plan. Screening for bacteriuria early in pregnancy may be indicated. The most common pathogens in pyelonephritis are *Escherichia coli, Klebsiella, Enterobacter,* or *Proteus.* Staph, strep group B, and *Enterococcus* are less common.

► Diagnosis

Rule out vulvovaginitis and intrauterine infection.

► Clinical Therapeutics

If colony count is > 100,000 colonies/mL of a single pathogen, a 3-day treatment of amoxicillin, ampicillin, or cephalexin, 250 to 500 mg PO q6–8h, with a repeat colony count 10 days later. Positive bacteria after 3-day course of therapy or recurrent infection later in the pregnancy is indication for suppressive prophylaxis with a once-daily dose of antibiotics.

► Clinical Intervention

Asymptomatic bacteriuria, lower UTI, and, in some cases, mild pyelonephritis early in pregnancy may be effectively treated on an outpatient basis. Outpatient management requires that the patient be able to take medications orally. Hospitalization is indicated for patients with moderate to severe pyelonephritis or > 24 weeks' gestation.

► Health Maintenance Issues

Preventive measures include increased water intake, frequent voiding, and proper hygienic practices (wiping from front to back, empty bladder before and after intercourse).

E. Third-Trimester Complications

1. Abruptio Placenta

► Scientific Concepts

Defined as premature separation of the placenta prior to delivery, may be graded as follows (Sher's grades):
1. Minimal or no bleeding, detected as retroplacental clot after delivery of a viable fetus
2. Delivery of viable fetus with bleeding and tender irritable uterus
3a. Delivery of nonviable fetus and no coagulopathy
3b. Delivery of nonviable fetus and coagulopathy

Risk factors include hypertension, cocaine use, trauma, maternal cigarette smoking and alcohol use, uterine decompression, and previous history of abruption.

► History & Physical

Acute-onset vaginal bleeding in the second or third trimester, painful contractions, moderate to severe abdominal or back pain, uterine tenderness, hypertonia, and fetal distress. Blood loss may be concealed; clinical signs of shock may not correlate with degree of vaginal bleeding.

► Diagnostic Studies

Diagnosis is made on clinical suspicion. CBC, platelet count, PT/PTT and fibrinogen levels useful in management. Ultrasound may show sonolucent retroplacental clot, but it is not often definitive; external fetal monitoring to assess fetal well-being.

► **Diagnosis**

Uterine rupture, placenta previa, or labor.

► **Clinical Therapeutics**

Severe abruptio is best managed with rapid delivery via cesarean section. Tocolytics such as terbutaline or oxytocin may be used to manage contractions in mild cases.

► **Clinical Intervention**

Management depends on Sher's grade, with maternal and fetal hemodynamic stabilization of prime importance. If hemodynamically stable, mild abruptio may be monitored, with bedrest until fetus is mature, and vaginal delivery.

► **Health Maintenance Issues**

Abruptio placenta is a medical emergency that requires prompt intervention, maternal stabilization, and assessment of the fetus.

2. Placenta Previa

► **Scientific Concepts**

Characterized by placental implantation in the lower uterine segment, either partially covering the cervical os (partial previa and marginal previa), totally covering the cervical os (total previa), or low-lying placenta where the placental edge is in the lower uterine segment but does not encroach on the internal cervical os. Placenta previa is related to poor uterine vascularization or large placental mass (multiple gestation or hydrops). Incidence increases with previous uterine surgery, leiomyoma, previous placenta previa, multiparity, and advancing maternal age.

► **History & Physical**

Patients present with bright red, painless vaginal bleeding in the second or third trimester. Previa may be identified on routine, early sonogram. Spotting early in pregnancy may suggest previa.

► **Diagnostic Studies**

Transabdominal and transvaginal ultrasound are most useful in locating placenta and degree of previa.

► **Diagnosis**

Rule out abruptio placenta, vas previa, and infection.

► **Clinical Therapeutics**

Observation, education, bedrest, coital restriction, and serial sonograms for placenta position and fetal assessment may be indicated for mild previa. Digital vaginal and/or rectal examination must be avoided so as to avoid digital separation of placenta and uncontrollable hemorrhage. Vaginal delivery may be attempted after 36 weeks' gestation in patients with marginal previa. Hemodynamic stabilization and fetal assessment are primary. Prompt delivery via cesarean section may be indicated if uncorrectable fetal compromise is evident.

► Clinical Intervention

Third-trimester vaginal bleeding is a medical emergency that requires prompt evaluation and management.

► Health Maintenance Issues

Minimization of risk factors.

3. Unspecified Antepartum Hemorrhage

► Scientific Concepts

Obstetric hemorrhage is one of the three leading causes of maternal death and a major cause of perinatal morbidity and mortality. Extrusion of cervical mucus (bloody show) is the most common cause of bleeding late in pregnancy. Most blood loss from placental challenge is maternal, yet fetal loss is also possible. Nonobstetric causes of third-trimester antepartum hemorrhage include cervicitis, cervical erosion, polyps, vaginal laceration, and neoplasia. Obstetric causes include premature separation of placenta (abruptio), placenta previa, uterine rupture, and abnormal clotting mechanisms. Uterine rupture may be traumatic (high-impact accidents) or spontaneous (vigorous labor, version, or following uterine surgery).

► History & Physical

There are no reliable signs of impending uterine rupture. Symptoms of shock related to acute blood loss include pallor, syncope, thirst, dyspnea, restlessness, agitation, anxiety, and confusion. Consider rupture of the uterus with complaints of increased suprapubic pain and tenderness with labor, sudden cessation of uterine contractions, "tearing" sensation, vaginal bleeding, regression of presenting part, and disappearance of fetal heart tones. The abdomen may be firm, painful, or expanding. Palpation may evoke contraction. Fetal heart tone may be muffled, and fetal heart rate may be increased or decreased.

► Diagnostic Studies

Antepartum hemorrhage is a medical emergency that requires prompt evaluation and immediate life support intervention. If patient condition permits, ultrasound is useful in assessing placental position, presence of retroplacental clot, and fetal well-being.

► Diagnosis

Differential includes obstetric and nonobstetric causes of late-pregnancy vaginal bleeding. Uterine rupture may be diagnosed following delivery.

► Clinical Therapeutics

Evaluation of vaginal bleeding in late pregnancy should take place in setting equipped to manage maternal hemorrhage and a compromised neonate. Digital rectal and vaginal exams must not be performed until placenta previa has been ruled out. Acute management efforts include airway management, fluid replacement, and expansion and use of vasoactive drugs if indicated. Laparotomy, cesarean section, or hysterectomy may be indicated.

▶ Clinical Intervention
As above.

▶ Health Maintenance Issues
The complications of ruptured uterus and antepartum hemorrhage include shock, postoperative infection, uterine damage, thrombophlebitis, amniotic fluid embolus, disseminated intravascular coagulation, renal failure, pituitary failure, and death.

F. Other Complications of Pregnancy

1. Postpartum Hemorrhage

▶ Scientific Concepts
Postpartum hemorrhage (blood loss > 500 mL for vaginal delivery or > 1,000 mL for cesarean section) may result from uterine atony (loss of tone and contractility), genital tract laceration, or retained products of conception including placenta. Predisposing factors include prolonged labor, infection, macrosomic infant, uterine overdistention, instrumentation, or utero manipulation.

▶ History & Physical
If vaginal bleeding persists after delivery of the placenta, aggressive intervention should be employed. Signs and symptoms of acute blood loss should be monitored.

▶ Diagnostic Studies
Postpartum hemorrhage is a medical emergency that requires prompt evaluation and immediate life support intervention.

▶ Diagnosis
Cause of bleeding should be identified.

▶ Clinical Therapeutics
Fluid expansion and replacement should be initiated. Oxytocin, 20 to 40 U/L, or methylergonovine, 0.2 mg IM, may be administered if the patient is hypertensive. Intravaginal or rectal prostaglandin suppositories, intrauterine irrigation with prostaglandins, and intramyometrial injection of prostaglandins have been noted to control hemorrhage from uterine atony. Bimanual compression and massage of the uterus and careful exploration of the uterus, with immediate removal of any retained particles and repair of lacerations, should be initiated immediately. Curettage and uterine packing are no longer favorable interventions.

▶ Clinical Intervention
As above.

▶ Health Maintenance Issues
The complications of postpartum hemorrhage include shock, postoperative infection, uterine damage or loss, renal failure, and death.

2. Hypertension in Pregnancy

► Scientific Concepts

Hypertension in pregnancy is characterized by an increase in systolic and/or diastolic blood pressure, > 140/90 mm Hg. Hypertension in pregnancy is idiopathic in 80% of all cases and of real origin in 20%. Hypertension associated with proteinuria (300 mg/24 hours), edema, acute weight gain (> 5 lb/wk) in primigravidas and after 20 weeks' gestation is preeclampsia. Other risk factors for preeclampsia include teenage pregnancy, multiple fetuses, lower socioeconomic status, and positive family history. Eclampsia is preeclampsia with tonic-clonic seizures of no other etiology. Hypertension in pregnancy is more common in women with a prior history of hypertension, women over 30, obesity, multiparity, and those with diabetes or renal disease.

► History & Physical

In addition to elevated blood pressure, patients with preeclampsia as well as those with hypertension in pregnancy may complain of mild headache, visual disturbance, hyperreflexia, apprehension, papilledema, amnesia, oliguria, and epigastric pain. Eclampsia is characterized by worsening of the above symptoms, muscle twitching, seizures, and coma.

► Diagnostic Studies

Repeated blood pressure readings, physical examination to assess for edema, and 24-hour urine for protein are the primary diagnostic studies. Creatinine clearance, aspartate transaminase, bilirubin, and lactic dehydrogenase may also be elevated.

► Diagnosis

Rule out chronic hypertension, pregnancy-induced or worsening hypertension, and underlying renal or renovascular disease.

► Clinical Therapeutics

Methyldopa and hydralazine are the safest and most effective antihypertensives for use during pregnancy. Magnesium sulfate, 4 g IV over 20 to 30 minutes and a maintenance dose of 1 to 2 g IV, is standard therapy for inpatient management of preeclampsia and seizure prophylaxis.

► Clinical Intervention

The primary treatment of preeclampsia and eclampsia is delivery. Beta blockers, angiotensin-converting enzyme (ACE) inhibitors, calcium channel blockers, and thiazide diuretics are contraindicated in pregnancy. Bedrest, increased water intake, and regular blood pressure monitoring may facilitate delay of delivery to more viable fetal age.

► Health Maintenance Issues

Lower blood pressure is of benefit to the mother; there is no direct fetal benefit to blood pressure reduction. Maternal morbidity and mortality due to hypertension in pregnancy are rare in the United States but can cause hemorrhage, stroke, seizures, pulmonary edema, and renal failure.

3. Rhesus Factor (Rh) Incompatibility

► Scientific Concepts

Rh incompatibility or isoimmunization is characterized as incompatibility between the infant's blood type and that of its mother, resulting in destruction of the infant's red blood cells. After delivery, red blood cells of an Rh-positive fetus precipitate development of antibodies against the Rh-positive blood in an Rh-negative mother. In subsequent pregnancies, anti-Rh antibodies cross the placenta and may destroy fetal blood. The resulting anemia may be severe enough to cause fetal death (erythroblastosis fetalis).

► History & Physical

The diagnosis is often made after delivery. Maternal signs during pregnancy include decreased fetal growth and/or movement. Signs in the infant include pallor, jaundice beginning 24 hours after delivery, unexplained bruising, swelling, poor reflex response, and lack of normal movement.

► Diagnostic Studies

Parental history, maternal assessment of Rh factor, and antibody titering are most useful. Amniocentesis may be indicated if maternal antibodies are elevated.

► Diagnosis

Rule out minor group incompatibility.

► Clinical Therapeutics

Treatment generally involves serial measurement of indirect Coombs, antibody titering, fluid replacement, ultraviolet light, vitamin K, and transfusion.

► Clinical Intervention

Anti-Rh gamma globulin (RhoGAM) is given to mother at 28 weeks' gestation and within 72 hours of delivery, abortion, ectopic pregnancy, or miscarriage to prevent formation of antibodies that might affect subsequent pregnancies. Antibody titers may be drawn anytime during the pregnancy.

► Health Maintenance Issues

Infant care, feeding, and prognosis are excellent.

4. Trisomy

► Scientific Concepts

It is now known that spontaneous abortions occurring in the first 8 weeks have a 50% incidence of chromosome abnormalities. Translocation, deletions, and rearrangements during meiosis lead to the loss of chromatin material. Trisomy may occur with any chromosome, with 13, 18, and 21 being the most common trisomic conditions seen in living individuals. Trisomy 21 accounts for 95% of all Down syndrome patients. Seen in the young, incidence increases dramatically with advanced maternal age.

▶ History & Physical

Advanced maternal age, previous history of genetic disorder, or low maternal serum alpha-fetoprotein (MS-AFP) on routine screening suggest further investigation. Diagnosis is often made after delivery.

▶ Diagnostic Studies

Fetal sampling via chorionic villus sampling, amniocentesis, or percutaneous umbilical blood sampling (PUBS) is definitive. Maternal serum beta-hCG in patients with Down syndrome pregnancies is on average two times the value of unaffected pregnancies.

▶ Diagnosis

Rule out central nervous system (CNS) malformation. Elevated MS-AFP at 15 to 18 weeks' gestation (optimal time for assessment) suggests neural tube defect.

▶ Clinical Therapeutics

No specific treatment.

▶ Clinical Intervention

If identified during pregnancy, care should be nondirective and supportive of parental decisions within the legal, ethical, and professional framework.

▶ Health Maintenance Issues

Risk increases with maternal age. Support and individual as well as family counseling are recommended.

5. CNS Malformation in Fetus

▶ Scientific Concepts

Infants with disorders of the CNS, including spina bifida and neural tube defects, tend to have a positive family history, multifactorial inheritance, or recurrence risk. Anencephaly occurs in 50% of neural tube defects. Poor glycemic control increases risk in diabetic patients. Neural tube defects may be incidentally identified during routine sonogram.

▶ History & Physical

Degree of suspicion during pregnancy prompts further evaluation.

▶ Diagnostic Studies

Elevated maternal alpha-fetoprotein warrants further evaluation of amniotic fluid for acetylcholinesterase, which may also be elevated. Patients with increased risk (positive family history, advanced maternal age) are often encouraged to undergo amniocentesis between 16 and 18 weeks or chorionic villus sampling, which may be performed transcervically between 9 and 10 weeks' gestation.

► Diagnosis

Differentiate between nervous system malformations.

► Clinical Therapeutics

No specific treatment.

► Clinical Intervention

Diagnosis, nondirective genetic counseling, and consideration of options. Emergency care involves delivery via cesarean section. If pregnancy is maintained, monitoring for hydrocephalus is indicated.

► Health Maintenance Issues

Genetic and personal counseling are important in reaching future childbearing decisions. Dietary supplementation with folic acid and weight loss in obese patients may reduce the risk of neural tube defects.

6. Multiple Fetuses

► Scientific Concepts

The cause of multiple gestation is unknown in most cases. Women who have borne twins have a 10-fold increased chance of subsequent multiple births. Thirty percent of all twins are monozygotic (resulting from fertilization of a single ovum by a single sperm), and approximately 70% are dizygotic (fraternal twins produced from two separate fertilized ova). Complications of twinning include growth retardation, cord compression, entanglement, abruptio placenta, prematurity, and abnormal presentation and position.

► History & Physical

Diagnosis of twinning is possible in over 75% of cases by physical exam. Signs and symptoms include uterine enlargement greater than expected for dates, excessive maternal weight gain, multiplicity of body parts, polyhydramnios, and recording of multiple fetal heart tones.

► Diagnostic Studies

Most twins are identified by ultrasound. Early consideration of the possibility of multiple pregnancy aids in early diagnosis and early intervention, including glucose management and prevention of prematurity.

► Diagnosis

Multiple pregnancies must be distinguished from large, single pregnancy; date calculation error; polyhydramnios; hydatidiform mole; and abdominal tumors.

► Clinical Therapeutics

No specific medication. Close monitoring of maternal and fetal well-being decreases morbidity and mortality associated with multiple gestation. Premature labor with intact membranes may be effectively treated with tocolytics.

▶ Clinical Intervention

Iron supplementation; high-protein diet; less physical exercise; more bedrest; prompt evaluation of vaginal infections, preeclampsia, or glucose variability; and more frequent antenatal visits improve outcome.

▶ Health Maintenance Issues

Mortality rate of multiple pregnancy is only slightly higher than single gestation. Morbidity and complications (risk of hemorrhage, abnormal presentation, operative delivery, PROM, etc.) are increased. Reduction of the incidence of low-birth-weight infants is the goal in managing multiple gestation.

7. Fetotoxic Exposure

▶ Scientific Concepts

Drug-induced teratology accounts for 2 to 3% of all fetal congenital malformations; most result from genetic, environmental, and unknown causes. Drugs given during pregnancy may alter placental function, produce a lethal or toxic effect on the embryo, or change myometrial activity. Exposure to toxins before the 20th week of gestation may have an all-or-nothing effect (no effect to abortion), sublethal effect (anatomical defect), or metabolic effect, which may manifest later.

▶ History & Physical

History, risk factors, degree of exposure relative to gestational age precipitate investigation. Known teratogens are to be avoided: viruses (rubella); parasites (toxoplasmosis); bacteria (syphilis); heavy metals (mercury); medications such as cancer chemotherapeutic agents, antiepileptics, anticoagulants, antibiotics (tetracycline), as well as alcohol and radiation.

▶ Diagnostic Studies

Intrauterine evaluation is limited to high-resolution sonogram.

▶ Diagnosis

The diagnosis is specific to the condition evaluated.

▶ Clinical Therapeutics

Specific to exposure and evaluation.

▶ Clinical Intervention

Patient education toward avoidance of potential toxin is best intervention.

▶ Health Maintenance Issues

See Clinical Intervention above.

8. Gestational Diabetes

▶ Scientific Concepts

Defined as glucose intolerance identified during pregnancy or antecedent to pregnancy, due to insulin receptor deficiency, decreased response to increased insulin resistance commonly associated with pregnancy, or reduced insulin sensitivity. Maternal obesity is an important predictor of gestational diabetes mellitus as well as associated fetal and neonatal complications.

► History & Physical

Risk increases with maternal weight; higher risk among African Americans, Latinos, Asians, and Native Americans. Other risk factors include advanced maternal age, positive family history, history of previous stillbirth or delivery of an infant weighing over 4,000 g, or history of repeated spontaneous abortions. Fetal complications include fetal macrosomia, which may lead to shoulder dystocia or cephalopelvic disproportion, congenital malformations, neonatal hypoglycemia, hyperbilirubinemia, hypocalcemia, and polycythemia. Polyhydramnios is a common maternal complication that is associated with increased risk of abruptio placenta and preterm labor.

► Diagnostic Studies

Pregnant women at low risk should undergo modified glucose tolerance test (GTT) at 24 to 28 weeks' gestation (50-g oral glucose load with serum glucose testing after 1 hour). If normal, repeat at 28 weeks. Follow-up test for abnormal reading (above 135 to 140) includes 3-hour GTT with blood samples assessed immediately following the glucose load and at 1, 2, and 3 hours. One abnormal reading is suggestive, and two or more abnormal readings are diagnostic for gestational diabetes mellitus.

► Diagnosis

Hemoglobin A_{1c}, home glucose monitoring, ultrasound, 24 hours for protein and creatinine clearance, blood pressure monitoring, and maternal alpha-fetoprotein facilitate diagnosis and management.

► Clinical Therapeutics

Safe dietary habits, including restriction of simple sugars, ingestion of complex carbohydrates and protein, and regular exercise, may preclude the need for pharmacologic therapy. Insulin therapy is generally required in patients who cannot be regulated on diet and exercise alone.

► Clinical Intervention

Close monitoring and tight management of serum glucose levels improve clinical outcome. Blood sugar should be normalized in labor, and serum testing for hyperglycemia postpartum is recommended.

► Health Maintenance Issues

Prepregnancy weight loss in overweight women and prepregnancy screening for high-risk patients may reduce maternal or fetal risks. Patient education, empowerment, and lifestyle changes may improve maternal and fetal outcome.

XII. ROUTINE PRENATAL CARE

► Scientific Concepts

The goal of antenatal care is to achieve the best possible maternal and fetal outcome. Diagnosis of pregnancy with accurate dating, confirmation of intrauterine implantation, and comprehensive data collection including history, physical examination, and appropriate laboratory tests are the first order. Danger signs include any vaginal bleeding, swelling of face or fingers, severe headache, dimness or blurring of vision, abdominal pain, persistent vomiting, fever or chills, dysuria, escape of fluid from the vagina, or marked changes in frequency or intensity of fetal movements.

► History & Physical

Patient may have a variety of common, nonspecific complaints, including nausea, vomiting, fatigue, breast tenderness, urinary changes, and, most commonly, amenorrhea. On physical examination, uterine softening and enlargement, bluish discoloration of the uterus (Chadwick's sign), and softening of the cervix (Hegar's sign) may be evident. Auscultation of fetal heart tone, palpation of fetal parts, and movement are signs of pregnancy > 12 weeks' gestation.

► Diagnostic Studies

Documentation of a positive pregnancy test (serum beta-hCG), CBC, urinalysis, urine culture, blood group and Rh, antibody screen, rubella titer, serologic test for syphilis, hepatitis B surface antigen, sickle cell prep, Pap smear, and cultures for gonorrhea and chlamydia should be completed at the first visit. MS-AFP at 15 to 18 weeks and 50-g glucose screening at 24 to 28 weeks are also recommended. Fetal imaging via ultrasound early in pregnancy and in third trimester is most useful in assessing implantation, gestational age, and fetal growth.

► Diagnosis

Diagnosis of uncomplicated pregnancy versus high-risk pregnancy guides interventions and management.

► Clinical Therapeutics

Prenatal vitamins and iron supplementation are commonly prescribed throughout pregnancy and lactation.

► Clinical Intervention

Patient education; discussion of maternal nutrition, lifestyle adaptations, and exposure to medications, drugs, or other potential toxins; reassurance and surveillance for complications are the mainstay of routine prenatal care.

► Health Maintenance Issues

Uncomplicated pregnancy should be monitored every 4 weeks for the first 32 weeks, every 2 weeks from 32 to 36 weeks, and weekly from 36 weeks until delivery. Each prenatal visit should include assessment of maternal weight, blood pressure, measurement of fundal height, screening for peripheral edema, urinalysis, and assessment of fetal position, movement, and heart tones. Intervention is specific to pathologic change.

XIII. NORMAL LABOR AND DELIVERY

► Scientific Concepts

Labor may be caused by endogenous oxytocin production, prostaglandin release, progesterone withdrawal, or drop in fetal cortisol levels. It is characterized by progressive contractions that occur at decreasing intervals and at increasing intensity, associated with cervical dilatation and effacement (stage I). The second stage of labor begins will full dilatation of the cervix and ends with delivery of the fetus. The third stage involves separation and delivery of the placenta.

► History & Physical

Patient may complain of progressive abdominal, back, pelvic, or thigh pain and nausea/vomiting associated with uterine contractions that may last for 30 to 90 seconds and occur every 1 to 3 minutes. Cervical effacement and dilatation may last up to 20 hours in primigravidas.

► Diagnostic Studies

Evaluation includes history and physical examination; fetal monitoring of heart rate; detection of ruptured membranes; and pelvic exam for staging, fetal presentation, engagement, descent, and assessment of amniotic fluid (nitrazine test and ferning).

► Diagnosis

Diagnosis is made on serial examinations and assessment of normal progression of labor.

► Clinical Therapeutics

Interventions are supportive. Ineffective contractions and failure to progress may be treated with oxytocin. Cephalopelvic disproportion and maternal complications may be treated with cesarean section.

► Clinical Intervention

The benefit of episiotomy to mother or infant has not been proven. Supportive measures during labor such as ambulation, positioning, and deep breathing offer relief to some.

► Health Maintenance Issues

Pregnancy is a normal physiologic process. Efforts toward maintaining a well-balanced diet, moderate exercise, precautions against exposure to toxins, patient education, early and regular prenatal care, and attention to patient and family psychosocial needs improve fetal and maternal outcome and patient's sense of well-being.

BIBLIOGRAPHY

Beckmann C, Ling F, Herbert W, et al. *Obstetrics and Gynecology,* 3rd ed. Philadelphia: Williams & Wilkins; 1998.

Crump W. UTIs in pregnancy: A case-based report, *Family Practice Recertification* 21(10):45–52; 1999.

Dambro M. *Griffith's 5-Minute Clinical Consultant.* Philadelphia: Lippincott/Williams & Wilkins; 1999.

DeCherney AM, Pernoll ML. *Current, Obstetric and Gynecologic Diagnosis and Treatment,* 8th ed. East Norwalk, CT: Appleton & Lange; 1994.

Dixon D, Rayz S, White G. Gestational diabetes mellitus: An update and review for primary care providers. *Physician Assistant.* (March):28–35; 1999.

Goldberg J. *The Instant Exam Review for the USMLE Step 3,* 2nd ed. Stamford, CT: Appleton & Lange; 1997.

Goroll A, May L, Mulley A Jr. *Primary Care Medicine: Office Evaluation and Management of the Adult Patient,* 3rd ed. Philadelphia: JB Lippincott; 1995.

Gries-Griffin J. Abnormal Pap test results, *Advance/PA;* July 1995.

Hutchins FL Jr. Fibroids in Primary Care, *The Clinical Advisor;* September 1998.

Keene GF. Office gynecology, common reproductive disorders, *Clin Rev* 9(1):58–80; 1999.

Miller H, McEvers J, Griffith J. *Instructions for Obstetric and Gynecologic Patients,* 2nd ed. Philadelphia: WB Saunders; 1997.

Moyers-Scott P. Performing cervical polypectomy, *JAAPA* 12(6):81–91; 1999.

Raplin A, Laghlin D. Guidlines for diagnosis and treatment of premenstrual syndrome. *Family Practice Recertification.* 21(1):41–68; 1999.

Stoffey W. Using medications safely in pregnancy, *PA Today;* (September 28):11–15; 1998.

Endocrinology 10

Dana S. Martin, MS, PA-C

I. DISEASES OF THE THYROID GLAND

A. Hyperthyroidism

▶ Scientific Concepts

Autoimmune; cause unknown; 15% of patients have family members with same disorder. Peak age is 20 to 40 years. Female:male ratio is 5:1. Graves' disease is an autoimmune disorder found particularly in the young, which is responsible for 80% of hyperthyroidism cases. Toxic multinodular goiter is a common cause of thyrotoxicosis in the elderly. Iodine-induced hyperthyroidism may be precipitated by medications. Subacute thyroiditis is characterized by a painful, tender goiter with transient hyperthyroidism. Antibodies (TSH-R Ab [stim]) develop against thyroid-stimulating hormone (TSH) receptor site in the thyroid cell membrane and stimulate the thyroid cell to increase growth and function. Pregnancy, iodide excess, lithium therapy, glucocorticoid withdrawal, bacterial or viral infections may trigger the acute episode. In thyroid storm, the number of catecholamine binding sites may be increased in heart and nerve tissues, causing increased sensitivity to circulating catecholamines. The number of catecholamines may be elevated secondary to severe illness.

▶ History & Physical

Palpitations, nervousness, easy fatigability, hyperkinesia, diarrhea, excessive sweating, heat intolerance, weight loss without loss of appetite, mild tachycardia, dyspnea on exertion, tremor, thyroid enlargement, muscle weakness and atrophy, proptosis, onycholysis, and pretibial myxedema may be present. In thyroid storm, there is acute exacerbation of all symptoms of thyrotoxicosis marked by hypermetabolism and excessive adrenergic response, which may culminate in hyperpyrexia, heart failure, shock, coma, or death. This commonly occurs after surgery, radioactive iodine therapy, or parturition in a patient with inadequately controlled thyrotoxicosis or during a severe illness such as uncontrolled diabetes, trauma, acute infection, severe drug reaction, or myocardial infarction.

▶ Diagnostic Studies

Elevated free thyroxine (FT_4) and suppressed TSH and proptosis or pretibial myxedema support the diagnosis of Graves' disease. If proptosis or myxedema not present, continue evaluation by obtaining radioiodine uptake. If uptake is high, consider Graves' or toxic nodular goiter. If uptake is low, consider subacute thyroiditis, acute-phase Hashimoto's thyroiditis, Graves' disease, or toxic nodular goiter in iodine-loaded patient. In thyroid storm, serum thyroxine (T_4), FT_4, and triiodothyronine (T_3) are elevated. TSH is suppressed. Refer to Table 10-1 for further information concerning the diagnostic approach to the evaluation of hyperthyroidism.

▶ Diagnosis

Differential diagnosis of thyrotoxicosis:

Toxic adenoma (Plummer's disease): Benign neoplasm localized to one

DISEASES OF THE THYROID GLAND

► table 10-1

DIAGNOSTIC APPROACH TO EVALUATION OF HYPERTHYROIDISM

Condition	History or Physical Exam	Serum Free T$_4$	Serum-Sensitive TSH	Further Evaluation
Normal	Normal	Normal	Normal	
Hyperthyroidism 2° severe illness	Clinically hyperthyroid	↓	Normal or ↓	↓ T$_3$
T$_3$ thyrotoxicosis	Clinically hyperthyroid	↓	Normal or ↓	↑ T$_3$ and ↑ RAIU scan
Ingestion of liothyronine (Cytomel)	Clinically hyperthyroid	↓	Normal or ↓	↑ T$_3$ and ↓ RAIU scan
Hyperthyroidism	Thyroid gland enlarged or normal	↑	↓	
Thyrotoxicosis factitia	Thyroid gland not enlarged	↑	↓	↓ RAIU scan ↓ Serum thyroglobulin
Subacute thyroiditis	Thyroid gland tender	↑	↓	↓ RAIU scan ↑ Serum thyroglobulin

T$_4$, thyroxine; TSH, thyroid-stimulating hormone; T$_3$, triiodothyronine; RAIU, radioactive iodine uptake; ↑, increased; ↓, decreased.

lobe of the thyroid. "Hot" nodule on thyroid scan is easily treated with antithyroid medications.

Toxic multinodular goiter: Characteristically occurs in older patient with long-standing multinodular goiter.

Subacute or chronic thyroiditis: Tender, painful goiter is noted. Mild to severe thyrotoxicosis is caused by acute release of T$_3$ and T$_4$. Radioiodide uptake is diminished. The condition spontaneously subsides over 2 to 3 weeks.

Thyrotoxicosis factitia: Caused by the ingestion of excessive amounts of T$_4$ or thyroid hormone usually for weight control. Thyroid exam is normal.

► **Clinical Therapeutics**

Antithyroid drugs (propylthiouracil or methimazole) most useful in the young with small glands and mild disease. Give until spontaneous remission of disease occurs. Relapse rate is 60 to 80%. Monitor course of therapy with FT$_4$ and TSH levels. Duration of therapy is 6 months to 20+ years. Subtotal thyroidectomy is recommended for those with large thyroid glands or multinodular goiters. Complications are recurrent laryngeal nerve injury and hypoparathyroidism (~ 1% of cases). Use radioactive sodium iodide I^{131} for those older than 21. The thyroid gland shrinks and patient becomes euthyroid in 6 to 12 weeks. Eighty percent develop hypothyroidism. Follow serum FT$_4$ and TSH levels. Replacement therapy with levothyroxine PRN. In pregnancy, radioactive iodine is contraindicated. May use propylthiouracil and subtotal thyroidectomy. Beta-adrenergic blocking agents alleviate tachycardia, hypertension, and atrial fibrillation. Multivitamin, phenobarbital, ipodate sodium or iopanoic acid, and cholestyramine are indicated.

► **Clinical Intervention**

Thyroid storm: Administer propranolol to control arrhythmias or verapamil for severe heart failure in the presence of asthma or arrhythmia, propylthiouracil or methimazole, sodium or potassium iodide, acetaminophen, fluids, electrolytes, and nutritional support. Use a cooling blanket. Treat underlying and/or precipitating disease.

► Health Maintenance Issues

Frequent remissions and exacerbations over a protracted period of time result in the need for definitive treatment by thyroidectomy or radioactive iodine. Afterwards, most remain euthyroid for some time but eventually become hypothyroid.

B. Hypothyroidism

► Scientific Concepts

Hypometabolic state caused by decrease or lack of thyroid hormone. Hypothyroidism is divided according to the following classifications: primary (thyroid failure), secondary (pituitary TSH deficit), tertiary (deficient hypothalamic thyroid-releasing hormone [TRH]), peripheral (resistance to the action of thyroid hormones). Primary hypothyroidism causes 90% of cases. Chronic autoimmune (Hashimoto's) thyroiditis is the most common cause in the United States and occurs with or without goiter. Other common causes include I^{131} therapy and thyroid surgery. Congenital hypothyroidism occurs in 1:4,000 newborns. In adults > 65 years, the frequency is 2 to 4%. In the general population, the frequency is 0.5 to 1.0%.

► History & Physical

Fatigue, weakness, weight gain (> 15 lb.), hoarseness, constipation, depression, slowed mentation, muscle cramps, menstrual irregularities, and/or infertility occur. Firm goiter with multiple nodular or a nonpalpable gland; bradycardia and distant heart sounds; myxedema; slow, hoarse, husky speech; cool, dry, thick, yellow-colored skin (carotenemia) and loss of scalp hair and eyebrows; puffy face and hands; dull facial expression; shallow, slow respirations; delayed relaxation of deep tendon reflexes; cerebellar ataxia; diminished memory and hearing; peripheral neuropathy and parasthesias; carpal tunnel syndrome are physical examination findings.

► Diagnostic Studies

Elevated TSH and total or decreased FT_4 indicate primary hypothyroidism. Evaluate thyroid autoantibodies. Presence of antithyroglobulin antibodies is confirmatory for Hashimoto's.

Refer to Table 10-2 for further information concerning the diagnostic approach to the evaluation of hypothyroidism.

► Clinical Therapeutics

Initiate low doses of levothyroxine and titrate dosage from 25 to 100 µg/d every 4 to 6 weeks according to supersensitive TSH assay and clinical response. Use lower starting dose in cardiac disease since this may exacerbate angina. Concomitant administration of cholestyramine, antacids, and/or iron supplements interfere with absorption of levothyroxine.

▶ table 10-2

DIAGNOSTIC APPROACH TO EVALUATION OF HYPOTHYROIDISM

Condition	History or Physical Exam	Serum Free T$_4$	Serum-Sensitive TSH	Further Evaluation
Normal	Normal	Normal	Normal	
Primary hypothyroidism	Commonly mild symptoms, frank myxedema occurs rarely	↓	↑	
Hashimoto's thyroiditis, postpartum thyroid dysfunction or recovery from severe illness	Goiter noted frequently in Hashimoto's thyroiditis	Normal or ↓	↑	Antithyroglobulin antibodies detected in 90% of those with Hashimoto's thyroiditis
Secondary hypothyroidism (hypopituitarism)	Clinically hypothyroid	↓	Normal or ↓	
TSH suppression 2° to dopamine or corticosteroids	Clinically hypothyroid or euthyroid	↓	Normal or ↓	TRH test or serial monitoring of TSH and Free T$_4$

T$_4$, thyroxine; TSH thyroid-stimulating hormone; TRH, thyroid-releasing hormone; ↑, increased; ↓, decreased.

▶ Clinical Intervention

Be alert for altered mental status culminating in coma, compromised ventilation, hypothermia, cardiomyopathy, and/or ataxia.

▶ Health Maintenance Issues

Repeat T$_1$ and TSH every 6 weeks until therapeutic response to levothyroxine is achieved. Repeat T$_4$ and TSH annually. Average maintenance dosage is 100 to 150 μg/d in adults. Increase dose of levothyroxine by 25% for pregnant and lactating patients. Gradually decrease levothyroxine dosage in aging patients to 50 to 75 μg/d.

C. Neoplasms of the Thyroid

▶ Scientific Concepts

Thyroid cancer is rare. Incidence is 0.004% in the United States. Most thyroid nodules are benign. Female:male ratio is 4:1. Majority of cases occur in those > 60 years old. Common presentation is a single nodule in the thyroid or large nodule in multinodular gland. The four major types of thyroid carcinomas are papillary, follicular, medullary, and anaplastic.

Papillary carcinoma makes up 70% of cases and is more likely to be found in females in their second or third decade of life. It is slow growing.

Follicular carcinoma comprises 15% of all thyroid malignancies. It is more aggressive than papillary carcinoma and has an increasing incidence with age.

Medullary carcinoma comprises 5% of all thyroid malignancies. It occurs either as a sporadic unifocal lesion in the elderly or as a bilateral lesion in combination with pheochromocytoma and hyperparathyroidism (multiple endocrine neoplasia type II [MEN II]), which is an inherited and autosomal dominant disorder.

Anaplastic carcinoma comprises 1% of all thyroid malignancies and is the most aggressive form of thyroid cancer. It is differentiated into two histologic types: giant cell and small cell. Patients with small cell have a 20% survival rate at 5 years. In those diagnosed with giant cell, death occurs within 6 months after diagnosis.

► History & Physical

The typical benign thyroid nodule is found in the older female with a family history of goiter who resides in area of endemic goiter. On physical examination, soft thyroid nodules are noted in the presence of multinodular goiter. The typical malignant thyroid nodule is found in a patient with a family history of medullary cancer, history of recent thyroid growth, and/or head and neck irradiation as a child. On physical examination, a palpable, solitary, firm, or dominant nodule that is inconsistent with the remaining glandular tissue is noted. Late-stage findings include vocal cord paralysis, lymphadenopathy, and/or metastasis to lung or bone.

► Diagnostic Studies

Perform fine-needle aspiration. If cytology shows benign cells, no further evaluation is required. If tissue is malignant or suggestive of malignancy on histocytopathologic exam, evaluate with the following studies: T_4, TSH, and thyroid antibodies: used to rule out the "lumpy" thyroid of Hashimoto's thyroiditis. Ultrasound distinguishes cystic nodules (benign) from semicystic or solid (malignant). Scanning techniques with ^{123}I or [99]m TcO_4 differentiate "hot" nodules (benign) from "cold" nodules (malignant). Suppression therapy with T_4 causes regression of a benign nodule, while malignant nodules remain unchanged. Serum calcitonin is elevated in thyroid cancer. Serum thyroglobulin is elevated after total thyroidectomy for papillary or follicular thyroid cancer and suggests metastatic disease.

► Diagnosis

The only definitive way to diagnose carcinoma of the thyroid is histologically, since every other test has limitations in accuracy.

► Clinical Therapeutics

Hashimoto's thyroiditis requires lifelong replacement of thyroid hormone. Use levothyroxine, 2 to 3 µg/kg/d (average dose 150 to 200 µg/d), to correct and prevent hypothyroidism.

► Clinical Intervention

In malignancy, lobectomy or thyroidectomy is performed. If nodule is < 2 cm, lobectomy is performed. Thyroidectomy is performed if nodule > 2 cm along with modified neck dissection for lymph nodes if metastasis is suspected. Postoperative radioiodide scan for nodule is > 2 cm or intra- or extrathyroid extension suspected. Initiate Cytomel, 50 to 100 µg/d × 4 weeks. Discontinue medication for 2 weeks and then decrease iodide in the diet. Using radioactive iodide, rescan. If residual radioactive iodine uptake occurs, then radioactive iodine is an effective treatment. If tumors fail to concentrate radioactive iodine, use local radiotherapy. Repeat scan annually until no further uptake is observed. Maintain on levothyroxine, 0.15 to 0.3 mg daily, to suppress TSH to undetectable levels. Medullary cancer is treated similarly. Follow serum calcitonin or carcinoembryonic antigen (CEA) levels. Screen family members for receptor tyrosine kinase (RET) oncogene. Anaplastic cancer is treated with isthmectomy and palliative radiotherapy. Staging predicts outcomes.

▶ Health Maintenance Issues

Levothyroxine given for TSH suppression. Evaluate supersensitive TSH to determine if the patient is receiving enough hormone replacement. Inquire about bone pain, headaches, and cough at 6-month to 1-year intervals. Examine for lymph node metastasis or recurrent thyroid mass. Monitor serum thyroglobulin level after thyroidectomy and rescan if increased levels are found since this may indicate cancer. Obtain a chest x-ray annually.

II. PARATHYROID DISEASE

▶ Scientific Concepts

Primary hyperparathyroidism caused by increased parathyroid hormone (PTH) secretion by single parathyroid adenoma (80%) or hyperplasia of all four glands (15%). Incidence is 42 per 100,000. Prevalence is 4 per 100 in females > 60 years of age. Female:male ratio is 4:1. Common feature of all hypercalcemic disorders (except for milk-alkali syndrome) is increased bone resorption of calcium. To a lesser extent, increased gastrointestinal (GI) absorption and decreased renal excretion of calcium contribute to disorders associated with hypercalcemia.

▶ History & Physical

Family history of hypercalcemia or renal stones and multiple endocrine neoplasia (MEN type I or IIa). Patients are usually asymptomatic; however, they may present with central nervous system complaints including fatigue, lethargy, difficulty concentrating, depression, personality changes, weakness, proximal neuropathy, psychosis, ataxia, or stupor. Renal complaints include nocturia, polyuria, polydipsia, or stones. GI complaints include nausea, vomiting, anorexia, or constipation. Be alert for cardiovascular complaints of bradycardia, which may lead to asystole. Mnemonic: stones, bones, abdominal groans, and psychiatric moans.

▶ Diagnostic Studies

Calcium (elevated), phosphorus (low to normal), alkaline phosphatase (increased or normal), renal function (decreased), urine calcium and parathyroid hormone levels with immunoradiometric assay (increased in primary hyperparathyroidism). Glomerular filtration decreased. Electrocardiogram (ECG) shows shortened QT interval. Radiographs show subperiosteal resorption of cortical bone in phalanges.

▶ Diagnosis

Metastatic carcinoma: Second most common cause of hypercalcemia. Sources of metastatic cancers in decreasing frequency are lung, breast, and multiple myeloma. They account for > 50% of tumors that cause hypercalcemia. The PTH assay is suppressed.

Familial benign hypocalciuric hypercalcemia: Autosomal dominant, life-long asymptomatic hypercalcemia detectable in cord blood. Marked by hypocalciuria. Diagnosis is unequivocal because serum calcium, phosphate, alkaline phosphatase, urine calcium, and parathyroid hormone levels overlap with those of primary hypoparathyroidism. Avoid unnecessary parathyroidectomy.

Multiple endocrine neoplasia types I and IIa: May occur as part of three different familial (autosomal dominant) endocrinopathies: MEN I, which includes tumors of the pituitary and pancreas (insulinoma, gastrinoma); MEN IIa, which includes hyperparathyroidism, pheochromocytoma, and medullary thyroid cancer; and isolated familial hyperparathyroidism.

Endocrine tumors: Uncomplicated pheochromocytoma produces parathyroid hormone-related peptide (PTHrp) from tumor. Tumors secreting vasoactive intestinal peptide (VIPoma) associated with hypercalcemia result from activation of PTH/PTHrp receptors.

Endocrinopathies:

- *Thyrotoxicosis:* Mild hypercalcemia occurs in 25% of thyrotoxic patients. PTH is suppressed.
- *Adrenal insufficiency:* Hypercalcemia is a feature of acute adrenal crisis.

Lithium therapy: Limits the inhibition of PTH secretion and causes hypercalcemia and hypocalciuria. Levels of PTH detectable or elevated. May unmask primary hyperparathyroidism. Psychiatric condition is not alleviated by parathyroidectomy.

Sarcoidosis and other granulomatous disorders: Ectopic production of $1,25(OH)_2D$ in macrophages of sarcoid tissue causes increased serum calcium. Serum phosphate, alkaline phosphatase, and urine calcium are normal or elevated. Level of PTH is suppressed. Other disorders include histoplasmosis, pulmonary eosinophilic granulomatosis, and untreated tuberculosis.

Thiazide diurectic therapy: Chlorthalidone, metolazone, and indapamide produce mild transient hypercalcemia not explained by hemoconcentration. Underlying primary hyperparathyroidism becomes persistent when exacerbated by thiazides.

Vitamin D and vitamin A excess: Vitamin D dosage > 50,000 IU daily causes increased calcium absorption and increased bone resorption. PTH is suppressed. Serum 25-hydroxyvitamin D levels are 5 to 10 times normal. Vitamin A, 50,000 to 200,000 IU qd, causes symptoms of lassitude, cheilitis, headache, anorexia, glossitis, scaly puritic rash, hepatomegaly and bone pain, elevated serum vitamin A and calcium.

Milk-alkali syndrome: This pure absorptive hypercalcemia is caused by ingestion of excessive amounts of milk, calcium supplements, or absorptive antacids. The chronic condition is associated with soft tissue calcification of kidneys and nephrocalcinosis. Renal insufficiency may ultimately occur.

► Clinical Therapeutics

Suppress PTH secretion to reduce bone resorption with calcitonin. More aggressive therapy may be indicated with pamidronate (bisphosphonates inhibit osteoclast bone resorption). Use plicamycin for refractory patients. Glucocorticoids are the first line for multiple myeloma, lymphoma, sarcoidosis, or intoxication with vitamin A or D. Medications for chronic hypercalcemia include glucocorticoids, oral phosphates, and indomethacin.

► Clinical Intervention

Hydrate with intravenous (IV) normal saline. Initiate diuresis with IV furosemide. Monitor and replace potassium and magnesium. Maintain a high daily intake of fluids (3 to 5 L/d) and of sodium chloride (> 400 mEq/d) to increase renal calcium excretion unless contraindicated. Decrease or discontinue digitalis dosage since hypercalcemia potentiates digitalis toxicity. Discontinue vitamins A and D, estrogens, antiestrogens, and thiazide diuretics. Decrease dietary calcium and vitamin D. Increase weight-bearing mobility of patients confined to bed.

Surgical parathyroidectomy is the definitive treatment of primary hyperparathyroidism. In the presence of a single large parathyroid gland, suspect adenoma and remove the enlarged gland and biopsy other glands. When multiple enlarged glands are present, suspect parathyroid hyperplasia and perform a 3 1/2-gland parathyroidectomy (this allows for a sufficient remnant to prevent hypocalcemia). Complications include damaged recurrent laryngeal nerve and inadvertent removal and/or devitalization of all parathyroid tissue, resulting in hypocalcemia. Treat hypocalcemia with IV or PO calcium and vitamin D if necessary.

► Health Maintenance Issues

Prevent osteoporosis, kidney stones, and compromised kidney function. High recurrence rates of hypercalcemia are associated with parathyroid hyperplasia.

III. DIABETES AND RELATED DISORDERS

A. Diabetes Type I (Insulin-Dependent Diabetes Mellitus)

► Scientific Concepts

Primarily affects juveniles (< 25 years of age), but occasionally nonobese adults. The majority of cases occur without genetic predisposition. A familial association is found in 10% of cases. There is a 30 to 50% concordance in monozygotic twins. Diabetes type I patients comprise 8% of all patients with diabetes in the United States. There is a paucity of insulin secondary to failure of pancreatic beta cells. Autoimmune component related to human lymphocyte antigen (HLA)-DR3 and HLA-DR4. Virus or environmental insult triggers immune response that alters pancreatic beta cell antigens or molecules of the beta cell. Beta cell function is affected by mumps and coxsackie B4 virus, toxic chemical agents, cytotoxins, or antibodies released by sensitized immunocytes.

► **History & Physical**

Sudden onset (1 to 3 weeks). Commonly symptomatic with polyuria, polydipsia, weakness or fatigue, polyphagia with weight loss, and nocturnal enuresis. May also present with recent blurred vision, vulvovaginitis or pruritus, peripheral neuropathy, or diabetic ketoacidosis (DKA).

► **Diagnostic Studies**

Fasting blood sugar $\geq$ 140 mg/dL on two occasions or sustained increase of plasma glucose $\geq$ 200 mg/dL after 75 g oral glucose load and one other value $\geq$ 200 prior to 2 hours following oral glucose load. Insulin levels measure none to low. Blood glucose usually 300 to 500 mg/dL at presentation. Plasma glucagon levels are increased. Ketonemia and/or ketonuria present.

► **Diagnosis**

Other causes of diabetes include hormonal excess (Cushing's syndrome, acromegaly, glucagonoma, pheochromocytoma), medications (glucocorticoids, diuretics, or oral contraceptives), insulin receptor unavailability, pancreatic disease (pancreatitis, pancreatectomy, hemochromatosis), genetic syndromes (hyperlipidemias, myotonic dystrophy, lipoatrophy), or gestational diabetes.

► **Clinical Therapeutics**

Insulin therapy with split dosing of regular and neutral protamine Hagedorn (NPH) insulin bid. Adjust according to monitored values.

► **Clinical Intervention**

Follow American Diabetes Association diet, which allows calorie portion according to the following guidelines: 50% carbohydrates, 30% fat, and 20% protein. Maintain cholesterol intake at < 300 mg/d and sodium intake at < 3,000 mg/d. Reduce animal and saturated fats. Consume smaller portions more frequently (6 to 7 small meals per day). Achieve and maintain ideal weight. Increase exercise cautiously to prevent hypoglycemic episodes. Monitor blood glucose at 5:00 P.M. and 9:00 P.M. Acceptable control:

80–130 mg/dL fasting blood sugar (FBS) and preprandial
< 180 mg/dL 1 hour postprandial
< 150 mg/dL 2 hours postprandial

Hemoglobin A_{1c} (HbA_{1c}) < 2% above upper limits of normal with slightly higher upper limits for elderly.

► **Health Maintenance Issues**

End-organ damage results in hypertension, renal failure, blindness, autonomic and peripheral neuropathy, lower extremity amputations, myocardial infarction, cerebrovascular accidents, and early demise. Forty percent develop end-stage renal disease, a major cause of death. Dyslipidemia is common. Provide patient education concerning maintenance of ideal weight, annual ophthalmologic exams, podiatric exams, blood pressure evaluations, serum blood urea nitrogen/creatinine (BUN/Cr), and urinalysis.

B. Diabetes Type II (Non–Insulin-Dependent Diabetes Mellitus)

▶ Scientific Concepts

Type II diabetes accounts for 85 to 90% of the diabetic population. Resistance to insulin is accompanied by decreased beta cell function, causing diminished insulin production. Chronic hyperinsulinemic state exists to work against the peripheral resistance. Eventually, beta cells are unable to maintain this state and decrease in function leading to diabetic state. Endogenous insulin production is usually adequate to avoid ketoacidosis; however, DKA may accompany intense stress. Environmental factors include obesity, diet, physical activity, intrauterine environment, and stress.

▶ History & Physical

Onset occurs typically at age > 40 years. Obesity present in 80 to 90% of affected individuals. Strong familial genetic predisposition exists with 100% concordance in monozygotic twins. No association with autoimmune disease. In decreasing frequency, ethnic groups show a predisposition: Native American, Mexican American, African American, white.

Gradual onset (weeks to months); presenting symptoms include polyuria, polyphagia, polydipsia, and/or blurry vision, and one or more neurological or vascular complications of the disease.

▶ Diagnostic Studies

Patients with type II diabetes are not ketosis prone under basal condition and do not require exogenous insulin for short-term survival. The following laboratory criteria must be met: FBS ≥ 140 mg/dL on two occasions or sustained increase of plasma glucose ≥ 200 mg/dL after 75 g oral glucose load and one other value ≥ 200 mg/dL prior to 2 hours following oral glucose load. Random blood sugar at presentation is typically 300 to 1,000 mg/dL. Insulin levels may be low, normal, or high.

▶ Diagnosis

Other causes of diabetes include hormonal excess (Cushing's syndrome, acromegaly, glucagonoma, pheochromocytoma), medications (glucocorticoids, diuretics, or oral contraceptives), insulin receptor unavailability, pancreatic disease (pancreatitis, pancreatectomy, hemochromatosis), genetic syndromes (hyperlipidemias, myotonic dystrophy, lipoatrophy), or gestational diabetes.

▶ Clinical Therapeutics

Initiate oral agents after failure of clinical intervention. Sulfonylureas stimulate insulin release from beta cells and may increase number of insulin receptors on hepatocytes, thus improving glucose uptake by skeletal muscle and adipose tissue. Expect reduction in blood glucose by 70 to 80 mg/dL. Side effects include severe hypoglycemia secondary to drug interactions with salicylates, sulfonamides, warfarin, phenylbutazone, and diphenylhydantoin. Sulfonylureas are contraindicated in pregnancy. Biguanides decrease hepatic gluconeogenesis. They are ideal for obese patients who have failed maximal sulfonylurea therapy. Fasting and postprandial hyperglycemia and hypertriglyceridemia is improved in the obese without the associated weight gain of insulin or sulfonylurea therapy. Side effects include GI upset, lactic acidosis, and decreased B_{12} absorption. Biguanides are contraindicated in insulin-dependent diabetes mellitus (IDDM); lactic acidosis prone; renal, cardiorespiratory, or hepatic insufficiency; alcoholics; and elderly. Alpha-glucosidase inhibitors decrease postprandial hyperglycemia by decreasing the rate of absorption of most carbohydrates by binding more readily to intestinal disaccharidases than digested carbohydrate products. They are insulin sparing. Common side effect is flatulence.

▶ Clinical Intervention

In crisis, insulin is used to treat severe hyperglycemia, hypertriglyceridemia, ketosis, or hyperosmolarity. If patients fail to achieve fasting plasma glucose of 140 mg/dL; become symptomatic with a postprandial plasma glucose > 250 mg/dL; experience major trauma, stress, or surgery, insulin is often required. Insulin is indicated for pregnant diabetics who are not diet controlled.

Lifestyle changes involve decreasing calorie intake in order to achieve and maintain ideal weight. Portion calories accordingly: 50% carbohydrates, 30% fat, 20% protein. Reduce cholesterol intake to < 300 mg/d and sodium intake to < 3,000 mg/d. Reduce animal and saturated fats. Exercise after meals or snacks with attention to blood glucose monitoring. Medications are second-line therapy after dietary changes and weight reduction fail to normalize blood glucose levels.

▶ Health Maintenance Issues

End-organ damage results in hypertension, renal failure, blindness, autonomic and peripheral neuropathy, atherosclerosis, and triglyceridemia. Dyslipidemia is common. Provide patient education concerning maintenance of ideal weight, annual ophthalmologic exams, podiatric exams, blood pressure evaluations, serum BUN/Cr, and urinalysis. Follow HbA_{1c} values after adequate glucose control is achieved.

C. Hyperosmolar Hyperglycemic Nonketotic Coma

▶ Scientific Concepts

More common in middle-aged or elderly with or without mild or occult type II diabetes. Coexisting congestive heart failure or renal insufficiency is common. Episodes are precipitated by infection (pneumonia, urinary tract infection, or gram-negative sepsis), cerebrovascular accident, myocardial infarction, severe burns, subdural hematoma, acute pancreatitis, use of concentrated glucose solutions, or medications (thiazides, furosemide, phenytoin, diazoxide, glucocorticoids, propranolol, or azathioprine). Associated with endocrine disorders (Cushing's disease, acromegaly, thyrotoxicosis).

Hyperglycemia, hyperglucagonemia, and increased hepatic glucose occur secondary to partial or relative insulin insufficiency. Glycosuria and osmotic diuresis with obligatory water loss ensues. Insulin levels are high enough to prevent lipolysis and ketogenesis but fail to prevent hyperglysuria. Fluid intake is inadequate. Renal insufficiency develops as plasma volume contracts, resulting in increased serum glucose and osmolarity leading to altered state of consciousness.

► History & Physical

Onset is insidious (days to weeks). Weakness, polydipsia, polyuria, weight loss, progressively diminishing level of consciousness, and hyperreflexia and/or generalized areflexia may occur along with evidence of dehydration.

► Diagnostic Studies

Blood glucose 600 to 2,000 mg/dL; serum osmolality > 350 mOsm/L; elevated BUN; sodium and potassium normal, high, or low; ketones normal or mildly increased.

► Diagnosis

Distinguish from DKA, which generally occurs in younger, more acidotic patients with type I diabetes. Those with hyperosmolar hyperglycemic nonketotic coma (HHNC) are less dehydrated and rarely comatose in comparison to those with DKA.

► Clinical Therapeutics

Admit to intensive care unit (ICU) and monitor clinical and laboratory response to therapy, recording fluid type and amount, urine output, blood pressure, pulse, central venous pressure, and ECG.
Fluid replacement: Isotonic saline for circulatory collapse, then use 0.45% saline. When blood glucose falls to 250 mg/dL, use 5% dextrose in 0.45 or 0.9% saline.
Insulin: If fluid replacement alone is inadequate to decrease glucose, initiate regular insulin, 15 units IV or IM. Subsequently, give regular insulin, 10 to 25 units q4h IM or IV until stable. Then give insulin subcutaneously until oral hypoglycemics are tolerated.

► Clinical Intervention

Evaluate underlying cause with chest x-ray, cardiac enzymes, and serial ECGs. Perform a sepsis evaluation and provide empiric coverage.

► Health Maintenance Issues

Mortality in HHNC is 10 times that of DKA since it primarily occurs in the elderly. Manage chronic diabetes and recognize and prevent predisposing factors and/or conditions.

D. Hypoglycemia

► Scientific Concepts

Hypoglycemic unawareness: Chronic IDDM patients lose counterregulatory hormone secretion, especially glucagon and epinephrine, in response to hypoglycemia. Glucose levels at which a patient perceives symptoms can change. Patients under tight glucose control tend to experience symptoms at lower levels, which gives them less time to respond between onset of symptoms and loss of consciousness. Autonomic neuropathy leads to loss of sympathoadrenal response. *Fasting hypoglycemia* may result from increased insulin, sulfonylureas, or as a side effect of beta blockers, salicylates, or ethanol. In the presence of nonbeta cell tumors, hepatic failure, chronic renal failure, adrenal insufficiency, renal failure, insulin autoantibodies, insulin receptor autoantibodies, hormonal deficiency (epinephrine, growth hormone, and glucocorticoids), and/or sepsis, hypoglycemia may occur. *Postprandial hypoglycemia* occurs after gastrectomy and in malabsorption syndromes.

▶ History & Physical
Reactive hypoglycemia occurs in response to a meal, specific nutrients, or a drug. It is the most common type of hypoglycemia. Symptoms occur 2 to 4 hours after a meal. The adrenergic response causes symptoms of sweating, tremor, palpitations, anxiety, and hunger. The neuroglucogenic response causes symptoms of headache, dizziness, blurry vision, confusion, decreased fine motor skills, abnormal behavior, seizure, and loss of consciousness. **Spontaneous hypoglycemia** occurs in the fasting state. **Nocturnal hypoglycemia** causes violent nightmares, vivid bizarre dreams, night sweats, and/or headache on awakening in morning, poor sleep, feeling unrested, seizure, and/or coma. **Hypoglycemic unawareness** in type I diabetics is particularly dangerous because it is asymptomatic.

▶ Diagnostic Studies
Hypoglycemia is diagnosed when the fasting plasma glucose is < 60 mg/dL or nonfasting plasma glucose is < 50 mg/dL, accompanied by symptoms consistent with hypoglycemia that improves upon administration of IV glucose or ingestion of food (Whipple's triad).

▶ Diagnosis
Evaluate for hypothyroidism, adrenal insufficiency, nephropathy, and malabsorption syndrome. Insulinoma is likely when C peptide level is elevated.

▶ Clinical Therapeutics
Carbohydrate ingestion alleviates symptoms. Frequent blood glucose self-monitoring is recommended.

▶ Clinical Intervention
Give IV glucose immediately or carbohydrates.

▶ Health Maintenance Issues
Permanent brain damage may result from prolonged severe hypoglycemia.

IV. DISORDERS OF THE ADRENAL GLAND

A. Adrenal Insufficiency

▶ Scientific Concepts

Primary adrenal insufficiency results from the destruction of adrenal gland through autoimmune, infiltration, or infectious processes.

▶ History & Physical

Weakness, hypoglycemia, weight loss, GI discomfort, salt craving, mucocutaneous hyperpigmentation of lips and buccomucosal membranes, multiple freckles, generalized tan along with areas of vitiligo, decreased axillary and pubic hair, overt or orthostatic hypotension, and/or volume depletion occur.

▶ Diagnostic Studies

Adrenocorticotropic hormone (ACTH) stimulation test (cosyntropin [Cortrosyn] test) shows decreased morning serum cortisol, and increased aldosterone ACTH. Metabolic acidosis, hyperkalemia, hyponatremia, hypercalcemia, decreased glucose, and increased melanocyte-stimulating hormone (MSH) occur.

▶ Diagnosis

A normal response to administration of cosyntropin (increase in plasma cortisol of at least 6 g/dL above baseline, unless baseline or post-ACTH levels already exceed normal range) rules out primary adrenal insufficiency. Baseline levels of ACTH are high in primary adrenal insufficiency and low or normal in secondary adrenal insufficiency. Baseline aldosterone levels are low or normal in primary adrenal insufficiency, and there is no response to cosyntropin. Aldosterone levels are low or normal but increase at least 4 ng/dL over baseline after administration of cosyntropin.

▶ Clinical Therapeutics

Replace glucocorticoids using prednisone 5 mg in A.M. and 2.5 mg in P.M. Increase dose for obese or active persons and with concomitant use of barbiturates, phenytoin, and rifampin. Decrease dose in the elderly and those with liver disease, diabetes mellitus, peptic ulcer disease, and/or hypertension. Replace mineralocorticoids using fludrocortisone 0.05 to 0.30 mg/d. Increase dose if hypotension, orthostatic hypotension, and/or hyperkalemia occurs. Decrease dose if hypertension, hypokalemia, and/or edema occurs. Increase sodium intake.

▶ Clinical Intervention

Chronic renal insufficiency may evolve into acute adrenal crisis in the presence of severe infection, trauma, or surgery. Treat fever, dehydration, nausea, and vomiting. Avoid circulatory shock. Give hydrocortisone, 100 mg IV bolus, and repeat q8h. Taper daily during recovery by one-third of daily dose until maintenance dosage is reached.

Initiate dextrose 5% in normal saline solution (D_5NSS) IV and add fludrocortisone after hydrocortisone is tapered to < 100 mg/d.

► Health Maintenance Issues

Medic Alert bracelets inform of steroid dependency. Adjust glucocorticoid dosage for mild illness or stress (double dose until resolved). Patients should not self-adjust mineralocorticoid dose.

B. Cushing's Syndrome

► Scientific Concepts

Cushing's syndrome results from chronic glucocorticoid excess. Endogenous causes include disorders of the pituitary (68%), adrenal (17%), and ectopic sources (15%). **Pituitary adenoma (Cushing's disease)** causes increased random and episodic ACTH secretion, resulting in hypersecretion of cortisol and the absence of the normal circadian rhythm, primarily in women of childbearing age. Female:male ratio is 8:1. **Adrenal tumors** cause autonomous production of cortisol. Plasma ACTH levels are low. These tumors occur primarily in children. **Ectopic** causes result from autonomous ACTH production from extrapituitary malignancy (commonly brochogenic carcinoma). Plasma ACTH levels are elevated. Adult males aged 40 to 60 years are primarily afflicted. **Exogenous** cause is steroid use.

► History & Physical

Common findings are central obesity (increased intraperitoneal fat with relatively thin extremities), hypertension, glucose intolerance, plethoric moon facies, purple striae, hirsutism, menstrual dysfunction, sexual dysfunction, general and proximal muscle weakness, dorsocervical and supraclavicular fatty deposition, bruising, and/or osteoporosis. Uncommon findings are mental changes, hyperpigmentation, acne, poor wound healing, superficial fungal infections, and hypokalemic alkalosis.

► Diagnostic Studies

Confirm hypercortisolism: Overnight dexamethasone suppression test or urinary steroid excretion tests (urinary free cortisol, 17-hydroxycorticosteroids [17-OHCS]) are performed.

Differentiate the form of Cushing's: Administer high-dose dexamethasone with concomitant measurement of 24-hour urinary 17-OHCS. Evaluate plasma ACTH level. Perform corticotropin-releasing factor (CRF) stimulation test.

Localization of lesion: When pituitary lesion is suspected, perform petrosal sinus sampling. Obtain sellar x-ray and computed tomographic (CT) scan. When adrenal lesion is suspected, perform ultrasound, CT scan, or magnetic resonance imaging (MRI). When ectopic lesion is suspected, perform chest x-ray and CT of the chest.

► Diagnosis

High-dose dexamethasone test: If urinary 17-OHCS is suppressed to > 50% of baseline, pituitary origin of Cushing's syndrome is likely. Failure to suppress 17-OHCS implies adrenal or ectopic Cushing's syndrome. Plasma ACTH levels measurable in a patient with hypercortisolemia implies ectopic or pituitary Cushing's. Undetectable ACTH levels in the presence of hypercortisolemia establishes the diagnosis of adrenal Cushing's syndrome. Patients with pituitary Cushing's syndrome (90%) increase ACTH and cortisol levels upon administration of CRF, while those with ectopic and adrenal Cushing's syndrome have no ACTH or cortisol response. This test differentiates ACTH-dependent from ACTH-independent Cushing's syndrome; however, pituitary may not be distinguished from ectopic if the pituitary fails to respond. Further evaluation with inferior petrosal sinus sampling is warranted.

▶ Clinical Therapeutics
Pituitary: Mitotane is used for symptom control.
Adrenal: Avoid hypoadrenalism.
Ectopic: Use adrenal enzyme inhibitors (metyrapone, aminoglutethimide, ketoconazole).

▶ Clinical Intervention
Pituitary: Treatment of choice is transsphenoidal adenomectomy or hypophysectomy. Pituitary microadenomas may be removed selectively; however, the remission rate is 85%. Consider pituitary x-irradiation for the young. The lag period is 12 to 18 months before hypercortisolism is corrected.
Adrenal: Surgically remove adenomas or carcinoma.
Ectopic: Surgically remove ACTH-secreting tumor if possible (usually not feasible). Consider adrenalectomy or adrenal enzyme inhibitors (metyrapone, aminoglutethimide, ketoconazole) or medical adrenalectomy with mitotane.

▶ Health Maintenance Issues
Failure to reduce hypercortisolism results in hypertension, cardiovascular disease, stroke, thromboembolism, susceptibility to infection, and ultimately death. While treatment of Cushing's disease (pituitary adenoma) improves survival, these patients experience increased mortality secondary to cardiovascular disease. Excellent prognosis for adrenal adenomas. Poor prognosis for adrenal carcinoma (life expectancy is 4 years). Poor prognosis for ectopic ACTH syndrome due to malignant tumor (life expectancy is days to weeks).

C. Hirsutism

▶ Scientific Concepts
Overproduction of androgens (increased concentration of free testosterone) results from hyperplasia or tumor of adrenal glands and/or ovaries. Hypersensitivity of hair follicles to normal levels of androgens may occur. Increased 5-alpha-reductase activity results in increased conversion of androgens, especially testosterone from steroid precursors in peripheral tissues. Exogenous sources and certain drugs may induce terminal hair growth.

► History & Physical

Determine age of onset, rate of progression, and family history. Terminal hair growth occurs on upper lip, chin, neck, chest, lower abdomen, back, and inner thighs. Increased sebaceous gland activity causes acne. Anovulation, oligomenorrhea, and amenorrhea may occur. In severe cases, defeminization (breast atrophy, loss of body contours), virilization (frontal balding, increased muscularity, deepened voice, and clitoromegaly), and ovarian enlargement occur.

► Diagnostic Studies

Measure dehydroepiandrosterone sulfate (DHEA-S), testosterone (total or free), cortisol levels, prolactin level, luteinizing hormone (LH), and follicle-stimulating hormone (FSH) levels and thyroid function tests. Obtain CT of abdomen and ultrasound of ovaries.

► Diagnosis

Polycystic ovary syndrome (Stein–Leventhal syndrome): Functional disorder of the ovaries that accounts for half the cases of clinical hirsutism. LH:FSH ratio is > 2.0. DHEA-S is normal or minimally elevated. Testosterone or androstenedione are moderately elevated. Serum free testosterone is elevated. Suppress testosterone with combination oral contraceptive.

Idiopathic or familial: Strong familial predisposition with or without elevated androstanediol glucoronide, a metabolite of dihydrotestosterone, which is produced in skin. Hirsutism may be normal in view of genetic background. DHEA-S is normal or minimally elevated. Testosterone, serum free testosterone, and androstenedione are normal.

Adrenal enzyme defects: Deficiency of 21-hydroxylase causes congenital genitalia ambiguity. Without corticosteroid replacement, virilization occurs. Salt wasting may occur. Adult onset of partial defect in 21-hydroxylase occurs without salt wasting. Evaluate serum 17-hydroxyprogesterone at baseline and after cosyntropin injection.

Rare causes: ACTH-induced Cushing's syndrome, acromegaly, and ovarian luteoma of pregnancy are rare. Adrenal carcinoma and ovarian tumors may result in elevated testosterone and androstenedione. If DHEA-S is elevated, consider adrenal source. Continue evaluation with pelvic exam and ultrasound and adrenal CT.

► Clinical Therapeutics

Suppress androgen production with oral contraceptives or progestins, glucocorticoids (dexamethasone), finasteride, flutamide, and spironolactone. Do not give antiandrogen therapy to pregnant women.

► Clinical Intervention

Laparoscopic bilateral oophorectomy is indicated for postmenopausal women with severe hyperandrogenism. Discontinue drugs that could potentially induce hair growth: androgens, cyclosporine, danazole, diazoxide, minoxidil, and phenytoin. Cosmetic treatment includes waxing, depilatories, shaving, bleaching, or electrolysis.

► Health Maintenance Issues
Evaluate and treat infertility.

V. OTHER ENDOCRINE DISEASES

A. Electrolyte Disorders

1. Hypocalcemia

► Scientific Concepts

Most common cause is renal failure. Other causes include decreased intake or absorption (malabsorption, vitamin D deficit), increased loss (alcoholism, chronic renal insufficiency, diuretic therapy), endocrine causes (hypoparathyroidism, sepsis, pseudohypoparathyroidism, medullary thyroid carcinoma), and physiologic causes (decreased serum albumin, hyperphosphatemia, drug induced).

► History & Physical

Patients complain of paresthesias of lips and extremities, muscle cramps, and abdominal pain. Physical examination reveals laryngospasm with stridor, convulsions, ventricular arrhythmias, heart block, Chvostek's sign, and Trousseau's sign.

► Diagnostic Studies

Serum calcium is < 9 mg/dL. Correlate serum calcium with simultaneous concentration of serum albumin. Evaluate serum magnesium. ECG shows prolonged QT interval.

► Diagnosis

Renal failure causes decreased production of active vitamin D_3 and hyperphosphatemia.

► Clinical Therapeutics

Administer calcium gluconate, 10% (4.7 mEq/10 mL) IV 10 to 20 mL over 10 to 15 minutes, for tetany, arrhythmia, or seizures. Then decrease to 10 to 15 mg/kg over 4 to 6 hours. If asymptomatic, give oral calcium carbonate preparations and vitamin D.

► Clinical Intervention
Correct underlying defect.

► Health Maintenance Issues
Chronic hypocalcemia causes cataracts.

2. Hypomagnesemia

► Scientific Concepts

Decreased absorption or intake occurs secondary to malabsorption, prolonged GI suction, malnutrition, and/or alcoholism. Increased loss occurs secondary to DKA, diuretics, hyperaldosteronism, and/or renal magnesium wasting. Unexplained causes include hyperparathyroidism, postparathyroidectomy, vitamin D therapy, and/or medications. Consider hypomagnesemia in patients who are hypokalemic and refractory to potassium replacement and/or hypocalcemic and refractory to calcium replacement.

▶ History & Physical

Patients describe weakness, muscle cramps, and tremor. Neurologic exam reveals athetoid movements, jerking, nystagmus, positive Babinski, hyperreflexia, fasciculations, tremors, convulsions, confusion, disorientation, delirium, and coma. Cardiovascular exam shows tachycardia and ventricular arrhythmias.

▶ Diagnostic Studies

Reduced serum magnesium (< 1.1 mEq/dL), calcium, and potassium are noted. ECG manifestations include prolonged QT interval due to lengthened ST segment, T wave flattening, prolonged PR interval, atrial fibrillation, and Torsade de pointes.

▶ Diagnosis

Determined by history and evaluation of underlying disease process.

▶ Clinical Therapeutics

For mild chronic hypomagnesemia, restore deficits with magnesium oxide, 250 to 500 mg PO bid or qid.

▶ Clinical Intervention

Correct magnesium deficiency: In severe hypomagnesemia (serum magnesium < 1.0 mg/dL) with accompanying symptoms (seizures, tetany), use 2 g of magnesium chloride or sulfate in 20 mL dextrose 5% in water (D_5W) IV over 1 hour. Monitor ECG, blood pressure, pulse, respiration, deep tendon reflexes, and urine output. Replace potassium and calcium as needed.

▶ Health Maintenance Issues

Correct underlying cause or condition(s).

3. Gout

▶ Scientific Concepts

Excessive serum uric acid from underexcretion of uric acid by kidneys causes 90% of all gout. The remaining 10% of cases result from overproduction of uric acid. Deposition of monosodium urate crystals from supersaturated extracellular fluids occurs in soft tissue, causing gouty tophi. Deposition in joints causes inflammation known as gouty arthritis.

Initial presentation of acute gouty arthritis occurs primarily in males aged 30 to 60 years. Presentation in females is usually after menopause. Ninty-five percent of all cases of gout are found in men.

▶ History & Physical

Episodic attacks may be preceded by dehydration secondary to trauma, foods high in proteins and purines, alcohol, drugs (diuretics), surgery, acute medical illness, or renal failure. A monoarticular joint (first metatarsophalangeal joint—podagra) suddenly becomes severely painful. The midtarsal and ankle are also commonly affected. Other sites include the instep, knee, ankle, and elbow. Sudden onset of asymmetric polyarthritis is atypical for gout. A warm, tender, swollen erythematous joint is noted on physical exam. When multiple joints are affected, patient may be febrile.

► Diagnostic Studies

Serum uric acid level is normal or elevated at onset of acute attack and may rise when symptoms resolve. Aspirate synovial fluid of affected joint and observe joint fluid for birefringent crystals under polarized light miscroscopy.

► Diagnosis

Monosodium urate crystals (needle-shaped, strongly negative birefringent crystals) and therapeutic response to colchicine within 24 to 48 hours is pathognomonic for gout. Synovial fluid of pseudogout shows calcium pyrophosphate dihydrate crystals that are rhomboid or polymorphic shaped, weakly positive, and birefringent.

► Clinical Therapeutics

Gout prophylaxis agents include indomethacin, naproxen, sulindac, and other nonsteroidal anti-inflammatory drugs (NSAIDs). Allopurinol may be used in combination with colchicine or probenecid as prophylactic therapy for patients with recurrent attacks despite dietary restriction of proteins, purines, and alcohol.

► Clinical Intervention

For acute attacks, give colchicine, 1 to 2 mg diluted in 20 mL of 0.9% sodium chloride IV initially, followed by 0.5 mg IV q 6 to 12 h. IV administration should be slow to avoid extravasation. The maximum IV dose is 4 mg/24 hr. Colchicine may also be administered, 0.5 to 1.2 mg PO initially, then 0.5 to 0.6 mg q 1 to 3 h until pain is relieved. The maximum total dose is 8 to 10 mg. For those who cannot tolerate colchicine or oral medications, consider glucocorticoids (IV or IM ACTH). Those with monoarticular involvement may be treated with intra-articular administration of methylprednisone or betamethasone.

► Health Maintenance Issues

Avoid foods high in purines (anchovies, sweetbreads) as well as alcohol, aspirin, and diuretics. Evaluate for renal failure.

B. Clinical Lipoprotein Disorders

1. Type II Hyperlipoproteinemia

► Scientific Concepts

Familial hypercholesterolemia is an autosomal dominant genetic defect causing deficient or defective low-density lipoprotein (LDL) receptors, leading to delayed catabolism of LDL and increased plasma

LDL. LDL receptor mutation(s) occurs. Lipoprotein pattern IIa and IIb are detected in 1:500 in general population. **Familial defective apo B-100** results from apolipoprotein B (apo B)-100 mutation. Lipoprotein pattern IIa occurs. 1:500 in general population are affected. The condition is associated with excess dietary cholesterol, hypothyroidism, nephrosis, multiple myeloma, porphyria, and obstructive liver disease.

► History & Physical

Family history of coronary artery disease (CAD) prior to age 55 may be present. Often, patients are asymptomatic. Corneal arcus (juvenile) may be present. Tendinous xanthomas of the Achilles, patellar, and digital extensor tendons may occur in juveniles.

► Diagnostic Studies

LDL and cholesterol are elevated. Measure intermediate-density lipoprotein (IDL) and very low-density lipoprotein (VLDL) and triglycerides.

► Diagnosis

Familial hypercholesterolemia: Characteristically, cholesterol is 300 to 400 mg/dL or greater. Triglycerides, IDL, and VLDL are elevated.
Familial defective apo B-100: Cholesterol is typically 250 to 300 mg/dL. Triglycerides are normal. IDL and VLDL are not elevated.

► Clinical Therapeutics

Initiate niacin, cholestyramine, hydroxymethylglutaryl coenzyme A (HMG CoA) reductase inhibitors alone or in combination. Use gemfibrozil in combination with HMG CoA reductase inhibitors.

► Clinical Intervention

Low-fat and low-cholesterol diet is recommended. Exercise should be encouraged.

► Health Maintenance Issues

By age 40, one of six males with type II hyperlipoproteinemia will have myocardial infarction. By age 60, two of three afflicted males will have a myocardial infarction.

2. Type III Familial Dysbetahyperproteinemia

► Scientific Concepts

Genetic apolipoprotein E_3 deficiency occurs in 1:10,000 in general population. Precipitating factors include obesity, diabetes, hypothyroidism, and/or inherited lipid disorder.

► History & Physical

Physical exam reveals obesity, tuberous and tendinous xanthomas, palmar and plantar xanthomatous streaks. Premature CAD is common.

► Diagnostic Studies

Cholesterol and triglycerides are equally elevated. VLDL and IDL are elevated. VLDL-cholesterol and plasma triglyceride ratio is below 0.30. Evaluate for hypothyroidism and glucose intolerance.

► Diagnosis

Electrophoretic pattern is "broad beta" and may be confused with hypothyroidism and resolving lipemias. Confirm diagnosis by absence of the E-3 and E-4 genes on allele-specific screening of genomic deoxyribonucleic acid (DNA) or of the corresponding proteins on isoelectric focusing of VLDL proteins.

► Clinical Therapeutics

Initiate niacin or gemfibrozil in low doses.

► Clinical Intervention

Achieve and maintain ideal weight. Low-cholesterol and low-saturated-fat diet is recommended. Avoid alcohol.

► Health Maintenance Issues

Patients have a very strong risk for atherosclerosis, especially in peripheral and coronary arteries. Control underlying condition(s).

3. Type IV Familial Hypertriglyceridemia

► Scientific Concepts

Heterogeneous genetic predisposition occurs in 1:500 in general population. Severity of hypertriglyceridemia correlates with associated conditions such as obesity, diabetes, hypothyroidism, uremia, alcohol abuse, oral contraceptive, estrogen, and/or glucocorticoid use.

► History & Physical

Atherosclerosis, obesity, and glucose intolerance may occur.

► Diagnostic Studies

VLDL and triglycerides are elevated. Cholesterol is normal or elevated. High-density lipoprotein (HDL) is low proportionally to elevated triglycerides. Evaluate for underlying condition(s).

► Diagnosis

Those with familial type V hyperlipoproteinemia characteristically have elevated chylomicrons and larger increase in triglycerides in comparison to type IV familial hypertriglyceridemia.

► Clinical Therapeutics

Initiate niacin or gemfibrozil.

► Clinical Intervention

Achieve and maintain ideal weight. Low-cholesterol and low-saturated-fat diet is recommended. Avoid alcohol and estrogen. Exercise should be encouraged.

► Health Maintenance Issues

Prevent CAD. Control underlying conditions.

4. Type V Hyperlipoproteinemia

▶ Scientific Concepts

Condition is familial with various defects. Poor clearance of exogenous and endogenous triglycerides occurs. Severity of hypertriglyceridemia correlates with associated conditions such as obesity, diabetes, uremia, alcohol abuse, oral contraceptive, estrogen, and/or glucocorticoids. No significant increase in CAD.

▶ History & Physical

Onset occurs in early adulthood. Eruptive xanthomas of extensor surfaces of extremities, lipemia retinalis, hepatosplenomegaly, abdominal pain, and recurrent pancreatitis may be present. Symptoms are exacerbated with ingestion of fats.

▶ Diagnostic Studies

Triglycerides are markedly elevated. Cholesterol elevation is modest. Cloudy plasma with creamy top layer may be visualized. Chylomicrons and VLDL are increased. Evaluate for underlying conditions.

▶ Diagnosis

In type IV familial hypertriglyceridemia, chylomicrons are not elevated. There is a milder increase in triglycerides in comparison to type V hyperlipoproteinemia.

▶ Clinical Therapeutics

Start niacin or gemfibrozil.

▶ Clinical Intervention

Achieve and maintain ideal weight. Low-cholesterol and low-saturated-fat diet is recommended. Avoid alcohol and estrogen. Exercise should be encouraged.

▶ Health Maintenance Issues

Control underlying conditions.

5. Familial Combined Hyperlipidemia

▶ Scientific Concepts

Most common form of hyperlipidemia (1:250 in general population). Transmission is autosomal dominant. Apo B-100 overproduction is associated with overproduction of VLDL. Lipoprotein pattern type IIa, IIb, IV, or V presents. Diabetes is often associated.

▶ History & Physical

Onset occurs at adulthood. Central obesity and insulin resistance occur. Xanthelasma as well as tendinous and tuberous xanthomas are absent.

▶ Diagnostic Studies

Triglycerides and cholesterol are normal or modestly elevated. LDL, VLDL, and IDL are elevated. Evaluate for underlying diabetes.

► **Diagnosis**

In type II familial hypercholesterolemia, xanthomas are present along with a large increase in cholesterol. In type IV familial hypertriglyceridemia, xanthomas are present along with a moderate increase in triglycerides. LDL and IDL are not elevated.

► **Clinical Therapeutics**

Initiate therapy with bile acid sequestrants (cholestyramine or colestipol) or HMG CoA reductase inhibitors to reduce LDL. HMG CoA reductase inhibitors may cause VLDL to increase. Niacin may be added.

► **Clinical Intervention**

Achieve and maintain ideal weight. Low-cholesterol and low-saturated-fat diet is recommended. Exercise should be encouraged.

► **Health Maintenance Issues**

Control underlying condition. Prevent and evaluate for CAD.

6. Decreased High-Density Lipoprotein

► **Scientific Concepts**

Possible genetic disorder.

► **History & Physical**

Cigarette smoking, obesity, decreased exercise androgen, anabolic steroid, and beta-androgenic antagonists have been implicated as predisposing/exacerbating factors.

► **Diagnostic Studies**

Lipid profile electrophoresis with low alpha region. LDL-cholesterol is < 35 mg/dL.

► **Diagnosis**

May occur secondary to familial hypoalpha lipoproteinemia and primary hypertriglyceridemias.

► **Clinical Therapeutics**

Niacin increases LDL levels. Postmenopausal women should be given replacement estrogen unless otherwise contraindicated.

► **Clinical Intervention**

Achieve and maintain ideal weight. Low-cholesterol and low-saturated-fat diet is recommended. Exercise would be encouraged.

► **Health Maintenance Issues**

Control underlying condition. Patient with cholesterol: HDL ratios > 4.5 have an increased risk of CAD. Discontinue smoking, androgen, anabolic steroid, and beta-androgenic antagonists.

BIBLIOGRAPHY

Andreoli TE, Carpenter CCJ, Plum F, Smith LH, eds. *Cecil's Essentials of Medicine,* 2nd ed. Philadelphia: WB Saunders; 1990.

Begany T. When to screen, when to treat thyroid disease. *JAAPA* 11:72–87; 1998.

Carey CF, Lee HH, Woeltje KF, eds. *The Washington Manual of Medical Therapeutics,* 29th ed. Philadelphia: Lippincott-Raven; 1998.

Ferri FF, ed. *Practical Guide to the Care of the Medical Patient,* 2nd ed. St. Louis, MO: Mosby-Year Book; 1991.

Greenspan FS, Strewler GJ, eds. *Basic and Clinical Endocrinology,* 5th ed. Stamford, CT: Appleton & Lange; 1997.

Largay J. Exercise recommendations for diabetic patients. *JAAPA* 11:22–36; 1998.

Lavin N, ed. *Manual of Endocrinology and Metabolism,* 2nd ed. Little, Brown and Company; 1994.

McTigue J. Cutaneous manifestation of thyroid disorders. *JAAPA* 11:12–17; 1998.

Sadler C, Einhorn D. Tailoring insulin regimens for type 2 diabetes mellitus. *JAAPA* 11:55–71; 1998.

Tierney LM, McPhee SJ, Papadakis MA, eds. *Current Medical Diagnosis and Treatment,* 37th ed. Stamford, CT: Appleton & Lange; 1998.

Rheumatology and Orthopedics 11

Roderick S. Hooker, PhD, PA

I. DIFFUSE CONNECTIVE TISSUE DISEASES

A. Rheumatoid Arthritis

▶ Scientific Concepts

Etiology is unclear, but rheumatoid arthritis (RA) is related to cell-mediated immune response (T cells) and loss of normal apoptosis function. Response is initially an inflammatory one against soft tissue and later cartilage, with subsequent bone loss and osteoarthritis due to bone reabsorption and bone-on-bone arthritis. Lymphokines and other inflammatory mediators initiate the cascade that leads to cartilage destruction. Functional impairment in activities of daily living may be more significant than pain. Systemic involvement of extra-articular systems such as lung and skin (nodules) may occur, but usually in late stages. Rheumatoid nodules occur in one-third of cases and tend to predict a severe course. Nodules are seen later, rather than earlier, in the course of the disease.

▶ History & Physical

Characteristically, a patient presents with morning stiffness of more than 1-hour duration with symmetrical swelling of wrists, metacarpals (MCPs), and proximal interphalangeal (PIP) joints but spares the distal interphalangeal (DIP) joints. May involve the elbows, knees, and metatarsal phalangeal (MTP) joints. Spares the spine and only very rarely involves the hips. Patients may complain of dysfunction more than pain. Incidence increases with each decade, but a typical picture is of a woman between 20 and 40 presenting with early RA within 1 year of parturition.

▶ Diagnostic Studies

Laboratory studies and hand radiographs are rarely helpful initially. Rheumatoid factor (RF) positive in 70% of cases but also present in normal population five times more frequently. Erythrocyte sedimentation rate (ESR) is often elevated, and a mild normochromic, normocytic anemia may be present.

▶ Diagnosis

Diagnosis is made clinically. Look for synovitis of the wrists, MCPs, and PIPs. Weak grip strength and the inability to touch fingertips to distal palmar crease.

► **Clinical Therapeutics**

Aimed at controlling the inflammation with nonsteroidal anti-inflammatory drugs (NSAIDs) and disease-modifying drugs such as hydroxychloroquine, methotrexate, gold, etanercept, leflunomide, and corticosteroids initiated early in the course of the disease (the window of opportunity), hopefully affecting the downstream effect of the disease before an irreversible effect takes place.

► **Clinical Intervention**

Moderately affected joints can be injected, braced, and splinted. Severely destroyed joints of the hands often have a surprising amount of function. Hips and knees may require joint replacement surgery. Arthrocenteses and intra-articular injections can be a useful therapy to calm inflamed joints.

B. Juvenile Chronic Arthritis

► **Scientific Concepts**

Etiology is unclear but is related to cell-mediated immune response (T cells) and loss of normal apoptosis function. Response is initially an inflammatory one against soft tissue and later cartilage, with subsequent bone loss and osteoarthritis due to bone resorption and bone-on-bone arthritis. Lymphokines and other inflammatory mediators initiate the cascade that leads to cartilage destruction.

► **History & Physical**

Under age 10, children may move slowly in the morning getting dressed as a result of joint stiffness more than joint complaints. A limp in a child of more than 1-week duration may be an early sign of juvenile-onset chronic arthritis and should be investigated.

► **Diagnostic Studies**

Three subsets of juvenile arthritis are classed depending on joints involved: pauciarthritis—small joints of the hands and < five; polyarthritis—more than four joints, often involving the knee; oligoarthritis—one to three large joints, virtually always knees. Laboratory studies help to categorize the type of arthritis.

► **Diagnosis**

Multifactorial depending on presence or absence of fever, systemic signs, rheumatoid factor and antinuclear antibody (ANA).

► **Clinical Therapeutics**

Aimed at controlling the inflammation with NSAIDs and disease-modifying drugs such as hydroxychloroquine, methotrexate, gold, sulfasalazine, leflunomide, entanercept, and corticosteroids initiated early in the course of the disease (the window of opportunity), hopefully affecting the downstream effect of the disease before an irreversible effect takes place. Newer drugs not yet on the market but available within the next decade, will be even more beneficial.

► Clinical Intervention

Moderately affected joints can be injected, braced, and splinted. This requires a close working association with physical therapy and occupational therapy. Arthrocenteses and intra-articular injections can be a useful therapy to calm inflamed joints.

► Health Maintenance Issues

All children should have an optometric or ophthalmologic exam to rule out uveitis. Over 70% of all children will outgrow their disease by late teens.

C. Systemic Lupus Erythematosus

► Scientific Concepts

Autoimmune disease characterized by the production of autoantibodies to components of the cell nucleus. Inflammation, vasculitis, and immune complex deposition in organs such as the kidney and skin manifest pathological findings. Lupus arthritis is polyarticular in presentation, usually with mild synovitis, and no joint destruction. Disease activity can severely impair renal function, cause pulmonary infiltrates, and pericarditis. Neuropsychiatric manifestations common during disease attacks.

► History & Physical

Disease of young females 14 to 40 years old, with a 10:1 female:male ratio. Arthritis mimics RA but only occurs in 30% of cases, usually transient, lasting a few weeks, and rarely deforming or destructive. Multiple organs at risk including brain, kidneys, skin, liver, spleen, and hematopoietic system.

► Diagnostic Studies

Clinical symptoms of fever, fatigue, arthralgias, morning stiffness, and myalgias. ANA positive in > 98% of cases but ANAs frequently occur in normal people as well. Anti-DNA presence associated with glomerulonephritis. Complements C3 and/or C4 often low.

► Clinical Therapeutics

Treatment consists of rest, NSAIDs, corticosteroids, hydroxychloroquine, and avoiding sun exposure. More severe disease calls for azathioprine, methotrexate, and cyclophosphamide.

► Clinical Intervention

When vital organs are involved, aggressive cortisone treatment is required.

► Health Maintenance Issues

Most people with systemic lupus erythematosus (SLE) should be maintained on hydroxychloroquine to reduce frequency and severity of lupus flares.

D. Polymyositis and Dermatomyositis

▶ Scientific Concepts

Idiopathic autoimmune disease that affects the proximal limb muscles with inflammation.

▶ History & Physical

Proximal muscle weakness with difficulty ascending stairs, alighting from car seat, or rising from hands and knees. Physical examination shows diffuse symmetrical upper arm weakness, difficulty doing an abdominal curl, or rising from a chair without use of hands. Usually painless but can be painful in some instances. Onset usually insidious. Gait may be slow and wide-based. Clinical presentations of proximal and symmetrical muscle weakness. Dermatomyositis presents with periorbital lilac rash and Gottron papules on knuckles.

▶ Diagnostic Studies

Elevated serum creatinine kinase (CK), or lactate dehydrogenase (LDH). Characteristic electromyographic abnormalities. Muscle biopsy is imperative to making an accurate diagnosis. ANA may be present. May develop calcium deposits in muscle groups in late-stage untreated disease. In rare instances, heart, lung, and kidney may be involved.

▶ Clinical Therapeutics

Moderate-dose corticosteroids are the initial treatment. Methotrexate or azathioprine is used early to avoid steroid side effects. Graded exercises after the inflammation is controlled restore some strength and range of motion.

▶ Health Maintenance Issues

Patients should be warned about malignant hyperthermia if undergoing general anesthesia.

E. Polymyalgia Rheumatica

▶ Scientific Concepts

Inflammatory disease of unknown etiology. Common syndrome in elderly may affect up to 5% of people > 70. Natural history is for this condition to be resolved within 2 years for most patients.

▶ History & Physical

Occurs in men and women > 60. Often an abrupt onset of pain and stiffness with loss of function in shoulder and hip girdles. Morning stiffness and difficulty rolling over or doing normal daily activities. Physical examination reveals tenderness of proximal muscles and reluctance to fully extend or rotate shoulders. Elevated ESR and clinical impairment of activities are the hallmarks of this disease.

▶ Diagnostic Studies

High ESR usually found. Complete blood count (CBC), thyroid-stimulating hormone (TSH), CK, aspartate transaminase (AST), RF, and ANAs negative. Chest x-ray normal. Diagnosis is by history and response to prednisone within a few days. If response is not seen in 1 week, diagnosis should be questioned.

▶ Diagnosis

The diagnosis is made by the history of being still, sore, and gelling characteristic of inflammatory disease. The response to prednisone is usually diagnostic. Giant cell arteritis, fibromyalgia, and polymyositis are part of the differential.

▶ Clinical Intervention

Responds rapidly to prednisone, 10 to 20 mg in divided doses. Reduce to 7.5 to 10 mg in 1 month. Therapy may continue for more than a year, but most are on < 7.5 mg within 6 months of treatment. Taper prednisone if possible. Ten percent of all polymyalgia rheumatica (PMR) cases will eventually develop idiopathic hypothyroidism.

▶ Health Maintenance Issues

Some people may need to be on prednisone for > 6 months. Divided doses of prednisone recommended for easier tapering. Osteoporosis prevention should be considered in most patients on long-term corticosteroid therapy.

F. Vasculitis

▶ Scientific Concepts

The vasculitides are a heterogeneous group of clinical syndromes characterized by inflammation of blood vessels. These are rare diseases that often appear in widely varying patterns. The pattern of onset is also variable. The vasculitic lesions may be focal, segmental, or diffuse. Some have a prediction for certain organs such as the kidney, lung, or skin. Untreated, the clinical course can be benign in some diseases and fatal in others.

▶ History & Physical

Patients with vasculitis have symptoms and signs that range from those that are almost universal but nonspecific, to less frequent but more specific, in manifestation. Fever and other constitutional signs, such as weight loss and night sweats, occur in ≥ 90% of patients with all types of vasculitis. Arthralgias occur in 90% of patients, but arthritis is rare. Abdominal pain occurs in many patients, and symptoms range from vague, almost constant pain to symptoms of abdominal ischemia. Renal disease occurs in almost 50% and the urine sediment shows hematuria and proteinuria, but a nephrotic syndrome is rare. Renal biopsy may show a segmental glomerulonephritis, often with epithelial crescents. Skin lesions may range from nonspecific urticaria to palpable purpura to necrosis and ulceration of digits. Skin lesions are almost universal in some vasculitides, such as Henoch–Schönlein purpura and rheumatoid vasculitis, and offer promising sites for biopsy. Neurological lesions are seen in > 50% of patients. These range from peripheral sensory neuropathy to the highly specific mononeuritis multiplex of Churg–Strauss syndrome.

▶ Diagnostic Studies

Biopsy or arteriography confirms the diagnosis of vasculitis. Biopsy of specific lesions such as palpable purpura, an inflamed temporal artery, or renal biopsy in a patient with active urine sediment. Sural nerve biopsy with concomitant gastrocnemius muscle biopsy is a useful procedure with high yield if there is neurological involvement. Blind muscle biopsies may yield 50 to 80% results if classical polyarteritis nodosa (PAN) is suspected. Arteriography can be very useful in certain circumstances when the mesentery or the aorta is involved.

Disease severity depends on classification of the vasculitis, size of vessels involved, depression of complements, organs involved, and duration of disease without treatment. Leukocytoclastic vasculitis (small vessel disease) has the best prognosis.

▶ History & Physical

The history and physical examination is highly variable, but usually vasculitis occurs over days or a few weeks. Fever and rash are common. Mild synovitis occurs in up to 20% of patients. Altered arterial pulses may be abnormal and multiple peripheral neuropathies may occur, especially in lower extremities.

▶ Diagnostic Studies

Biopsy of arteries or arterial imaging studies are usually confirmatory. In Churg–Strauss syndrome, presence of eosinophils in peripheral blood is suggestive. Antineutrophil cytoplasmic antibody (ANCA) is present in most cases of Wegener's granulomatosis. Skin biopsies often diagnostic of hypersensitivity vasculitis.

▶ Clinical Therapeutics

Mainstay of treatment for most forms of vasculitis is empiric. Corticosteroids and immunosuppressives such as azathioprine and cyclophosphamide are mainstays of treatment. Methotrexate has a role in chronic suppression of many of the vasculitides.

▶ Health Maintenance Issues

Most systemic vasculitides need long-term therapy while hoping the underlying disease will go into an extended remission or be self-limited. Examples of monophasic vasculitic syndromes are hypersensitivity vasculitis, Henoch–Schönlein purpura, PAN, giant cell arteritis, and Takayasu's arteritis. Relapsing diseases can be Wegener's granulomatosis, Churg–Strauss syndrome, and Behçet's disease.

II. SERONEGATIVE SPONDYLOARTHROPATHIES

A. Ankylosing Spondylitis

▶ Scientific Concepts

An inflammatory disease of the spinal joints and sacroiliac joints. If left untreated, there can be complete loss of spinal motion from occiput to coccyx. Treatment is to preserve motion through exercise and control inflammation with medication.

► History & Physical

Rare disease that presents in young men aged 15 to 30. Often presents as diffuse low back pain that fails to improve with rest. Gelling phenomenon or stiffness on arising after resting is common. Usually responds to NSAIDs. May present with effusions of large joints. Restriction on lumbar flexion, neck rotation, chin-on-chest deformity, inability to touch occiput to wall when standing with heels touching the wall, restriction of chest expansion.

► Diagnostic Studies

History, physical examination, and single radiographic view of sacroiliac joints demonstrating sclerosis makes the diagnosis. Later in the course of the illness, spine films demonstrate progressive ankylosis. Restriction of chest expansion and limitation of the normal excursion of the lumbar spine (Schober maneuver). Elevated ESR will confirm presence of inflammation.

► Clinical Intervention

Initial flare is treated with rest and NSAIDs. Mobilization and flexibility exercises are started as the inflammation is controlled. Favored medications are NSAIDs, sulfasalazine, and methotrexate.

► Health Maintenance Issues

Avoiding thoracic kyphosis and maintaining a straight spine are hallmarks of health maintenance in ankylosing spondylitis.

B. Reiter's Syndrome

► Scientific Concepts

Although early description of Reiter's syndrome (RS) described a triad of arthritis, conjunctivitis, and urethritis, the presence of a seronegative oligoarthritis in a young man plus one other extra-articular feature may be sufficient for diagnosis.

► History & Physical

Recent exposure to an enteric pathogen (e.g., a diarrheal illness after travel) or a sexually transmitted disease (usually in a new sexual partner). Prior history of low back pain or recurrent tendinitis is not uncommon. Fever, if present, is usually low grade. Mucous membranes can be ulcerated. RS is the leading cause of inflammatory knee disease in young men when trauma is excluded. In most cases, there is significant improvement with NSAID therapy over a 3- to 4-month period. In 25 to 40%, however, there is a chronic course with sustained activity or intermittent flares. Long-term disability may occur in some patients.

► Diagnostic Studies

The cardinal feature is an asymmetric arthritis, typically oligoarticular and predominantly below the waist. Most common are knees, ankles, and metatarsophalangeal joints, but upper extremity involvement may occur. Plantar fasciitis and Achilles tendinitis are quite specific for RS. Mucocutaneous involvement may include urethritis, proctitis, cervicitis, cystitis, stomatitis, or uveitis. Elevated ESR is present in an acute episode. Human lymphocyte antigen (HLA)-B27 is not a diagnostic test but is present in 70% of cases.

▶ Diagnosis

The history and physical examination make the diagnosis. The clinical triad of arthritis, uveitis, and nongonococcal urethritis is no longer required to make the diagnosis because many cases include only two of the three parts of the syndrome. *Chlamydia trachomatis* should be suspected and perhaps treated empirically. Gonococcal arthritis and human immunodeficiency virus (HIV) infection should be suspected. Psoriatic arthritis, gout, RA are part of the differential diagnosis.

▶ Clinical Intervention

X-rays are rarely helpful in the acute phase of RS. Intra-articular injections following arthrocentesis is the therapy of choice for most patients. If patients fail to respond to potent NSAIDs within 2 months, methotrexate or sulfasalazine may be considered. Oral steroids are used less frequently. An ophthalmologist and a rheumatologist should manage uveitis. Generally, local steroids will suffice. Chest x-ray will rule out intrathoracic sarcoidosis.

▶ Health Maintenance Issues

For patients with chronically active disease, medication such as methotrexate, sulfasalazine, or other, newer drugs may be necessary for long-term suppression of flares.

C. Psoriatic Arthritis

▶ Scientific Concepts

Of people with psoriasis, 5 to 7% have psoriatic arthritis (PsA), a form of inflammatory joint disease. Why this association occurs is not clear since a shared epitope has not been found. Degree of arthritis does not correlate with skin involvement.

▶ History & Physical

There are five types of PsA:

1. **Oligoarthritis** (70% of cases) affects scattered DIPs and PIPs of hands and feet. Dactylitis occurs when two or more joints of a finger or toe are involved, presenting as a "sausage digit."
2. **Classic PsA** is actually rare and involves all DIPs and usually nail beds, producing pits and onycholysis. Often initially confused with Heberden nodes.
3. **Arthritis mutilans** is a disabling form of PsA (5% of cases) and is identified by osteolysis of affected joints and foreshortening of the digits.
4. **Symmetric polyarthritis** of PsA resembles RA, is seronegative, and constitutes 15% of cases.

5. **Psoriatic spondyloarthritis** occurs in up to 5% of patients with PsA and presents with clinical and radiographic features that may be indistinguishable from those of idiopathic sacroiliitis or ankylosing spondylitis. The histocompatibility antigen HLA-B27 is found in 40% of this group, but this test need not be ordered since it is not diagnostic or specific. Gross destruction of joints and changes in the spine and/or sacroiliac portend a worsening course.

▶ Diagnostic Studies

Diagnosis is clinical and there are no criteria. Joints such as fingers and toes are most commonly affected; larger joints such as knee and ankle may be involved. Constitutional symptoms such as malaise, morning stiffness, and fever can occur and are more commonly seen with symmetrical polyarticular pattern. Back pain may be indicative of spondylitis or sacroiliitis. RF is usually negative. ESR and other acute-phase reactants are elevated and parallel the activity of the arthritis. Radiographic features of digits can be diagnostic when ankylosis or destructive changes take place. "Fluffy" periostitis of bones and joints is sometimes seen.

▶ Clinical Therapeutics

Management goals and therapeutic efforts applied to PsA are the same as RA. Methotrexate tends to be the disease-modifying drug of choice along with NSAIDs. Sulfasalazine and gold salts are also used. Two new drugs, entanercept and leflunomide, have been used but await formal approval. Intra-articular injections of corticosteroids such as triamcinolone hexacetonide can interrupt an otherwise destructive course of disease in a joint.

III. BONE AND CARTILAGE DISORDERS

A. Osteoarthrosis/Osteoarthritis

▶ Scientific Concepts

Osteoarthrosis or osteoarthritis (OA) disease is characterized by progressive loss of articular cartilage, followed by formation of new bone and cartilage at joint margins (osteophytes). Incidence increases with age, obesity, repetitive occupational activity (carpenters, coal miners, jackhammer operators, etc.). Pathology of OA reflects damage to joint and reaction of surrounding tissues. Increase in water content of cartilage occurs with increased proteoglycan synthesis. As disease progresses, joint surface thins and becomes fibrillated. Apposition bone growth in subchondral region leads to sclerosis seen on radiographs. With further degeneration, progression of clefts and fractures of subchondral plate occur, with formation of subchondral cysts. Growth of bone and cartilage at joint margins form osteophytes. Synovitis and joint effusions may be present.

OA is the most common musculoskeletal problem in people > 60. Characterized by focal degeneration of joint cartilage and new bone formation (hypertrophy) at base of cartilage and at joint margins, giving rise to osteophytes. Peripheral OA (Heberden and Bouchard types): a Heberden node at the DIPs of fingers is the most common form of primary OA. Bouchard nodes at the PIPs of fingers are the next most common. Both follow familial lines. Generalized OA is defined by three or more joints or joint groups (DIPs count as one group). The DIPs, PIPs, first carpometacarpal (CMC) joint, spine, hip, knee are commonly involved.

► History & Physical

Symptomatic patients are usually > 40 and complain of pain of insidious onset in one or a few joints. The pain is aching and poorly localized in the hands but more distinct in the CMC, hips, and knees. Pain occurs after normal joint uses but can be relieved by rest. Morning stiffness lasts < a half hour. Joints may be tender, especially if swelling and warmth are present. Pain on weight bearing may be present without pain on passive range of motion. Joint enlargement may result from presence of joint effusion, synovial hyperplasia, or osteophytes. In later disease stages, there may be crepitus, gross deformity, and subluxation (caused by cartilage loss, collapse of subchondral bone, bone cysts, and gross bony overgrowth). Joint loss of motion occurs with disease progression, muscle spasms, and contractures or mechanical blockage by osteophytes.

► Diagnostic Studies

History and physical can make the diagnosis, but radiographs are diagnostic as well. The main features are joint space narrowing, osteophyte formation, periarticular ossicles, subchondral bone cysts, and an altered shape of bone end. No specific laboratory abnormalities are seen in primary OA. CBC, ESR, RF, chemistries, and urinalysis are normal. Radiographic grading has been described that tends to correlate with symptoms:
Grade I: Possible OA.
Grade II: Minimal OA.
Grade III: Moderate OA.
Grade IV: Severe OA.

► Clinical Intervention

Generally, amount of joint destruction cannot be reversed. Heberden and Bouchard forms of OA theoretically may be prevented from worsening if heavy hand labor is reduced. If joint is undergoing a particularly inflammatory phase of arthritis, intra-articular injections may be helpful. NSAIDs and acetaminophen are helpful for pain. Capsaicin cream is helpful in reducing pain in ~ 50% of patients. Advanced OA changes of the hips and knees usually require joint replacement surgery.

► Health Maintenance Issues

Protection of joints from excessive force and chronic overuse. Supportive splints and use of ambulatory aids (cane, crutches, walker) are protective. Avoidance of repetitive impact loading (jumping, running) in lower-extremity OA. Weight loss is beneficial. Physical therapy to increase joint motion and strength is beneficial. Drug therapy consists of analgesics (acetaminophen), aspirin, and NSAIDs. Narcotics should be used only as short-term measures. Intra-articular corticosteroids may be helpful in management of acute flares of knees. Viscosupplement agents include Synvisc and Hyalgan. Surgery is reserved for cases in which conservative therapy fails. Options include arthroscopic lavage and debridement, osteotomy, arthroplasty, and fusion. Orthotics may help knee OA.

B. Lumbar Disk Disease

▶ Scientific Concepts

Nuclear material bulges, protrudes, or extrudes from the disk space to put pressure on the ligaments and nerve roots. Molecular changes in the disk with aging alter structural properties of disk and the annulus fibrosis that contains the disk. The disk loses water and becomes dry and friable, decreasing its ability to withstand axial loads. With sudden loading or repetitive loading in flexion and rotation, disk material is extruded beyond confines of the annulus, resulting in neurological symptoms.

▶ History & Physical

Low back pain with radiation below the knee; leg pain is usually greater than the back pain. Ten percent of backaches are related to some sort of nerve root irritation. Altered sensation, paresthesias, numbness may be present in lower extremity. Pain increases with coughing, sneezing. Weakness may be present. Central disk bulge may cause bilateral symptoms. Signs of limited spine motion, antalgic gait, sciatic list. Hip and knee flexed with standing, extended with sitting, absent or diminished reflexes, diminished sensation in a dermatome pattern. Positive tension signs with straight leg raising or sitting root tests.

▶ Diagnostic Studies

Radiographic evaluation may demonstrate disk space narrowing or may be normal. Computed tomographic (CT) scan and magnetic resonance imaging (MRI) allow visualization of the disk and neural elements. Electromyogram (EMG) will show changes only after several weeks of symptoms. Dense paresthesias with complete motor impingement. Progressive loss of motor function and sensation an indication for early surgical intervention. Loss of bowel and bladder function (cauda equina syndrome) requires emergency treatment with surgical decompression of neural elements to prevent permanent dysfunction.

▶ Clinical Intervention

Early intervention with short period of bedrest (3 to 5 days), in conjunction with NSAIDs and ice. This is followed by mobilization with back rehabilitation exercises. While no patients will obtain relief in 4 weeks, 90% will in 3 months, and 96% in 6 months. Surgical intervention is required for progression of symptoms and for those unresponsive to conservative management.

► Health Maintenance Issues

There are many strong advocates for flexion exercises, extension exercises, isotonic exercises, and combination exercises. Most studies show benefit when any of these exercises are done consistently (usually daily). Most studies done in the 1990s advise returning to work within a few days of onset of symptoms, even before complete remission.

C. Osteoporosis

► Scientific Concepts

Losses in bone mineral content leading to spontaneous fractures of spine, hip, and wrist. Commonly postmenopausal women. Other risk factors include heredity, drug use (steroids, heparin, thyroid), nutritional factors, sedentary activity, cigarette smoking, and alcohol. Disuse osteoporosis results when bones are not stressed normally (e.g., paralysis, prolonged bedrest, immobilization).

► History & Physical

Osteoporosis is not a painful condition. Fractures and deformities as a result of the disease are painful. Progressive loss of height and thoracic kyphosis may suggest vertebral fractures. Bone pain in axial skeleton suggests recent vertebral collapse. Caucasian and Asian postmenopausal females at greatest risk. Disease severity is suggested by multiple compression fractures with thoracic kyphosis. Fractures of femoral neck, wrist, ribs, and ankles also suggest advanced disease.

► Diagnostic Studies

Plain radiographs may show osteopenia but not as reliably as bone densitometry such as dual-energy x-ray absorptiometry (DEXA). Other imaging methods such as ultrasound of calcaneus and x-ray carpal studies are being used. Laboratory screen should consider thyroid abnormalities, hematological disorders, and malignant disease.

► Health Maintenance Issues

Goal is to prevent fractures. This preventive strategy includes exercise, calcium, estrogen, alendronate, calcitonin, or roloxifene. Other drugs are under study. Fall prevention education with avoidance of sedatives, alcohol, slippery rugs, high-heeled shoes, unprotected bathrooms, and possibly loop diuretics may decrease incidence of fractures.

IV. INFECTIOUS ARTHRITIS

A. Gonococcal Arthritis/Synovitis

► Scientific Concepts

Presentation of systemic gonococcal infection, gram-negative intracellular and extracellular diplococcus, produces a septic arthritis to hands, wrists, elbows, ankles, and, rarely, the axial skeleton.

► History & Physical

Acute loss of joint motion with fusiform swelling of digit or knee. Erythema, redness, fevers, migratory polyarthritis, multiple arthralgias. Highest finding is in sexually active women between 16 and 35 years old. Palmar pustules may be most important clue. Multiple-location presentations means present for > 6 days.

► Diagnosis

History and physical diagnosis confirmed by aspiration and culture of pustule or effused joint. Radiographs for the first week are normal. Frequent presentation in sexually active 15- to 30-year-old with 5 to 7 days of fever, shaking, chills, multiple skin lesions (petechiae, papules, pustules, hemorrhagic bullae, or necrotizing lesions), migratory polyarthritis, and tenosynovitis in the fingers, wrists, toes, and ankles. Operational rule for diagnosis is to culture all orifices and plate at the bedside on chocolate agar or Thayer–Martin medium (synovial fluid, blood, cervix, urethra, rectum, pharynx, and skin lesion fluid).

► Clinical Intervention

Presentation of systemic gonococcal infection (*Neisseria gonnorrhoeae*) requires urgent attention and prompt use of antibiotics. Current treatment recommendations are initial ceftriaxone, 1 g/d × 7 days; if found to be sensitive, penicillin, 10 to 20 million units/d, or ampicillin, 4 g/d × 7 days. Daily needle aspiration of synovial fluid should be performed as long as it continues to accumulate. Gonococcal infections usually do not require surgical debridement and drainage, and most often do not produce permanent damage.

B. Osteomyelitis

► Scientific Concepts

In children, osteomyelitis is usually hematogenous. Seeding occurs in the small arterioles of the metaphysis where there is sluggish blood flow. Infection elevates pressure, creating pain. Pus lifts the periosteum and may cause cortical necrosis, resulting in a sequestrum. The most common organism is *Staphylococcus aureus,* except in neonates, in whom *Streptococcus* B is most common. *Haemophilus influenzae* is seen most often in the 6-month to 5-year range. In adults with septic arthritis or osteomyelitis, ~ 40% are > 60. In this group, 75% of the infections occur in joints with prior arthritis or joint damage.

► History & Physical

More common in children and elderly than healthy adults and young people. May be associated with trauma; usual seeding is hematogenous. Presents with refusal to bear weight or move extremity. Fever 100 to 102°F may be present. Disease severity is associated with worsening symptoms in spite of treatment, pain at rest, elevated white blood count (WBC), chronic disease comorbidities (diabetes, renal failure, etc.). Rising ESR may be helpful for monitoring disease activity.

▶ **Diagnostic Studies**

WBC, ESR, blood cultures. Radiographs may show soft tissue swelling early, followed by periosteal elevation and finally bone infarct and collapse. Bone scan (shows focal increased activity) and MRI are usually diagnostic.

▶ **Diagnosis**

Clinical suspicion and an extra-articular focus of infection should prompt a search for septic arthritis. Positive Gram stain and culture of the synovial fluid are the fundamental criteria for diagnosis of any bacterial arthritis. Synovial fluid analysis is the most important test in acute septic arthritis.

▶ **Clinical Intervention**

Aspiration is useful to recover organisms for antibiotic selectivity. Blood cultures may substitute if positive. Intravenous (IV) antibiotics followed by oral medication after temperature normalized for 6 weeks or until WBC and ESR normalize. Immobilization for symptomatic relief. Surgical debridement for refractory cases.

▶ **Health Maintenance Issues**

Current recommendations to prevent infection of joint prosthesis are:
1. Search for and eradicate any foci of infections in dental, genitourinary, gastrointestinal, or cutaneous sites before joint surgery.
2. Discontinue corticosteroids and immunosuppressive drugs or reduce to the lowest possible dose.
3. Administer preoperative antibiotics.
4. Treat any infection promptly and aggressively.
5. Use prophylactic antibiotics for procedures likely to produce bacteria in patients with high risks.

C. Lyme Disease

▶ **Scientific Concepts**

Disease caused by *Borrelia burgdorferi*, a spirochete borne by the deer tick (*Ixodes dammini*). Disease occurs in three stages: rash, neurological symptoms (neuritis, neuropathy, encephalopathy), arthritis. Immune complexes and cryoglobulin accumulate in the synovial fluid and tissues of the host.

▶ **History & Physical**

Highly variable presentation: joint effusions, arthralgia, myalgia, fatigue, occasional cardiac arrhythmia, central nervous system (CNS) involvement (Bell's palsy, headaches). May have characteristic rash, erythema chronicum migrans ("bull's-eye" rash). Knee effusion may be asymptomatic. Cardiac and CNS symptoms indicate disease severity.

▶ **Diagnostic Studies**

Joint aspirates negative by culture, radiographs normal; serological testing: enzyme-linked immunosorbent assay (ELISA) screen, confirmatory Western blot.

► Clinical Intervention

Treatment with oral doxycycline, 100 mg bid, or amoxicillin, 2 g/d × 3 weeks. Recalcitrant cases: ceftriaxone, 2 g/d IV × 6 weeks.

► Health Maintenance Issues

Vaccine is available for prevention in at least 70% of cases.

V. CRYSTAL-ASSOCIATED ARTHRITIS

A. Gout

► Scientific Concepts

Tissue deposition of monosodium urate crystals from supersaturated extracellular fluids. Recurrent attacks of severe articular and peripheral inflammation: gouty arthritis. Accumulation of crystalline deposits in the soft tissue: gout tophi. Renal impairment: gouty nephropathy. Causes: overproduction of serum uric acid, 10%; underexcretion of serum uric acid, 90%. Age, alcohol, dehydration, trauma/surgery, diuretics, and high-purine diet may precipitate attacks.

► History & Physical

Acute onset of painful, swollen, erythematous joints, deposition of crystals in soft tissue, tophi. Trauma, alcohol, diuretics, surgical stress, or acute medical illness may precede attacks. Occurs in great toe in 70% of cases, followed by ankle, knee, tarsals, wrists, fingers, and elbow. Polyarticular attacks, soft-tissue tophus formation, joint destruction, and associated renal failure are indications of disease severity and warrant aggressive treatment.

► Diagnostic Studies

Aspiration of joint fluid for phagocytosis of crystals. Birefringence confirms monosodium urate crystal.

► Clinical Intervention

Treatment with NSAIDs; indomethacin, 25 to 50 mg tid. Chronic management for those with ≥ three attacks per year; colchicine, probenecid, sulfinpyrazone, and allopurinol.

B. Calcium Pyrophosphate Deposition Disease (Pseudogout)

► Scientific Concepts

Genetic defects are believed to contribute to metabolic disorders that enhance deposition of calcium pyrophosphate dihydrate (CPPD) crystals. Crystals are shed into the joint and phagocytized by leukocytes, which release lysosomal enzymes, resulting in acute inflammatory response. Diseases associated with CPPD include hyperparathyroidism, hemochromatosis, hypophosphatasia, hypomagnesemia, gout, neuropathic arthropathy, and osteoarthrosis.

► History & Physical

Acute-onset painful, swollen, or achy, red, large joints seen in 25% of patients, mimicking gout. Knee most commonly involved, followed by hips and wrists. Attacks usually self-limited from a few days to a few weeks. Rare involvement of small joints of hands and feet. Chondrocalcinosis found on radiographs in majority of cases.

► Diagnostic Studies

No known biochemical abnormalities on routine laboratory screen. Aspirated synovial fluid requires confirming diagnosis. CPPD crystals are rhomboid shaped and exhibit weakly positive birefringence. Differential: gout, septic arthritis, and hydroxyapatite crystal deposition disease. Radiographs demonstrating widespread chondrocalcinosis. Knee menisci, symphysis pubis, and triangular cartilage of wrist. Subchondral bone cysts and hooklike osteophytes of metacarpal joints.

► Clinical Intervention

Arthrocentesis alone removes a significant quantity of inciting crystals and chemical mediators, thereby allowing the synovitis to subside. Intra-articular injections of triamcinolone hexacetonide (Aristospan) or other long-acting corticosteroid preparations is the treatment of choice. NSAIDs have little benefit except for acute pain management.

VI. NEUROVASCULAR DISORDERS

A. Peripheral Entrapment (Carpal Tunnel Syndrome)

► Scientific Concepts

The median nerve and common flexors pass through the common tunnel in the wrist, bound volarly by the transverse carpal ligament. Any process that impinges upon the median nerve may create symptoms.

► History & Physical

Night symptoms are common with paresthesias in the median nerve distribution (index and long fingers, sometimes the radial half of the ring finger). Progressive median nerve dysfunction with loss of two-point discrimination and weakness of thumb abduction and thenar atrophy suggest disease severity.

► Diagnostic Studies

Other associated conditions, including RA, diabetes, pregnancy, amyloidosis, and thyroid disease, need to be excluded. Examination is usually diagnostic. Diminished sensation in median nerve distribution. Positive Tinel's sign in carpal canal or positive Phalen's test. Nerve conduction velocity delays across carpal tunnel is confirmatory.

▶ Clinical Intervention

Primary treatment is rest and with a cock-up resting splint. Injection of a corticosteroid may be effective, especially if there is an inflammatory component of the cause. Surgical decompression for those not responding to conservative treatment.

B. Spinal Stenosis

▶ Scientific Concepts

Maturing of the skeleton results in degenerative changes and hypertrophy of spinal canal and facet joints. Bony overgrowth constricts the nerve roots. Ligamentous thickening and diskogenic protrusions may exacerbate this.

▶ History & Physical

Elderly patients with complaints of difficulty walking the length of a mall. History is often not specific, but note that they cannot walk the distance they once could for unclear reasons. Sometimes history suggests claudication. When pain in back is present, rest often relieves it. Paresthesias and weakness of legs is uncommon. Back pain may be aggravated by hyperextension of spine and relieved with flexion of spine. Sensory sensations are vague but descriptions of water or candle wax dripping down the leg is common. Clinical impairment of activities with neurogenic claudication. Pain increased with any activity that causes hyperextension of the spine.

▶ Diagnostic Studies

Radiographs may show degeneration of facet joints. CT is best noninvasive test for bony stenosis. Myelograms are used less often to confirm findings.

▶ Clinical Intervention

Adjustment to the limitations of the disease in conjunction with pain medications, stretching, and an exercise program will decrease pain. Laminectomy to decompress the nerve root will provide good relief for many patients.

VII. EXTRA-ARTICULAR DISORDERS

A. Rotator Cuff Tear

▶ Scientific Concepts

The rotator cuff of the shoulder comprises the tendons of the supraspinatus, infraspinatus, teres minor, and subscapularis muscles and attaches at the humeral tuberosities. A tear anywhere in the rotator cuff presents as pain or loss of some function.

▶ History & Physical

Generally, an acute tear of a rotator cuff after trauma is easily recognized. Shoulder pain, weakness on abduction, and loss of motion occur in varying degrees, ranging from severe pain and mild weakness to no pain and marked tenderness. Positive "arm drop sign" and inability to actively maintain 90° passive shoulder abduction is present in large tears.

▶ Diagnostic Studies

An abnormal arthrogram showing communication between the glenohumeral joint and the subacromial bursa establish the definitive diagnosis of a ruptured rotator cuff. Diagnostic ultrasound or MRI helpful in identifying small or incomplete tears.

▶ Diagnosis

Imaging makes the diagnosis. In trauma, especially falls, resulting in a ruptured cuff, fractures of the humeral head and dislocation of the joint should be considered.

▶ Clinical Therapeutics

Small tears and incomplete tears are treated conservatively with rest, physical therapy, and NSAIDs.

▶ Clinical Intervention

Subacromial injections of a steroid may be of benefit in relieving pain.

▶ Health Maintenance Issues

Specific range-of-motion and strengthening exercises should be incorporated as soon as tolerated.

B. Shoulder Tendinitis

▶ Scientific Concepts

Tendinitis is inflammation of the tendon sheath secondary to overuse. This may be due to acute overload with partial tearing of the tendon as a result of repetitive stress. A sudden change in use or sporting activity that exceeds the body's reparative capabilities will result in "overuse" tendinitis.

▶ History & Physical

Soft-tissue swelling or pain over bicipital or supraspinatus tendon near insertion. May be acute in onset or a result of repetitive overload, often seen after a sudden change in activity.

▶ Diagnostic Studies

Physical signs of localized inflammation may be rare. Point tenderness over tendon and painful arc in abduction. Weakness usually secondary to pain.

▶ Clinical Intervention

Local treatment with ice massage and oral analgesics. NSAIDs provide pain relief but do little to reduce the inflammation of tendons. A corticosteroid injection alongside tendon sheath is often curative.

Restoration of normal motion through gentle stretching program followed by strength exercises and endurance training can reduce recurrence. Return to sports and activity is gradual.

▶ Health Maintenance Issues

Assessment of work activity and sports intensity with adaptation of program will reduce recurrence.

C. Bursitis

▶ Scientific Concepts

Bursae form whenever two tissue planes move in opposite directions or where tissues travel over a bony protuberance. Normal bursal locations are in the subacromial space of the shoulders, over the olecranon of the elbow, over the tibial tubercle, and in the prepatellar space. This normal structure allows skin, tendon, muscle to slide over each other easily. If the bursa becomes infected, injured, or inflamed, fluid will accumulate in the bursa and produce visible swelling. Fibrinous loose bodies may also be formed in the bursa. After inflammation subsides, adhesions and fibrosis may occur in the bursa, resulting in crepitation and sometimes pain.

▶ History & Physical

Soft-tissue swelling that may be either painful or painless, usually over a bony prominence. Swelling may occur spontaneously or as a result of trauma or part of an inflammatory event (gout, RA). Bursal fluid aspiration with high WBC indicates disease severity.

▶ Diagnostic Studies

Clinical evaluation. Technically, a bursa is a fluid-filled sac that a needle can be inserted into and fluid exchanged. The diagnosis is often made incorrectly when tendinitis or enthesis is present but not a bursitis (e.g., shoulder bursitis, trochanteric bursitis). Bursa should be palpable and fluctuant to confirm presence of inflammatory fluid in the bursa.

▶ Clinical Intervention

Acute treatment consists of rest, ice, aspiration, and corticosteroid injections. Aspirate should be analyzed for elevated WBC, bacteria, and crystals. Use of protective padding, elbow and kneepads can prevent recurrence. Surgical excision is sometimes needed if the size or the location interferes with activities of daily living.

▶ Health Maintenance Issues

Avoidance of repetitive motions and trauma will prevent bursal inflammation. Treatment of any underlying collagen vascular disease or crystalline arthritis will control the bursal swelling.

D. Fibromyalgia

▶ Scientific Concepts

Etiology is unknown. Fatigue is felt to be due to sleep disturbance (nonrestorative sleep) and loss of sustained periods of deep sleeping (delta wave sleep). Alpha intrusions into the delta wave pattern may be part of the pathology. At least one-third of patients have a temporal association of an event with onset of the condition.

► History & Physical

Patients present with diffuse achiness, stiffness, fatigue, associated with multiple areas of clinical tenderness. Ninety percent are female, with an age distribution of 20 to 60 years. Virtually all will have pain of more than 3 months' duration and most with more than 2 years' duration at time of diagnosis. Pain is most pronounced in the axial distribution such as the neck and lower back. Upper trapezius is common location of pain. Tenderness is present with moderate pressure in the occiput, trapezii, infrascapularis, lower back, L-4, lateral epicondyles, and pes anserine area. No correlation with subjective pain perceptions and outcome or limitations.

► Diagnostic Studies

Clinical examination makes the diagnosis; there are no exclusion lab tests. Thyroid tests and CK may be helpful, but ESR, RF, ANA, and Lyme tests are not indicated in chronic, nonprogressive pain disorders.

► Clinical Therapeutics

Patient education and reassurance that this is not an inflammatory disease nor the prodrome of a more serious debilitating disease. Recovery is possible. Aerobic exercise is more beneficial than stretching alone. NSAIDs and narcotics are not effective. Soporific doses of tricyclic antidepressants (doxepin, imipramine, amitriptyline, protriptyline) and trazodone may be helpful for sleep and pain reduction.

VIII. DISORDERS OF THE BACK AND SPINE

► Scientific Concepts

Back pain is usually a self-limiting condition resulting from an acute strain or repetitive overload. The resulting pain is usually of ligaments pulled, muscles and tendons shortened by contracture, and sometimes short-term disability from the pain. Signs of inflammation are not present and steroids do not seem to help. NSAIDs offer some analgesic benefit.

► History & Physical

Predisposing factors include age 30 to 50, repetitive movements such as lifting, pulling, bending, and twisting. Exposure to chronic vibration and prolonged sitting. Contributing factors include sedentary life-style, cigarette habituation, poor posture, emotional stress, and obesity. Physical evaluation of spine motion in all planes. Perivertebral muscle spasm. Presence of radicular pain below the knee suggests neurological involvement or sciatica.

► Diagnostic Studies

Imaging such as radiographs, MRI, and CT are rarely necessary for initial evaluation but indicated when symptoms persist and radicular neurological symptoms develop later.

► Clinical Intervention

Short period of rest (3 to 5 days). Treatment of muscle pain with ice massage and lumbar support. Acetaminophen, NSAIDs, or narcotics for analgesic effect. Education to prevent recurrence and in proper body mechanics.

► Health Maintenance Issues

Muscle strengthening for back and abdomen combined with back flexibility program should be strongly encouraged.

IX. OTHER MUSCULOSKELETAL PROBLEMS

A. Bruises and Contusions

► History & Physical

Most injuries involve some soft tissue, skin, skeletal muscle, or fascia (the fibrous tissue that encloses muscles). Injury may be closed or open. In closed injuries, there is no break in the skin. A bruise or contusion occurs when a blunt object strikes against the body with sufficient force to crush the tissue beneath the skin. Within this tissue, a contusion (bruise) develops. Subsurface damage may extend for varying depths beneath the skin. Generally, amount of contusion determines degree of severity. Pools of blood may collect under the skin (hematoma) suggesting greater severity of injury.

► Diagnostic Studies

When considerable amounts of tissue are damaged or torn, or when large blood vessels are disrupted at the site of the contusion, a lump may develop rather rapidly from a pool of blood collecting within the damaged tissue.

► Clinical Intervention

Small bruises require no special emergency medical care. With severe, closed soft-tissue injuries, extensive swelling and bleeding beneath the skin may cause shock. Applying local padding and a soft roller bandage for counterpressure can partially control this bleeding in extremities. Elevating extremity and applying ice locally to the area are also helpful in decreasing bleeding of injured tissue and preventing initial tissue swelling. If athlete has suffered extensive soft-tissue damage, fractures should be considered.

B. Muscle and Tendon Strains

► Disease Severity

It is often difficult to differentiate between mild and moderate strains. Knowing the extent of the pain, spasm, and weakness is useful in estimating the extent of the injury and the time lost from normal activities. Severe strains often result in palpable deformities and absence of function. The clinician must be careful not to misinterpret the actions of synergetic muscles in examination of severe strains.

▶ History & Physical

A strain is a tear in the muscle and tendon fibers. This is due to sudden overload on the musculoskeletal unit. Knowing the type of injury (sports, falling, other accidents) helps to define the most common of strains.

▶ Diagnostic Studies

Signs and symptoms of muscle strain (tearing of muscles) include pain over the site of injury, muscle spasms, and loss of strength. Careful examination may find muscle and tendon deficits. Timely examination is essential so a treatment and rehabilitation plan can be established.

▶ Clinical Intervention

Initial management of strains is rest, ice, compression, and elevation (RICE). This treatment reduces the tissue damage from bleeding and swelling. An ice compress held in place with elastic bandage should be administered 15 to 30 minutes q1–2. Strains of the lower extremity that are too painful for walking should be protected and rested. Crutches, slings, and commercial supports should be employed.

C. Ligament Sprains

▶ History & Physical

Sprains are the stretching and tearing of ligaments. They differ from strains in that sprains involve a joint while strains involve tendons and muscles. Sprains more specifically refer to the joint injury in which a dislocation has not taken place but the ligaments are damaged.

▶ Diagnostic Studies

Ligament tears may be seen with an open wound, but more commonly they are based on the following signs:
- *Tenderness:* Point tenderness is elicited over the injured ligament.
- *Swelling and ecchymosis:* There is typically swelling and bruising at the point of ligament laxity.
- *Instability:* Gently stressing the injured ligament will increase pain and demonstrates an increased abnormal range of motion. Comparing the injured limb to the uninjured limb helps to determine the diagnosis and extent of the injury.
- *Inability to use the extremity:* Because of the pain of the injury, it is often very difficult to use the limb normally.

Ligament sprains are graded according to the following classification:

Grade I (mild): The ligament is stretched, but there is no loss of continuity of its fiber.

Grade II (moderate): The ligament is partially torn, resulting in some increased laxity to the joint.

Grade III (severe): The ligament is completely torn, resulting in laxity (instability) of the joint which it stabilizes.

▶ Clinical Intervention

The management of ligament sprains depends on the degree of injury. First-degree sprains are treated with RICE until acute symptoms subside. A rehabilitation program will help prepare for a return to normal activity sooner than without. Second-degree sprain is treated similarly but may require additional immobilization and analgesics. Depending on location and severity of the injury, a third-degree sprain may require prolonged immobilization or surgical intervention to restore continuity of the ligament.

X. FRACTURES

A. Closed Fractures and Dislocations of the Hand and Phalanges

▶ History & Physical

In general, fractures of the hand require physical assessment and radiographic evaluation. Treatment is often complex, and the functional result may depend on the experience of the person with these injuries.

▶ Diagnostic Studies

Clinical diagnosis is obvious if there is any gross deformity. However, in many occult and nondisplaced fractures, clinical diagnosis may be difficult. Most reliable sign of injury is localized tenderness, but this does not specifically localize the injury to soft tissue or bone. Radiographs are essential for confirmation of the fracture and the degree of displacement of the fractures. The types of common hand fractures include:

- *Gamekeeper's thumb:* This results from the forceful abduction of the thumb away from the hand. Local tenderness is on the ulnar side of the metacarpophalangeal joint. Diagnosis is confirmed by stressing the joint laterally in extension. A radiograph may reveal fractures or volar subluxation of the joint.
- *Dislocation of the MCP joint:* MCP dislocations usually follow hyperextension injuries and dislocation dorsally in respect to the metacarpal head. The joint remains hyperextended and foreshortened with obvious deformity.
- *Metacarpal fractures:* Metacarpal fractures, particularly of the neck of the fifth metacarpal, are relatively common. Usually caused by a direct blow to the MCP joint with a clenched fist, as when striking a hard object. Usually there is tenderness, swelling, and angulation on the back of the hand. Radiographs determine if the fracture is oblique, multiple, or complicated.

► Clinical Intervention

Management of fractures and dislocations is with splinting, immobilization, casting, and sometimes surgical intervention. Minimum of 4 to 6 weeks is needed for fracture healing in proper alignment.

B. Fractures of the Foot and Leg

► History & Physical

Direct trauma to the foot or leg may cause fractures of the bones of the foot or lower leg. All 26 bones of the foot and the two long bones of the lower leg are vulnerable, and the site of the fracture depends on the amount of force and its direction. A fractured phalanx is usually a minor injury, but an open comminuted fracture of the tibia is a major problem. If injured toe is in good alignment, it can be taped to adjacent toe. Open comminuted tibial fracture requires surgical intervention. Pain, swelling, and localized tenderness are noted at the site of injury. X-rays are used to confirm diagnosis. Most foot injuries are not emergencies, with the exception of open dislocations and fracture–dislocations of the hindfoot.

► Diagnostic Studies

Clinical diagnosis is obvious if there is any gross deformity. However, in many occult and nondisplaced fractures, clinical diagnosis may be difficult. Most reliable sign of injury is localized tenderness, but this does not specifically localize the injury to soft tissue or bone. Radiographs are essential for confirmation of fracture and degree of displacement of fractures.

► Clinical Intervention

Closed nondisplaced fractures of the foot usually respond to conservative treatment. The tibia usually requires a cast while the fibula can be managed without a cast. Fractures of the first and fifth metatarsal take a long time to heal and need to be relieved of weight bearing. Fractures of the metatarsal and midtarsal bones may require short walking cast or hard-soled shoe.

C. Cervical Fractures

► History & Physical

Violent force in flexion or extension may cause fractures of cervical vertebrae. Perhaps the most frequent cause of spinal cord injury is that of axial loading of the cervical spine in football and other contact sports.

► Diagnostic Studies

A cervical fracture or dislocation is a medical emergency. With head injury, the clinician should always consider possibility of cervical spine fracture or injury and protect conscious patient from random movements. The conscious patient with a cervical spine injury can assist the examiner in assessing movement, sensation, and muscle power. Cervical spine fracture can be diagnosed only by imaging studies.

- Fracture of first cervical vertebra (Jefferson's fracture) is a burst fracture of the ring of C1 when the condyles of the occiput are driven down against the ring of the atlas, splitting this fragile bone. This fracture may be difficult to detect and overlooked with ordinary x-rays.
- Fracture of second cervical vertebra (hangman's fracture) results in altered alignment between first two cervical vertebrae. Odontoid process of second cervical vertebra may rupture transverse ligaments of first cervical vertebra, allowing the atlas to slide forward on second cervical vertebra and encroach on the space occupied by spinal cord.
- Fractures of lower cervical spine are often seen in motor vehicle accidents and contact sports injuries. These occur often at the fourth, fifth, and sixth cervical levels. These injuries may be associated with varying degrees of damage to neural elements and can cause transient or permanent damage. Potential for neurological damage is high.

A fracture, subluxation, or dislocation of the normal alignment of the cervical vertebrae results in loss of the normal anatomic alignment with associated ligament, tendon, muscles, disk, bone, and neural elements. Only appropriate imaging studies can determine extent and severity of injury.

▶ Clinical Intervention

If x-rays are positive for cervical fracture, the neck must be stabilized to prevent further neurological damage and determine if surgical intervention is necessary. Paralysis and even sudden death can occur almost any time in the course of stabilization and management.

XI. SPINE CONDITIONS

A. Upper Back and Thoracic Spine Injuries

▶ History & Physical

Soft-tissue injuries to the upper back are usually blunt injuries and cause contusions. When severity of the blow is sufficient, rib fractures can occur. Because they often result in bleeding, swelling, and tenderness at the site of the injury, they are confused with muscle contusions. Thoracic or dorsal spine fractures can result from either direct or indirect force. The nature of thoracic spine injuries differs from that of cervical and lumbar spine injuries because of the protective effects of the rib cage. Fractures from direct blows are rare and are usually the result of vertical loading of the spine or a rotational force. Spinal fractures are classified as stable or unstable depending on their potential to shift and cause further injury to spinal cord or nerve roots. The vertebral body compression or wedge fracture is the most common thoracic fracture. Although bone is compressed, ligamentous structures are intact, making this a stable fracture. In the unstable slice or chance fracture, there is horizontal disruption of the vertebral body and ligamentous structures.

► Diagnostic Studies

Thoracic pain referred to the site of injury from pressure over an uninvolved portion of the same rib is indicative of a fractured rib. Sometimes only an x-ray can differentiate between a fracture and a contusion. Correct diagnosis is important because a rib fracture can puncture the pleural lining of the chest cavity or even the lung.

► Clinical Intervention

Treatment of any vertebral fracture is rest from activity for 3 to 5 days, then gradual rehabilitation. The fracture will require 4 to 6 weeks of analgesic management until it stabilizes and begins healing. If there is intrinsic bone loss due to osteoporosis or other metabolic disorders, these will need to be investigated and treated.

B. Spondylolysis and Spondylolisthesis

► Scientific Concepts

Chronic pain confined to the lumbar spine may be caused by segmental instability and associated with lumbar pars interarticularis defects.

- **Spondylolysis** is a defect in the pars interarticularis. Cause of this defect is unknown. It may be congenital or a result of sustained repetitive stress to the area as from an unhealed stress fracture. If both the right and left pars interarticularis of a vertebra are defective, the affected vertebra can slip anterior to the one below it.
- **Spondylolisthesis** is actual displacement of one vertebra on another through the spondylitic defect on the pars, which usually occurs at L5–S1. Spondylolisthesis, or slippage, occurs in 5% of people with spondylolysis.

Symptoms of either of these pathologies are seen in athletes in whom the spine is repetitively loaded in a flexion or extension mode (football players, gymnasts, ice skaters).

► Diagnostic Studies

Most people with these spinal defects are unaware that they have them. The defects are frequently noted on routine films taken for some other reason. In a few individuals, degree of spondylolisthesis is progressive during teen years and results in a narrowed neural canal (spinal stenosis). An acute pars defect can be differentiated from a chronic one by bone scan.

► Clinical Intervention

If pain in low back is from spondylolisthesis or spondylolysis, rest is the cornerstone of treatment. Usually for a few weeks depending on the severity of the condition. Sometimes a splint is used for severe cases. In rare situations, surgical treatment is employed.

BIBLIOGRAPHY

Hoppenfeld S. *Physical Examination of the Spine and Extremities.* New York: Appleton-Century-Crofts; 1976.

Kelley WN, Ruddy S, Harris ED, Sledge CB, eds. *Textbook of Rheumatology,* 5th ed. Philadelphia: WB Saunders; 1997.

Magee DJ. *Orthopedic Physical Assessment.* Toronto, ON: WB Saunders; 1992.

Schumacher RH, ed. *Primer on the Rheumatic Diseases,* 11th ed. Atlanta, GA: Arthritis Foundation; 1997.

Neurology 12

Ricky E. Kortyna, MMS, PA-C

I. INFECTIOUS DISEASES

A. Brain Abscess

▶ **Scientific Concepts**

About 25% with no discernible etiology. Most arise as the result of local extension or hematogenous spread from other infections with eventual localization to the gray-white junction. The most frequent sites for spread are sinusitis with *Staphylococcus aureus* and *Streptococcus*, otitis or mastoiditis with gram-negative bacilli and *Streptococcus*, dental infections with *Streptococcus* and *Bacteroides*, pulmonary infections with *Streptococcus* and mixed flora, endocarditis with *Streptococcus* and *S. aureus*, and head wound/surgical with *S. aureus* and gram-negative bacilli. Needs to be considered with those with acquired immune deficiency syndrome (AIDS) and intravenous (IV) drug abusers. Mortality is about 20%; morbidity is near 50% with residual neurological deficits and seizure disorders.

▶ **History & Physical**

Most do not present with signs of acute infection such as fever, nuchal rigidity, or leukocytosis. Most common symptoms in descending order are headache, focal deficit that corresponds to the lobe involved, altered mental status such as drowsiness or confusion, seizure, fever, vomiting, papilledema, nuchal rigidity.

▶ **Diagnostic Studies**

Either computed tomography (CT) or magnetic resonance imaging (MRI). Ring enhancing lesion with central focal necrosis and edema; "Daughter lesions" or satellite lesions may be seen. Definitive diagnosis via CT-guided stereotaxic brain biopsy. Lumbar puncture contraindicated as it may lead to rapid neurological deterioration if patient has increased intracranial pressure. After positive scan, workup needs to include chest x-ray, electrocardiogram (ECG), dental films, sinus CT, etc. to find etiology.

▶ **Diagnosis**

Certain tumors such as glioblastomas, metastases, infarctions, resolving hematoma, and radiation necrosis may be confused with brain abscess on CT or MRI.

▶ **Clinical Therapeutics**

Antibiotics tailored to the cultures obtained via biopsy. If empiric therapy needed, broad-spectrum antibiotic regimen such as penicillin G, 4 million units IV q4h, plus ceftriaxone, 4 g IV q12h, plus metronidazole, 500 mg IV q6h, is suggested therapy. Antibiotic treatment alone may be successful for those lesions < 3 cm. Duration of treatment is 6 to 8 weeks. Follow lesions with serial CT/MRIs.

▶ **Clinical Intervention**

CT-guided stereotaxic biopsy important to obtain exact infecting organism(s) and drain abscess.

► Health Maintenance Issues

Prompt and complete treatment of upper respiratory infections (URIs). About 50% left with neurological sequelae that may be focal in nature. Use of anticonvulsants after abscess treatment common as up to 50% have seizures.

B. Meningitis

► Scientific Concepts

Inflammation of the meninges caused by an infective agent such as a virus, bacteria, tuberculosis, fungus, chemical agent, or tumor infiltration. Incidence is 3/100,000. Often a history of preceding URI. Most common community-acquired organisms: *Streptococcus pneumoniae, Neisseria meningitidis,* and *Listeria monocytogenes.* Most common nosocomial: gram-negative bacilli, *Staphylococcus aureus,* and coagulase-negative staphylococci. Nosocomial is on the increase secondary to trauma and neurosurgical procedures. Damage due to cytokines such as interleukin-1, interleukin-6, and tumor necrosis factor (TNF), with secondary brain edema, increased intracranial pressure, and altered cerebral blood flow. Mortality varies with causative organism—gram-negative the highest at 36% in one study.

► History & Physical

Fever, headache, and cognitive dysfunction in 75%. Positive Kernig's and/or Brudzinski's. Nausea, vomiting, rigors, sweats, weakness, myalgias, and photophobia. One-third with seizures. Signs of meningismus such as nuchal rigidity in 90%, positive Kernig's and/or Brudzinski's on examination. Focal deficits such as cranial nerve palsies, hemiparesis, aphasia in up to 20% of patients. Papilledema rare. Petechial rash with meningococcemia. Symptoms subtle in elderly.

► Diagnostic Studies

If no papilledema, do lumbar puncture. If papilledema, CT scan first to eliminate intracranial mass or abscess. Also need blood cultures, complete blood count (CBC) and differential. Nuclear scans sensitive but not specific for cerebrospinal fluid (CSF) leak post-surgery/trauma.

► Diagnosis

CSF with increased neutrophils, decreased glucose, and increased protein. Any or all of these studies may be normal in up to 30% of bacterial infections. High opening pressure in 75%. CSF cultures positive in > 70%. Obtain stat Gram stain. Rapid tests such as counterimmunoelectrophoresis (CIE) and latex agglutination specific but sensitivity may be variable.

► Clinical Therapeutics

Antibiotics must penetrate blood–brain barrier. Culture-specific treatment preferred but often must treat empirically. For adults, community-acquired: ampicillin, 2 g IV q4h, and ceftriaxone, 2 to 3 g IV q12h. For adults, nosocomial: vancomycin, 1 g IV q12h, and ceftazidime, 2 g IV q8h. Duration 10 to 21 days. Use of steroids controversial in adults but decreases morbidity in *Haemophilus influenzae* meningitis in children.

► Clinical Intervention

Remove hardware (shunt, ventriculostomy, etc.) in neurosurgery patient if possible.

► Health Maintenance Issues

Close contacts of documented cases of *N. meningitidis* or *H. influenzae* treated with rifampin immediately. Health care workers also should be treated if in contact with secretions. Dose: 600 mg bid for adults, 10 mg/kg for children. Pneumococcal vaccine helpful.

II. DEGENERATIVE DISEASES

A. Alzheimer's Disease

► Scientific Concepts

Affects up to 10% of Americans over the age of 65, but accounts for only ~ 60% of all cases of dementia. Increased in head injury patients, Down syndrome, prolonged exposure to solvents, lower educational levels, epilepsy, exposure to anesthetics, and depression. More frequent in women. Life expectancy reduced by 5 to 10 years.

► History & Physical

The initial or *mild stage* lasts 2 to 4 years. Patients repeat words, misplace objects, forget words, become passive and apathetic, and become lost on familiar routes. The *moderate stage* lasts 2 to 10 years and is highlighted by increasing confusion, belligerence, pacing, and wandering. Personal grooming habits deteriorate, hallucinations or delusions occur, and full-time supervision is needed. The *severe stage* lasts 1 to 3 years and patients cannot function independently, cannot recognize themselves or their family, cannot use or understand language, and have no capacity for self-care. They are susceptible to malnutrition and infections.

► Diagnostic Studies

Stereotaxic biopsy or postmortem samples needed for definitive diagnosis. These show senile plaques and neurofibrillary tangles. CSF normal. Nonspecific enlargement of the lateral ventricles, atrophy of the cortex, and widening of the sulci on CT/MRI. Biochemical reduction of choline acetyltransferase is seen.

► Diagnosis

Dementia established by neuropsychometric examination, deficits in two or more areas of cognition, progressive worsening of memory, no disturbance of consciousness, onset between ages of 40 and 90, and absence of other disease. Diagnosis by biopsy. Other considerations: cerebrovascular dementias, Parkinson's, Huntington's, Pick's, HIV dementia.

► Clinical Therapeutics

Cholinesterase inhibitors such as tacrine and donepezil; calcium channel blockers such as nimodipine; anti-inflammatory drugs such as aspirin, colchicine, and ibuprofen; estrogen; antioxidants such as vitamins C and E. There are varied new medications under trial.

► Clinical Intervention

None.

► Health Maintenance Issues

Education of families necessary. Social service, day care programs, elder care, institutionalization. Aluminum intake not an issue, although it has been demonstrated in the neurofibrillary tangles.

B. Parkinson's Disease

► Scientific Concepts

Prevalence is 120/100,000 in the United States. Incidence increases with age. Etiology undetermined but is probably multifactorial. In young-onset patient, correlation with rural residence, drinking well water, and exposure to pesticides. Reduced risk in cigarette smokers.

► History & Physical

The principal features are bradykinesia, rigidity, and tremor. Bradykinesia (slowness of movement) is often the presenting sign. Patients lose dexterity for fine motor movements and have difficulty getting up from a chair. Rigidity is of a cogwheeling nature. Tremor is 3 to 5 cycles/sec and is known as pillrolling. Other findings include masked facies, seborrhea, micrographia, shuffling gait, flexed posture, dysarthria, drooling, depression, sleep disorders, psychosis, and dementia.

► Diagnostic Studies

Pathologically: pallor of the substantia nigra and presence of Lewy bodies. Biochemically: a deficiency of dopamine in the striatum.

► Diagnosis

Parkinsonian syndrome may be secondary to encephalitis, trauma, toxic or metabolic disease, or may be drug induced by neuroleptics or antipsychotics. Similar symptoms also seen with vascular disease, hydrocephalus, tumors, Creutzfeldt–Jakob disease, and Wilson's disease.

► Clinical Therapeutics

Selegiline, 2.5 mg bid and titrate up (for neuroprotection). Carbidopa-levodopa (Sinemet) 25/100 and titrate up. Vitamins C and E to prevent toxic effects of Sinemet. Levodopa helps about 75%, but because of side effects, was combined with carbidopa to make Sinemet. Trihexyphenidyl (Artane) and benztropine mesylate (Cogentin) may also help.

► Clinical Intervention

Stereotaxic thalamotomy reduces or eliminates tremor and rigidity but not bradykinesia. Transplantation of fetal tissue shows hope for some.

► Health Maintenance Issues

Avoid monoamine oxidase (MAO) inhibitors with patients on Sinemet as the combination may produce hypertensive crisis. Sinemet contraindicated in patients with glaucoma. Patients show lessening effects of improvement after about 5 years of pharmacological treatment. Physical and speech therapy helpful early on in the disease.

C. Multiple Sclerosis

► Scientific Concepts

Afflicts 250,000 Americans. Symptoms from recurrent attacks of inflammation on the nervous system leading to demyelination. Etiology is autoimmune. Female:male ratio is 2:1. Generally strikes at ages 20 to 40, especially Caucasians and those living in northern latitudes. Not inherited but it does cluster in families. Seldom fatal and life expectancy is not significantly shortened. Good prognosis with younger age, sensory symptoms only, rapid resolution, and benign course for the first 5 years.

► History & Physical

Findings separated by time and space. Any neurological complaint can be multiple sclerosis (MS). Most common are weakness/numbness in one limb, optic neuritis, tremor, incoordination, diplopia, dysarthria, vertigo, bowel and bladder dysfunction, and fatigue. Most symptoms are focal; diffuse symptoms are rare. Usually, symptoms occur abruptly and then disappear after 1 to 2 months, but repeated attacks leave residual deficits, and the course is one of remission–relapse with eventual progressive deterioration. Symptoms may occur after exercise, shower. Lhermitte's sign (electrical sensations that spread down the body with flexion of the neck) present with MS and with cervical spinal cord lesions.

► Diagnostic Studies

MRI highly sensitive for periventricular plaques but not specific. CSF with increased immunoglobulin G (IgG) and oligoclonal bands, slight increase in white blood cells (WBCs) and protein. Evoked potentials may help to diagnose.

► Diagnosis

Diagnostic criteria: two separate central nervous system (CNS) lesions; two or more separate episodes; involvement of the white matter; objective findings on exam; patient between 10 and 50 years old; no other disease accounting for symptoms. Also may have two attacks with one lesion and abnormal CSF or one attack with two lesions and abnormal CSF. The course is one of remission–relapse. Differential includes hysteria, encephalomyelitis, vasculitis, Lyme disease, syphilis, sarcoidosis, AIDS, stroke, tumors, and syringomyelia (cavitation of the spinal cord).

▶ Clinical Therapeutics

Steroids: prednisone, 60 mg qd × 7 to 10 days for mild symptoms, methylprednisolone, 500 to 1,000 mg IV × 3 to 4 days for more severe symptoms. Beta-interferon decreases the frequency of the attacks but not practical for most patients. Relief of spasicity via baclofen, diazepam, and dantrolene. Clonazepam to decrease tremor; propranolol or primidone less effective for this. Amantadine to combat fatigue.

▶ Clinical Intervention

No surgical intervention.

▶ Health Maintenance Issues

Supportive measures for neurogenic bladder, decubiti, etc. Psychological support.

III. DISEASES OF THE PERIPHERAL NERVES

A. Diabetic Neuropathy

▶ Scientific Concepts

Also known as distal sensorimotor polyneuropathy–autonomic neuropathy. Diabetic polyradiculopathy is a separate entity. Usually related to duration and severity of hyperglycemia; may be presenting symptom of occult diabetes. Increased incidence of carpal tunnel syndrome and ulnar neuropathy.

▶ History & Physical

Loss of feeling, lower-extremity paresthesias, dysesthesias (burning), hyperesthesias, and pain. These sensory symptoms are often accentuated at night. Symptomatology with a slow evolution. Tends to begin unilaterally but becomes bilateral and symmetric. Begins in toes and feet with distal to proximal involvement. Pain may resolve. Bilateral footdrop in severe cases. Autonomic involvement may lead to lower-extremity anhidrosis (lack of sweating). Exam with decreased sensation to light touch, pinprick, and temperature in stocking distribution. Proprioception, vibratory and reflexes preserved. Rarely ataxia. Other findings include increased heart rate secondary to reduced vagal function, constipation, gastric atony, erectile dysfunction with retrograde ejaculation.

▶ Diagnostic Studies

Abnormal nerve conduction studies. CSF normal. Biopsy seldom done. Workup to rule out differentials as below.

▶ Diagnosis

Uremia, alcoholic/nutritional deficiencies, connective tissue, vasculitis, B_{12} deficiency, hypothyroidism, toxic, paraneoplastic, amyloidosis must be ruled out.

► Clinical Therapeutics

Optimal control of diabetes. Phenytoin, carbamazepine, tricyclic antidepressants, and mexiletine to treat pain. Less effective are capsaicin, clonazepam, and clonidine. Pain tends to resolve after months even without treatment.

► Clinical Intervention

No surgical intervention.

► Health Maintenance Issues

Tight control of diabetes needed (ideal fasting glucose < 70 to 100; ideal 1 hour postprandial < 160). Aggressive foot care.

B. Other Metabolic Neuropathies

► Scientific Concepts

Notoriously difficult to diagnose secondary to the myriad of possible etiologies.

► History & Physical

B_1 *deficiency* with paresthesias, numbness, dysesthesias, pain and cramps in calves. Distal weakness and depressed ankle jerk; graded sensory loss. B_{12} *deficiency* with paresthesias, loss of proprioception, sensation and reflex loss. *Vitamin E deficiency* with loss of deep tendon reflexes, sensory loss and ataxia, muscle weakness and atrophy. *Uremic polyneuropathy* with decreased vibration, depressed Achilles reflex, ascending sensory loss. *Porphyria* with extremity pain/weakness. *Hypothyroidism* with paresthesias of the hands. *Acromegaly* with carpel tunnel syndrome. *Hyperparathyroidism* with generalized weakness, easy fatigability, atrophy, and hyperreflexia.

► Diagnostic Studies

Extremely varied. Thiamine level, Schilling's test for B_{12}, CBC, and for megaloblastic characteristics with B_{12} indices, acanthocytes with vitamin E deficiency. Electromyograms (EMGs) positive in uremic polyneuropathy. Urine alpha-aminolevulinic acid and blood porphobilinogen levels for porphyria. Calcium for parathyroid, thyroid function tests, erythrocyte sedimentation rate (ESR), blood urea nitrogen (BUN), and creatinine.

► Diagnosis

B_1, B_6, B_{12}, B_2, vitamin E deficiencies; hypophosphatemia; uremia; diabetes mellitus; hypo- and hyperthyroidism; hyperparathyroidism; porphyrias; critical illness polyneuropathy.

► Clinical Therapeutics

B_1 *deficiency:* Thiamine, 10 to 100 mg/d IV × 3 days, then 2.5 to 25 mg/d PO until symptoms resolve.
B_{12} *deficiency:* Cyanocobalamin, 1,000 μg IM daily × 1 week, then weekly × 4, then monthly.
Vitamin E deficiency: Vitamin E, 50 to 100 mg IM.

Hypothyroidism: Symptoms may improve with replacement therapy.
Porphyria: Hematin, 2 mg/kg/d IV as this reduces porphyrin precursor excretion.
Thyroid and parathyroid: Treat underlying disease.

► Clinical Intervention

No surgery other than the removal of a parathyroid adenoma.

► Health Maintenance Issues

Aggressive follow-up of nutritional disorders. Renal transplant reverses uremic polyneuropathy, but dialysis does not. Tight follow-up of thyroid and parathyroid patients. Avoid provocative factors such as estrogens, phenytoin, and alcohol in porphyria.

C. Toxic Peripheral Neuropathies

► Scientific Concepts

May be pharmacological, iatrogenic, or environmental with exposures to arsenic, lead, mercury, acrylamide, cyanide, methyl bromide, thallium.

► History & Physical

Findings widespread and symmetric. Signs and symptoms begin at the feet. Signs and symptoms usually occur shortly after exposure. Should affect all in an exposed group.
Arsenic: Hyperkeratosis, hyperpigmentation, Mee's lines (horizontal white lines on the nails), distal pitting edema, weakness, malaise, anorexia, vomiting, later numbness and burning of the hands and feet, stocking–glove sensorimotor neuropathy. Subacute exposure with abdominal pain, diarrhea, tachycardia, hypotension, vasomotor collapse, and death.
Lead: Weight loss, anorexia, fatigue, constipation, and abdominal pain. Microcytic, hypochromic anemia. Predominantly motor, arms are involved. Weakness with distal atrophy, reflex loss, and fasciculation.
Mercury: Tremor, ataxia, hearing loss, dysarthria, chorea, myoclonus, hyperreflexia, and Babinski.

► Diagnostic Studies

Arsenic: Electrodiagnostic studies with axonal degeneration and denervation yet normal nerve conduction velocity (NCV). Lab normal. Arsenic found in nails, hair, urine. Sural nerve biopsy with decreased myelinated fibers.
Lead: EMG with denervation, NCV spared. Anemia with basophilic stippling, elevated urine coproporphyrin, positive urine lead levels.
Mercury: Anemia, proteinuria, and glycosuria.

► Diagnosis

Commonly overdiagnosed. All environmental toxins to which the patient may have been exposed must be eliminated as possible etiologies.

► Clinical Therapeutics

Arsenic: Chelation. Therapy with British Anti-Lewisite (BAL) or penicillamine.

Lead: Chelation with edetate calcium disodium (EDTA), BAL, and penicillamine.

► Clinical Intervention

No surgical intervention.

► Health Maintenance Issues

Avoid exposure. Secure chemicals to prevent children from obtaining access.

D. Entrapment Neuropathies of the Arm

► Scientific Concepts

Carpal tunnel syndrome: Median nerve compression frequently associated with repetitive motions. Also seen in acromegaly, hypothyroidism, rheumatoid arthritis, wrist fractures, and pregnancy.

Ulnar neuropathy: Cubital tunnel syndrome, trauma, may occur postoperatively after malpositioning.

Thoracic outlet syndrome: Congenital abnormalities such as cervical rib and tight scalene muscle.

► History & Physical

Carpal tunnel syndrome: Nocturnal paresthesias, possible radiation to the forearm and arm, decreased tactile sensation over fingertips, weakness, atrophy of thenar muscles, positive Phalen's and Tinel's. Patient awakes at night and shakes hand to relieve symptoms.

Ulnar neuropathy: Paresthesias in small finger and weakness of hand, positive Tinel's.

Thoracic outlet syndrome: Numbness, tingling, and hand pain dependent on shoulder position; weakness and wasting of the hand, especially median distribution; positive Adson's maneuver. See Table 12-1.

► table 12-1

MOTOR, REFLEX, AND SENSORY LEVELS OF THE EXTREMITIES

	Motor	Reflex	Sensation
C5	Deltoid	Biceps	Lateral upper arm
C6	Wrist extension	Brachioradialis	Lateral forearm
C7	Wrist flexion	Triceps	Middle finger
	Finger extension		
C8	Finger flexion	None	Medial forearm
T1	Interosseous	None	Medial upper arm
L4	Anterior tibialis	Patellar	Medial foot
	Foot inversion		
L5	Extensor digitorum longus	None	Midfoot
S1	Peroneus longus and brevis	Achilles tendon	Lateral foot

► Diagnostic Studies

Carpal tunnel syndrome: Electrophysiologic studies with slowing or mixed nerve conduction at the wrist.

Ulnar neuropathy: Electrophysiologic studies with slowing at the elbow.

Thoracic outlet syndrome: Reduced sensory action potentials in the small finger and denervation in the intrinsics. X-ray with possible beaking of C7 transverse process, cervical rib.

► Diagnosis

Carpal tunnel syndrome: Cervical radiculopathy, thoracic outlet syndrome, and transient ischemic attacks (TIAs).

Ulnar neuropathy: Carpal tunnel syndrome, thoracic outlet syndrome.

Thoracic outlet syndrome: Rotator cuff injury.

► Clinical Therapeutics

Carpal tunnel syndrome: Extension splinting of the wrist, steroid injection, cessation of symptom-producing activity, nonsteroidal anti-inflammatory drugs (NSAIDs).

Ulnar neuropathy: Restriction of flexion.

Thoracic outlet syndrome: Treatment of muscle spasm.

► Clinical Intervention

Carpal tunnel syndrome: Volar carpal tunnel release.

Ulnar neuropathy: Cubital tunnel release, epicondylectomy, transposition of the nerve.

Thoracic outlet syndrome: Removal of brachial plexus band, resection of first rib, scalene section.

► Health Maintenance Issues

Avoidance or limitation of repetitive actions, especially for carpal tunnel syndrome.

E. Entrapment Neuropathies of the Leg: Tarsal Tunnel Syndrome

► Scientific Concepts

Uncommon, caused by compression of the tibial nerve or any of its branches. Etiology is trauma, tenosynovitis, thrombophlebitis, mass lesion in the tunnel.

► History & Physical

Burning pain of the foot and ankle that worsens after prolonged walking or standing. Paresthesias in the sole occasionally, positive Tinel's behind lateral malleolus, muscle atrophy in the sole, weakness unusual, reflexes normal.

► Diagnostic Studies

Slowing on nerve conduction tests.

► Diagnosis

Stress fracture, bursitis, arthritis, plantar fasciitis, lumbosacral radiculopathy. Also consider reflex sympathetic dystrophy.

► Clinical Therapeutics
Correct-fitting shoes, elevation, arch support, oral steroids or NSAIDs, local injection with steroids.

► Clinical Intervention
Rarely need for surgical decompression.

► Health Maintenance Issues
Avoidance of repetitive movements, proper footwear.

IV. CENTRAL NERVOUS SYSTEM TRAUMA

► Scientific Concepts
Epidural hematoma: Collection of blood between the inner table of the skull and the dura. Generally arises from the middle meningeal artery secondary to laceration via the temporal bone. Rare in the very young and old secondary to dural adhesion to the skull.
Subdural hematoma: Collection of venous blood between the dura and arachnoid. An asymptomatic small clot may lyse and form membrane—a chronic subdural. May be from an insignificant head injury in the elderly, especially if they are on warfarin.

► History & Physical
Epidural hematoma: Expanding mass that may lead to transtentorial herniation. *Triphasic* injury with loss of consciousness, "lucid interval" in which patient is conscious, and then loss of consciousness again as mass expands. The triphasic response, although classically taught, is often not clinically seen.
Subdural hematoma: Varied presentation—may be rapid or slow changes or a waxing and waning course. Altered mental status, focal deficit, headache, or other changes from a mass effect.

► Diagnostic Studies
Epidural hematoma and *subdural hematoma* both diagnosed with CT. MRI may be used but takes longer and is more expensive. Suspect either if a fracture is present on skull x-ray.

► Clinical Therapeutics
No pharmacological treatment for either.

► Clinical Intervention
Surgical removal after radiographic localization for epidural or subdural. If the patient has a unilaterally enlarged pupil, most often the lesion is on the same side as the pupillary abnormality. A burr hole done at the bedside may be all that is needed for a chronic *subdural hematoma* since it is liquefied.

► Health Maintenance Issues
Generalized safety measures to prevent head injury, especially for those on anticoagulants.

V. VASCULAR DISEASE

A. Transient Ischemic Attacks

▶ Scientific Concepts

Temporary cessation of brain activity caused by inadequate perfusion. Occurs most frequently in older patients and those at risk for vascular disease. Sudden onset. Most last a few minutes but may be symptomatic for over an hour. TIAs usually correspond to a vascular distribution, either carotid or vertebral. Cardiogenic activity may produce emboli; cocaine may also be an etiologic factor. By definition they resolve. Usually occur with daily activities.

▶ History & Physical

Carotid artery TIAs: Contralateral hand/arm weakness with sensory loss; face and leg symptoms are less severe; may be ipsilateral visual symptoms or aphasia, amaurosis fugax, no carotid bruits if stenosis is > 95% secondary to low turbulence.

Vertebrobasilar TIAs: Diplopia, ataxia, vertigo, dysarthria, either unilateral or bilateral visual loss, cranial nerve palsies, leg weakness on either side, perioral numbness, hemiparesis and even quadriparesis, drop attacks. Fundoscopy may reveal cholesterol plaques.

▶ Diagnostic Studies

Cardiac workup to exclude arrhythmias and new murmurs; hematologic workup to exclude coagulopathies; ESR to rule out temporal arteritis; cholesterol, prothrombin time/partial thromboplastin time (PT/PTT), antiphospholipid antibodies, ECG, transthoracic two-dimensional echocardiogram, CBC and differential, carotid Dopplers, magnetic resonance angiography. Arteriogram is the gold standard.

▶ Diagnosis

Seizures with loss of consciousness, migraine, transient global amnesia, syncope, mass lesions, multiple sclerosis.

▶ Clinical Therapeutics

Admission for IV heparin beginning at 1,000 U/h adjusted to keep PTT 1.5 × normal, aspirin (recommended dose not established), sulfinpyrazone, dipyridamole PO for long-term prophylaxis. Ticlopidine in women and in cases of aspirin failure.

▶ Clinical Intervention

Carotid endarterectomy for those with a proven > 70% stenosis.

▶ Health Maintenance Issues

Control hypertension, atrial fibrillation.

B. Cerebrovascular Accidents

▶ Scientific Concepts

There are 500,000 new cerebrovascular accidents (CVAs) each year; increases with age; higher in blacks. Risk factors include hypertension, elevated blood lipids, diabetes, obesity, family history, elevated fibrinogen, high hematocrit, coronary artery disease, congestive heart failure, atrial fibrillation, left ventricular hypertrophy, smoking, oral contraceptives, alcohol abuse, physical inactivity. If secondary to atherothrombosis of a major vessel, then termed *ischemic;* these often occur during sleep, the patient waking with a new neurological deficit. *Lacunar* infarcts are small infarcts of the branches of the major cerebral arteries with etiologies of lipohyalinosis (deposition of a hyaline substance within the arterial wall leading to occlusion and seen secondary to hypertension) or embolism. *Intracerebral hemorrhage* occurs with direct bleeding into the brain and primarily secondary to hypertension; these often occur with the patient awake. *Subarachnoid hemorrhage* from arteries/veins bleeding into subarachnoid space. Illicit drug use, especially cocaine and amphetamines, must be considered.

▶ History & Physical
Ischemic: Varies with location of the lesion.
- *Internal carotid:* Ipsilateral blindness, contralateral hemiparesis, hemianopia, aphasia.
- *Middle cerebral:* Main trunk; hemiplegia, hemianesthesia, hemianopia, aphasia. *Upper division:* hemiparesis and sensory loss with arm affected more than leg, Broca's aphasia. *Lower trunk:* Wernicke's aphasia.
- *Anterior cerebral:* Hemiparesis and sensory loss affecting leg more than arm, impaired responsiveness, tactile anomia.
- *Posterior cerebral:* Hemianopia, hemiballism (involuntary throwing or flinging movements of the limbs), amnesia, oculomotor palsy.

Hemorrhagic:
- *Putamenal:* Severe hemiparesis/hemiplegia, hemianopsia, and aphasia.
- *Caudate:* Abrupt headache, vomiting, nuchal rigidity, and less frequently hemiparesis/gaze palsy.
- *Thalamic:* Hemiparesis/hemiplegia immediately; conjugate horizontal gaze deviation toward the lesion; upward gaze palsy with miotic, unreactive pupils with larger lesions. Lobar varies with hemiparesis of arm in frontal, sensorimotor and visual deficit in parietal, homonymous hemianopsia in occipital, Wernicke's aphasia in dominant temporal.
- *Cerebellar:* Sudden onset of nausea, vomiting, dizziness, inability to stand, headache but rarely loss of consciousness, limb or gait ataxia, facial palsy, ipsilateral gaze palsy. These strokes often worsen after initial presentation.
- *Pontine:* Generally leads to deep coma within minutes and decerebrate rigidity, bilateral pinpoint pupils, ocular motility disorders, abnormal respirations.

Subarachnoid hemorrhage: "Worst headache of life," 30% with change in level of consciousness, cranial nerve III palsy, nuchal rigidity, subhyaloid hemorrhages on fundoscopy in 25%.

► Diagnostic Studies

Carotid Dopplers, CT, MRI, arteriogram is gold standard. *Ischemic stroke* with hypodensity on CT that follows vascular pattern. *Hemorrhagic* with hyperdensity that may be parenchymal, subarachnoid, intraventricular, subdural or a combination of these. Ischemic stroke on MRI with hypointensity in T1 and hyperintensity in T2. Hemorrhagic varies with date—if less than 24 hours may not be visible, thereafter hyperintense on T1 images. Arteriogram is optimal for evaluating arterial lesions such as aneurysms and arteriovenous malformations. Magnetic resonance angiography rapidly replacing standard arteriograms. *Subarachnoid* with blood in basal cisterns and sylvian fissures on CT acutely, intraparenchymal blood and hydrocephalus later; MRI not useful acutely but excellent after a few days for detecting aneurysms, etc. Angiography gold standard, nontraumatic lumbar puncture 6 to 12 hours after headache with xanthochromic CSF.

► Diagnosis

Embolism, hemorrhage, trauma, migraine, seizure, epidural or subdural hematoma, neoplasm, abscess.

► Clinical Therapeutics

Carotid endarterectomy for prevention of *ischemic stroke,* also antiplatelet drugs such as aspirin, ticlopidine. *Hemorrhagic* with ICU management, hyperventilation, mannitol and steroids now controversial, surgery usually ineffective. *Subarachnoid* with nimodipine and hypertension to prevent vasospasm, general ICU management as this is an emergency.

► Clinical Intervention

Angioplasty for ischemic. Clipping of aneurysm in first 3 days for subarachnoid.

► Health Maintenance Issues

Control hypertension, treat bacterial endocarditis, resect atrial myxoma, treat atrial fibrillation, cessation of smoking, increase physical activity. *Subarachnoid:* must follow closely as there is a risk of rebleeding, vasospasm, hydrocephalus, seizures, hyponatremia, Torsade de pointes, and ventricular fibrillation after event.

C. Seizures

► Scientific Concepts

A seizure is a single event, and epilepsy is a condition with recurrent seizures (20 to 70/100,000). Head trauma is a frequent cause of seizures in young adults; tumors and vascular disease are the most likely etiologies in the elderly. Seizures may occur with withdrawal of alcohol, barbiturates, benzodiazepines, anticonvulsants. Cocaine use may cause seizures. There is an association with neurofibromatosis, tuberous sclerosis, Sturge–Weber syndrome, and other neurological diseases.

► History & Physical

Fever, headache, cognitive dysfunction, Kernig's sign, nuchal rigidity in those with meningititis. Staring episodes seen in petit mal. Todd's postictal paralysis (limb weakness that occurs after a seizure and may last up to 48 hours). Left hemisphere seizures cause eye deviation to right. Auras may occur with temporal lobe seizures.

► Diagnosis

Need to eliminate metabolic abnormalities such as hypoglycemia, hypocalcemia, hyponatremia, and hypernatremia. Consider pseudoseizures in those patients whose seizures do not fit a classical pattern. Obtain a CT to rule out intracranial bleed/tumor. Electroencephalogram (EEG) helpful if positive. A lumbar puncture must be done to rule out infection. Syncope occurs without tonic-clonic movement or aura.

► Clinical Therapeutics

Phenytoin	Generalized/Partial	3–5 mg/kg/d
Phenobarbital	Generalized/Partial	2–3 mg/kg/d
Primidone	Generalized/Partial	10–25 mg/kg/d
Carbamazepine	Generalized/Partial	10–20 mg/kg/d
Valproic acid	Generalized/Partial	20–60 mg/kg/d
Ethosuximide	Absence	20–35 mg/kg/d
Clonazepam	Absence	0.05–0.2 mg/kg/d

► Clinical Intervention

Status epilepticus is a prolonged seizure lasting > 15 to 30 minutes. After drawing glucose, electrolytes, magnesium, BUN, give 50 mL of 50% dextrose and 100 mg thiamine IV. Then IV diazepam, 0.2 mg/kg, or lorazepam, 0.1 to 0.2 mg/kg, repeatedly until seizures stop plus loading dose of phenytoin (in saline as it precipitates in glucose solutions) or phenobarbital. When controlled, may start other anticonvulsants such as carbamazepine.

► Health Maintenance Issues

Treatment of choice is monotherapy. Valproic acid best for women on oral contraceptives but may cause neural tube defects. Phenytoin can cause gingival hyperplasia and hirsutism. Check CBC in patients on carbamazepine to rule out agranulocytosis or aplastic anemia. Check liver function tests in those on valproic acid to rule out hepatic dysfunction. Driving restrictions after a seizure vary from state to state. Titrate patient off anticonvulsants to prevent rebound seizures.

VI. VIRAL INFECTIONS

A. Polio

► Scientific Concepts

Because of immigration from underdeveloped countries, cases continue to come into the United States. It is spread by fecal–oral route, affects anterior horn cells, and is seen in outbreaks in the summer. It affects adolescents and young adults primarily. Incubation is 1 to 5 weeks.

► History & Physical

Subclinical: No symptoms.

Abortive: Malaise, fever, headache, sore throat, cough, diarrhea, nausea, vomiting.

Nonparalytic: Malaise, fever, sore throat, cough, diarrhea, nausea, vomiting, headache, meningismus, CSF pleocytosis and elevated protein.

Paralytic: Muscular stiffness, spasms, coarse fasciculations, focal weakness, urinary bladder dysfunction, respiratory failure, pharyngeal and facial weakness.

Postpolio syndrome: Muscle wasting that occurs years later.

► Diagnostic Studies

Isolation of virus from throat, stool, and CSF. CSF is rarely positive.

► Diagnosis

Consider Guillain–Barré, transverse myelitis, botulism, heavy metal poisoning, tick paralysis.

► Clinical Therapeutics

Supportive for symptoms.

► Health Maintenance Issues

Oral polio vaccine and formalin inactivated polio vaccine.

B. Rabies

► Scientific Concepts

Rhabdovirus spread via animal bites such as dogs, skunks, raccoons, foxes, wolves, and bats. Suspicion should be raised in unprovoked attacks. Animal saliva and CNS tissue only infectious tissue. Incubation period 30 to 90 days but may be as long as a year.

► History & Physical

Prodrome: Lasts 1 to 4 days, is nonspecific with symptoms such as low-grade fever, malaise, gastrointestinal upset, cough, and headache. Most patients will develop pain, paresthesias, and/or pruritis at the bite.

Acute neurologic period: Confusion and anxiety with progression to agitation and combativeness. Hallucinations may occur. Also with vocal paralysis, hyperreflexia, facial grimacing, contractures of the pharynx and larynx when attempting to swallow liquids (hydrophobia), optic neuritis, and facial nerve palsies. About 20% of patients with ascending paralysis as the primary symptom.

Final phase: Coma and brain stem respiratory death. Survival from the onset of neurological symptoms is < 21 days.

► Diagnostic Studies

Viral isolation from saliva or CSF requires at least 6 days. Direct fluorescent antibody staining for antigen detection on saliva and corneal impression or skin biopsy from nape of neck are best tests available. Brain biopsy shows Negri bodies.

▶ Diagnosis

Botulism, malaria, epilepsy, metabolic encephalopathy, illicit drug use, rickettsial disease, CVA, tetanus.

▶ Clinical Therapeutics

Preexposure vaccination—1 mL IM of human diploid cell rabies vaccine (HDCV) or rabies vaccine, absorbed (RVA) on days 0, 7, 21, and 28. Postexposure vaccination in unvaccinated patients—ASAP administer 20 IU/kg of rabies immune globulin (RIG) and, at a different site from the first dose of HDCV. Additional doses of HDCV should be given on days 3, 7, 14, and 28. If patient previously vaccinated, HDCV given on days 0 and 3 only.

▶ Health Maintenance Issues

Preexposure prophylaxis for veterinarians and others at high risk.

C. AIDS Dementia Complex

▶ Scientific Concepts

Pathological with cerebral atrophy and white matter degeneration and perivascular infiltration by macrophages and lymphocytes.

▶ History & Physical

Memory problems, slow verbal and motor responses, slow thinking, and apathy occur early. Frank psychosis may occur later. Eye movement disorders, weakness, ataxia, seizures, mutism, incontinence, apathy, and quadriparesis may occur.

▶ Diagnostic Studies

CT with cortical and deep atrophy, MRI with "fluffy" white matter changes. The CSF has oligoclonal bands, pleocytosis, increased protein, and low glucose.

▶ Diagnosis

Consider psychiatric illness, medication side effects, chronic meningitis, thiamine and cyanocobalamin deficiency.

▶ Clinical Therapeutics

Zidovudine (AZT) up to 1,000 mg/d. Treat thiamine and cyanocobalamin deficiencies.

▶ Health Maintenance Issues

Avoid IV drug use and sexual promiscuity.

VII. BRAIN TUMORS

► **Scientific Concepts**

There are 24,000 primary and an additional 24,000 metastatic tumors diagnosed each year in the United States. Gliomas are most common at 60% of primary tumors followed by meningiomas at 20%. More than 100 types of tumors known. Tumors are second only to stroke as neurological cause of death in adults. Etiologies varied: inherited with neurofibromatosis I, tuberous sclerosis, and bilateral retinoblastomas; environmental with ionizing radiation exposure possibly predisposing to meningiomas and gliomas.

► **History & Physical**

Headache in 35%: Frontal headaches are nonspecific, intermittent, dull, ipsilateral, supratentorial. Occipital headaches occur with tumors in the posterior fossa. Brain tumor headaches tend to wake the patient at night, improve during the day, and are worsened with coughing or exercise. Examination findings may include papilledema; seizures, especially in adults without a prior history; and an altered mental status. Tumors have signs/symptoms related to their location:

Frontal lobe: Personality changes, especially disinhibition, irritability, impaired judgment, abulia (lack of initiative); exam showing gaze preference, forced grasping, snout reflex (percussion above the lips causing puckering of the lips), anosmia, hemiparesis, seizures, aphasia, urinary frequency, gait difficulties.

Temporal lobe: Varied seizures, aphasia, and superior quadrantanopsia.

Parietal lobe: Contralateral sensory loss in proprioception, stereognosis, graphesthesia, aphasia, hemiparesis, homonymous field defects, agnosias, apraxias.

Occipital lobe: Homonymous hemianopsia, visual seizures.

► **Diagnostic Studies**

Skull x-ray is not needed as CT and MRI widely used. Angiography occasionally useful. Positron-emission tomography (PET) helpful but not usually available. Other study modalities include visual fields, EEG, audiometry, CSF analysis, and endocrine evaluation.

► **Diagnosis**

Consider subdurals, hydrocephalus, arachnoid cysts, benign intracranial hypertension, abscess, multiple sclerosis, infarcts, congenital abnormalities.

► **Clinical Therapeutics**

Anticonvulsants, usually phenytoin, if seizures present. Anticonvulsants not needed if tumor is small and infratentorial. Corticosteroids used to decrease edema. May need head elevation, fluid restriction, diuretics, and/or hyperventilation if corticosteroids not effective.

► Clinical Intervention

Observation if tumor "benign" on radiographic studies. Surgical resection or debulking to allow adjunct therapies to work better. Radiotherapy as either conventional beam therapy, stereotactic brachytherapy, stereotactic radiotherapy. Chemotherapy with varied agents. Being reviewed are immunotherapy, hormonal therapy, antiangiogenic agents, and gene therapy.

► Health Maintenance Issues

After diagnosis, physical therapy and rehabilitation, emotional and psychological support, hospice.

VIII. ILL-DEFINED PRESENTATIONS

A. Dizziness

► Scientific Concepts

Varied etiologies including imbalance of tonic vestibular signals; cerebral ischemia; low glucose or catecholamines; depression of CNS; loss of vestibulospinal, proprioceptive, or cerebellar function.

► History & Physical

Must be sure the patient and clinician are referring to the same problem as lightheadedness (feeling faint) is often confused with dizziness. A history of drug/medication usage including over-the-counter medications is needed, especially alcohol, tranquilizers, anticonvulsants, antihypertensives, and aminoglycosides. Spinning usually indicates a vestibular disorder. True vertigo is episodic, whereas situational dizziness may be psychogenic. Do a general exam plus doll's eye, iced calorics, Barany maneuver (having a seated patient lie down abruptly and tilt head backwards and to the side, both at 45°, watching for the development of nystagmus) and test gait, orthostatic blood pressures, and check for nystagmus.

► Diagnostic Studies

Electronystagmography, rotational testing, posturography, CT and/or MRI, and appropriate drug levels.

► Diagnosis

Consider benign positional vertigo, vestibulopathy, Ménière's disease, migraine, TIAs, hyperventilation, orthostatic hypotension, arrhythmias, alcohol, phenytoin, carbamazepine, aminoglycosides, syncope, epilepsy, otitis, hypoglycemia.

► Clinical Therapeutics

Antivertiginous medications such as scopolamine, meclizine (Antivert), dimenhydrinate (Dramamine), prochlorperazine (Compazine), and Metoclopramide (Reglan). Vestibular rehabilitation. Discontinue ototoxic agents. Low-salt diet for Ménière's. Removal of triggers and use of antimigrainous medications for migraine. Anti-platelet or anticoagulants for vertebrobasilar insufficiency.

▶ Health Maintenance Issues

Monitoring of drug and glucose levels. Elimination or titration of medications or causative agents if possible.

B. Headache

▶ Scientific Concepts

Usually benign. May result from distention, traction, or dilatation of intracranial or extracranial arteries; dural traction; compression or inflammation of cranial and spinal nerves; spasm; trauma or traction to cranial or cervical muscles; meningeal irritation; increased intracranial pressure; drug withdrawal; oral contraceptives. Also associated with medical diseases such as thyroid disorders, mononucleosis, systemic lupus erythematosus (SLE), inflammatory bowel disease, and hypertension.

▶ History & Physical

For all headaches, a detailed history is needed. Must ask about the age of onset, frequency, location, quality, duration, associated symptoms such as nausea and vomiting or auras, provocative and palliative factors, changes in behavior, postdrome, medication or drug use, and previous medical diagnosis.

Cluster: Peaks in men 30 to 50 years old, orbital or temporal in location, and occurs often in smokers. The headaches are made worse with alcohol ingestion. There are generally 1 to 2 attacks daily lasting < 1 hour, associated with red eye and nasal stuffiness homolaterally, possibly with ipsilateral Homer's. The cluster lasts ~ 6 weeks.

Tension: Occurs in all ages and is increased in females. Nondescript, "bandlike" discomfort with no particular pattern.

Brain tumor: Occurs in all ages/sexes. Unique in that it interrupts sleep; associated with nausea, vomiting, and visual changes; steadily increases in severity.

Arteritis: Located at the temporal or occipital area in patients of either sex > 55 years old. Examination shows scalp tenderness with a possible dilated temporal artery. Patients complain of "jabbing pain," fatigue, and morning stiffness in hip and shoulders. May last months.

Subarachnoid: Worst headache of life with level of consciousness changes.

▶ Diagnostic Studies

ESR possibly increased in arteritis; CT or MRI for mass or sinusitis.

▶ Diagnosis

Consider migraine, posttraumatic, facial pain, depression, tumors, arteritis, postherpetic, intracranial mass, infections, drug withdrawal, visual problems, menstrual, temporomandibular joint (TMJ) dysfunction.

► Clinical Therapeutics

Cluster: Prednisone, lithium, methysergide, ergotamine, and verapamil; oxygen.

Tension: Aspirin, NSAIDs, muscle relaxants, antidepressants.

Tumors: Perhaps corticosteroids.

Subarachnoid: None.

► Clinical Intervention

See Brain Tumors section. Surgical correction of vascular abnormality for subarachnoid.

► Health Maintenance Issues

Correction of underlying medical disease, refraction, avoidance of triggering factors, rapid treatment of arteritis to avoid blindness.

C. Malaise and Fatigue

► Scientific Concepts

Accompanies most medical and psychological diseases.

► History & Physical

A detailed history to discover emotional or psychological factors such as depression, change in occupation, divorce, etc.; endocrine disorders such as hypothyroidism, Addison's disease, diabetes mellitus; pulmonary disorders with complaints of shortness of breath as well as sleep apneas; fever, arthralgias, weight loss, and other signs of underlying malignancy or connective tissue disease; poor diet; various anemias; cardiac disease with arrythmias and congestive heart failure; renal disease; lymphadenopathy; medications; myasthenia gravis, multiple sclerosis, Parkinson's disease, and chronic fatigue syndrome.

► Diagnostic Studies

Thyroid function tests; blood glucose; search for underlying malignancy with stool for guaic, chest x-ray, urinalysis, prostate-specific antigen, carcinoembryonic antigen, etc.; rheumatoid factor, CBC and differential, ESR, BUN/creatinine, Monospot; purified protein derivative; liver enzymes.

► Diagnosis

Consider brown recluse spider bites, cat scratch disease, arteritis, Hodgkin's disease, infections, influenza, Lyme disease, rabies, tuberculosis, chronic anxiety disorders, depression, use of anticonvulsants or antifungals, hypothyroidism, apathetic hyperthyroidism in elderly, myasthenia gravis, opiate withdrawal, arthritides, SLE.

► Clinical Therapeutics

Treat underlying medical or psychological problem.

► Health Maintenance Issues

Need for close medical follow-up of underlying diseases.

D. Migraine

▶ Scientific Concepts

Occurs in women more than men, with an overall lifetime prevalence of ~ 16%. Onset in second and third decades, rarely after age 50. There is usually an associated prodrome.

▶ History & Physical

Without aura: Unilateral headaches 4 to 72 hours in length, moderate severity, aggravated with activity, associated with nausea, vomiting, photophobia, phonophobia.

With aura: Aura may be visual (scintillations [flashing lights], photopsias [flashes of light], or fortifications [jagged lines]) or sensory (tingling or numbness in the hand/mouth distribution). Headaches with throbbing pain, usually unilateral, photophobia, nausea but seldom vomiting. Headache severe lasting 4 to 72 hours, aggravated by physical activity, often relieved with sleep.

▶ Diagnosis

Consider cerebrovascular disease such as TIAs, CVA, subarachnoid hemorrhage, vasculitis; brain tumors or other mass lesions; epilepsy; posttraumatic headache; use of vasodilators; hypoxia or hypercarbia; hypoglycemia; fever; sinusitis; glaucoma; withdrawal from drugs including caffeine.

▶ Clinical Therapeutics

Mild: Aspirin, acetaminophen, NSAIDs.

Severe: Dihydroergotamine, sumatriptan, butorphanol nasal spray.

Prophylaxis: Propranolol, timolol, methysergide, calcium channel blockers, amitriptyline, valproate.

▶ Health Maintenance Issues

Avoidance of precipitating factors such as caffeine, chocolate, red wine, cheese, nuts and yogurts, stress, smoking, inadequate sleep, hunger, and some oral contraceptives.

E. Reye's Syndrome

▶ Scientific Concepts

Postinfectious encephalopathy affecting mostly children but occasionally adults. Pathology not completely defined but affects mitochondria of multiple organs.

▶ History & Physical

Prodrome: Illness such as influenza or varicella followed in 3 to 5 days by persistent vomiting.

Clinical: Oriented but irritable and possibly lethargic.

Encephalopathic: Hyperexcitable progressing to coma with posturing and finally flaccid paralysis. Occasional survivors. Hepatomegaly may be found.

► Diagnostic Studies

Prodrome: None.

Clinical: Serum glutamic oxaloacetic transaminase (SGOT) and serum glutamic pyruvic transaminase (SGPT) with up to 30-fold rise; bilirubin normal, and serum ammonia varied.

Encephalopathic: Ammonia level 3 to 20 times normal. CSF with < 8 leukocytes/cm³.

► Diagnosis

Consider CNS infections; hemorrhagic shock with secondary encephalopathy; toxin or drug ingestion; metabolic diseases such as organic acidemias, systemic carnitine deficiency (important in lipid metabolism).

► Clinical Therapeutics

Provide glucose via IV, maintain fluid and electrolyte balance, treat bleeding diathesis.

► Clinical Intervention

Temperature control and respiratory and hemodynamic support if needed. Monitor intracranial pressure.

► Health Maintenance Issues

Number of cases decreased since possible association with salicylates discovered. Avoid Pepto-Bismol since it contains bismuth subsalicylate.

F. Sleep Disturbances

► Scientific Concepts

Sleep apnea: Obstructive—respiratory effort without air flow; central—neither air flow nor effort, and mixed types; 2 to 4% of adult population affected, with 38,000 deaths a year from associated cardiac arrhythmias.

Narcolepsy: Unknown etiology manifested with excessive sleepiness; 2 to 16/100,000; abnormal rapid eye movement (REM).

Disordered sleep common in psychiatric disorders, especially depression, mania, and hypomania; vascular and endocrinopathies such as hyperthyroidism; Parkinson's disease, uremia, painful disorders such as arthritis and peptic ulcer disease; congestive heart failure; Alzheimer's and other dementias; asthma; cardiac ischemia; chronic obstructive pulmonary disease.

► History & Physical

Sleep apnea: Excessive daytime sleepiness, snoring, obesity, falling asleep while driving, verified apnea during sleep, morning headaches, depression, hypertension, nocturnal angina, impotence, nocturia, arrhythmias. Seen with congenital nasopharyngeal abnormalities and large necks. Cheyne–Stokes respiration with central sleep apnea.

Insomnia: Difficulty initiating and maintaining sleep; review for various medications, caffeine, alcohol, illicit drugs.

Narcolepsy: Excessive daytime sleepiness, cataplexy, hypnagogic hallucinations, and sleep paralysis. Laughter and anger may produce cataplexy.

► Diagnostic Studies

Polysomnography is gold standard. CBC will show secondary polycythemia.

► Diagnosis

Consider seizures, Neimann–Pick disease, bilateral medullary lesions, syringobulbia, diabetic neuropathy, phrenic nerve paralysis, myopathies, and myasthenia gravis for central sleep apnea.

► Clinical Therapeutics

Sleep apnea: Pharmacological treatment with anecdotal success.
Narcolepsy: Sleepiness treated with pemoline and methylphenidate, cataplexy with clomipramine and protriptyline.

► Clinical Intervention

Sleep apnea: Nasal continuous positive airway pressure (CPAP) or low-flow oxygen via nasal cannula and weight loss. Uvulopalatopharyngoplasty and oral appliances less effective.
Narcolepsy: Strategic napping, avoid stimulants.

► Health Maintenance Issues

For sleep apnea, decrease weight and compliance with CPAP.

G. Syncope

► Scientific Concepts

Varies depending on etiology but all with reduced cerebral perfusion.

► History & Physical

Vasovagal from stress, fear, fatigue, injury, or pain. Bradycardia, nausea, pallor and diaphoresis on exam. *Postural* with sudden arising from recumbent position. *Cardiac* with history of cardiac disease, arrhythmias, blood loss.

► Diagnostic Studies

ECG and/or Holter monitor for brady- or tachyarrhythmias; hemoglobin/hematocrit for blood loss and/or dehydration, echocardiogram to rule out atrial myxoma, valvular stenosis, infarction, tamponade; glucose to rule out hypoglycemia; arteriogram if cerebral vasculature problem is suspected; tilt testing for orthostasis; EEG if seizure is suspected.

► Diagnosis

Consider seizures, TIAs, hysterical fainting, hyperventilation, migraine.

► Clinical Therapeutics

Consists of correcting the underlying medical condition.

▶ Clinical Intervention

Consists of correcting the underlying surgical condition in the case of myxomas and valvular stenosis.

▶ Health Maintenance Issues

Primary concern is the sequelae from falling with fractures and other trauma, especially in the elderly.

BIBLIOGRAPHY

Adams RD, Victor M. *Principles of Neurology,* 1st ed. New York: McGraw-Hill; 1981.

Duss P. *Topical Diagnosis in Neurology,* 3rd rev. ed. Stuttgart: Thieme; 1998.

Gilman S, Newman S. *Manter and Gatzs Essentials of Clinical Neuroanatomy and Neurophysiology.* Philadelphia: FA Davis; 1996.

Haerer AF. *DeJong's The Neurological Examination,* 5th ed. Philadelphia: JB Lippincott-Raven; 1992.

Hoppenfeld S. *Orthopedic Neurology,* 1st ed. Philadelphia: Lippincott-Raven; 1997.

Perkin DG. *Mosby's Color Atlas and Text of Neurology.* Philadelphia: Mosby-Wolfe; 1998.

Samuels MA, Feske S, eds. *Office Practice of Neurology.* New York: Churchill Livingstone; 1996.

Snell RS. *Clinical Neuroanatomy for Medical Students.* Philadelphia: Lippincott-Raven; 1997.

Psychiatry | 13

Douglas R. Southard, PhD, MPH, PA-C, Anita Duhl Glicken, MSW

I. PSYCHOSES

A. Affective Psychosis: Mania and Psychotic Depression

► Scientific Concepts
Tend to cluster in families. Incidence increases with age.

► History & Physical
Family history, clinical features of mood disorder precede psychotic state. Illness generally episodic rather than continuous. Symptoms include: *Mania*—hyperactivity, pressured and rapid speech, labile affect with elation or irritability, flight of ideas, distractibility, impulsivity, grandiosity, paranoia. *Depression*—psychomotor retardation, agitation, slowed speech, changes in appetite or weight, poor self-care, somatic delusions, guilt, derogatory hallucinations, suicidal ideation. Alcohol abuse common.

► Diagnostic Studies
No pathognomonic signs or studies; rule out medical etiology through history and lab work (i.e., thyroid and adrenal dysfunction).

► Diagnosis
Differentiate from other psychiatric disorders including personality disorders (schizophrenia), attention deficit hyperactivity disorder (ADHD), substance abuse, and/or intoxication. Rule out medical etiologies (thyroid, adrenal dysfunction, medications, Parkinson's disease, multiple sclerosis, pancreatic and other malignancies, lupus, central nervous system [CNS] tumors, cerebrovascular accidents [CVAs], viral illness).

► Clinical Therapeutics
Acute mania: Neuroleptics or benzodiazepines to control agitation. Lithium titrated to serum levels of 1.0 to 1.5. Anticonvulsants (valproic acid, carbamazepine) effective. Electroconvulsive therapy (ECT) may be used for rapid control.
Psychotic depression: ECT most effective; antidepressants combined with neuroleptic also effective. Poor response from antidepressants alone.

► Clinical Intervention
Hospitalization for protection of self and others and diagnosis. Therapeutics as above. Ongoing low-dose neuroleptics; antidepressants for depression; supportive therapies; family support.

► Health Maintenance Issues
Monitor improvement in target symptoms. Maintenance doses of medications should be closely monitored. For mania and bipolar, mood stabilizers should be continued on an outpatient basis for at least 4 to 6 months, at dose required for control of acute symptoms. Indefinite continuation should be considered after three or more

manic episodes. Discontinuation of antipsychotics should be considered following symptom resolution. For psychotic depression, there is a 50% chance of relapse if antidepressants are discontinued before 6 months, so therapy should be continued for at least 6 to 12 months. Discontinuation should occur gradually and with longer prophylaxis considered if there is a history of recurrence, greater severity, long depressive episodes, and older age at onset. Support groups and therapy. Monitor possible alcohol and substance use.

B. Paranoid States

▶ Scientific Concepts

Paranoia is a nonspecific symptom that can be present in personality disorders, delusional disorder, schizophrenia, mania or depression with psychotic features, brief psychotic disorder, and substance-related disorders.

▶ History & Physical

Course and severity of paranoid ideation varies.

▶ Diagnostic Studies

Laboratory screening should include complete blood count (CBC); complete chemistry profile, including electrolytes, liver function tests, renal function tests, and tests for calcium and magnesium; urine drug test; thyroid function tests; blood concentrations for any medications being taken. Once substance-related disorders and general medical conditions are ruled out, complete psychiatric evaluation will reveal diagnosis. Neuropsychological testing, electroencephalogram (EEG), computed tomography (CT), and/or magnetic resonance imaging (MRI) may help identify underlying organic conditions.

▶ Diagnosis

Differential may include paranoid personality disorder and delusional disorder of the persecutory type, typically with paranoid ideation that has been constant over long periods. Absence of delusions in paranoid personality disorder; prominent delusions in delusional disorder. Paranoia in mania or depression is present only during acute episodes. Schizophrenia usually identified by presence of other symptoms, such as thought disorders or hallucinations.

▶ Clinical Therapeutics

If patient is already taking antipsychotic medications, give another dose of that medication. In general, psychotic paranoid patients can be given haloperidol, thiothixene, fluphenazine, or trifluoperazine, all at doses of 2 to 5 mg PO or IM as needed. Paranoid conditions caused by intoxication or withdrawal from drugs can be managed with lorazepam, 1 to 2 mg PO or IM. Severely anxious paranoid patients treated with lorazepam. Paranoia with agitation caused by delirium or dementia can be managed with haloperidol, 1 to 5 mg PO or IM.

► Clinical Intervention

History, lab work, clinical therapeutics as described above. Treat in emergency room or office according to diagnosis. Dangerous patient may need hospitalization, even involuntary commitment. Question regarding suicide or homicidal ideation. Directly ask patient what he or she would do to those perceived against him or her. Ask about previous acts of violence and suicide attempts.

► Health Maintenance Issues

Follow-up related to diagnosis. Monitor improvement in target symptoms and long-term medication use. Psychiatric referral and support groups.

C. Delusional Disorder (Formerly Paranoid Disorder)

► Scientific Concepts

Etiology unknown; genetically unrelated to schizophrenia and affective disorders; formerly called paranoia or paranoid disorder.

► History & Physical

Primary manifestation fixed, nonbizarre, systematized delusion; typically midlife onset; functioning variable; mental status exam typically normal except for delusional system; mood consistent with delusions.

► Diagnostic Studies

Toxicology screening, routine laboratory work, neuropsychological testing, EEG or CT scan for differential diagnosis.

► Diagnosis

Symptoms as above; the *Diagnostic and Statistical Manual*, 4th edition (DSM-IV) specifies seven subtypes based on predominant content of delusions; persecutory and jealous types most common, erotomanic and somatic types most unusual; also grandiose, mixed, and unspecified. Delusion can accompany many neurological and medical illnesses, including basal ganglia disorders, endocrinopathies, limbic system disorders, systemic disorders; differential diagnosis also to rule out malingering and factitious disorder with predominantly psychological signs and symptoms; delirium, dementia, substance-related disorders, schizophrenia, mood disorders, obsessive–compulsive disorder, somatoform disorders, and paranoid personality disorder.

► Clinical Therapeutics

In emergency, antipsychotic drug IM, followed by antipsychotic drugs like low-dose haloperidol, pimozide; maintenance doses typically low; some patients may receive no benefit; unresponsive patients to antipsychotic drugs may try antidepressants like lithium or anticonvulsants, particularly with family history of mood disorder; most common cause of drug failure is noncompliance.

► Clinical Intervention

Can generally be treated as outpatient; hospitalization for evaluation and differential; evaluation of patient's control over violent impulses; legal commitment may be necessary; individual psychotherapy, insight-oriented, cognitive, behavioral, and family therapy may be helpful. Stimulate continued motivation to receive help, emphasizing patient's management of anxiety and irritability. Do not support reality of delusions, but avoid making disparaging remarks about delusions.

► Health Maintenance Issues

Successful treatment may be satisfactory social adjustment rather than disappearance of delusions; continue to promote positive therapeutic alliance with patient; overgratification may increase patient's hostility and suspiciousness because not all demands can be met; avoid disparaging remarks about delusions, but emphasize that preoccupation with delusions interferes with daily life.

D. Psychosis Originating in Childhood

► Scientific Concepts

Developmental factors relevant to treatment and diagnosis. Nature of psychological and neurobiological processes underlying psychotic phenomena in children and adolescents remains largely unknown. Before the *Diagnostic and Statistical Manual*, 3rd edition (DSM-III), all severe childhood disturbance was equated with schizophrenia. Epidemiology of psychotic depression in children is very limited. Bipolar disorder develops in a sizable minority of children and adolescents who initially present with depression.

► History & Physical

Schizophrenia: *Childhood:* Early-onset (EOS) and very-early-onset (VEOS) frequency increases after 11 years. *Adolescence:* Conditions as above with increasing frequency, develops gradually over weeks or months; symptoms often denied until situation becomes emergent. Emergent constellation of symptoms consistent with adult disorder includes at least two characteristic symptoms (delusions, hallucinations, disorganized speech, grossly disorganized or catatonic behavior) as well as social–occupational dysfunction and duration of at least 6 months.

Mood disorders (*major depression with psychosis* and *bipolar disorder*): Source of greatest diagnostic confusion. Longitudinal information clarifies nature of disorder underlying initial psychotic presentation. Manic symptoms vary with age. Children < 9 more likely to present with aggressiveness, emotional lability, and irritability. Older children with euphoria, grandiosity, or paranoid ideation and flight of ideas. Pressured speech, overactivity, and distractibility noted in all ages. Mania in adolescence similar to adults with psychotic features more common.

► Diagnostic Studies

No pathognomonic signs or lab studies. Symptoms as described above. Psychological testing (IQ), communication assessments, projective testing, and adaptive behavior. Physical and neurological examinations, evaluate potential substance abuse.

► Diagnosis

Schizophrenia—EOS after 13 years; VEOS before 13 years, quite rare. Difficulties in diagnosis in younger children. Delusions and hallucinations are often less elaborate in childhood. Disorganized speech and behavior may characterize a number of other conditions. For schizophrenia and mood disorders, rule out substance-induced psychotic reaction; medical illness that produces delirium; coexisting antisocial behavior disorder; ADHD; brief psychotic disorder. Major depression with psychotic features must be differentiated from manic phase of bipolar disorder.

► Clinical Therapeutics

Schizophrenia: Major tranquilizers effective during the active psychotic phase, typically in range of 400 mg/70 kg; lower doses during maintenance phase. Therapeutic effect may not be apparent for some time after treatment is initiated. Some patients fail to respond; for those patients atypical antipsychotics should be considered.

Mood disorders: Pharmacologic treatments of adult mood disorders generally appropriate for children. Lithium in bipolar disorders and antidepressants in treatment of major depression associated with psychosis.

► Clinical Intervention

Treatment of child with psychosis will depend on nature of disorder, characteristics of the individual, stage of illness, and developmental level of the child. Often, multiple treatment modalities, including pharmacotherapy, educational and family interventions, and supportive psychotherapy. Inpatient treatment may be needed during acute phase. Excessive medication is common. Possible short- and long-term side effects should be monitored with planned reevaluation. Family intervention programs may help reduce relapse rates. Supportive psychotherapy, educational interventions, and social skills training may be indicated. Long-term treatment program should be flexible and well integrated.

► Health Maintenance Issues

Ongoing flexible and integrated treatment program as above. Monitor medication use for possible side effects; potential substance abuse; comorbid conditions (e.g., depression). Adolescents with bipolar conditions are more likely than adults to relapse. Family programs may reduce relapse.

E. Schizophrenia

► Scientific Concepts

Evidence that it runs in some families, path of transmission is unclear. Pathogenesis through stress diathesis model; constitutional factors determined by heredity (diathesis) interacting with environmental influences (stress) that precipitate overt expression of clinical symptoms. Pathological findings include nonspecific gliosis, cellular loss, and disordered orientation of the pyramidal cells in the hippocampus, suggesting developmental rather than degenerative disturbance.

► History & Physical

Family history; onset typically late teens through twenties; precipitated by stress. Often have premorbid schizoid features; begins gradually, duration of symptoms at least 6 months with at least two psychotic symptoms for at least 1 month. Constellation of symptoms rather than a single symptom; formal thought disorder; content of thought, perceptual disturbances, and alterations in emotions and behavior; loose associations, tangentiality, incoherence; mood-congruent and -incongruent delusions, paranoia, being controlled, thought broadcasting, grandiosity, religion and somatic delusions; visual and auditory hallucinations; bizarre and catatonic behavior; psychotic depression; may have soft neurologic signs, motoric abnormalities.

► Diagnostic Studies

No pathognomonic signs or lab studies; typically, patient must exhibit two or more of following symptoms for a significant portion of time during a 1-month period: delusions, hallucinations, disorganized speech, grossly disorganized or catatonic behavior, negative symptoms; impaired functioning during active phase. Symptoms for at least 6 months; schizoaffective and mood disorder exclusion.

► Diagnosis

Symptoms as above; DSM-IV subtypes; paranoid, disorganized, catatonic, undifferentiated, and residual based on clinical presentation. Positive and negative symptom classification. Positive: productive symptoms including delusions, hallucinations, and bizarre behaviors. Negative symptoms marked by absence of functioning including affective flattening, avolition, social withdrawal. Differential diagnosis includes a wide range of nonpsychiatric medical conditions and a variety of substances that induce symptoms of psychosis and catatonia, including psychotic or catatonic disorder due to general medical condition and substance-induced psychotic disorder.

► Clinical Therapeutics

Neuroleptic agents for controlling active symptoms of psychosis and prophylactic effect to prevent relapse; two major classes of dopamine receptor antagonists (i.e., chlorpromazine, haloperidol, sulpiride) and serotonin–dopamine antagonists (i.e., clozapine, risperidone, olanzapine); dopamine receptor antagonists appear to help only a small percentage of patients (25%) with annoying and serious adverse effects. Serotonin–dopamine antagonists appear to be effective with broader range of patients and cause few extrapyramidal symptoms; however, clozapine carries a 1 to 2% risk of agranulocytosis.

► Clinical Intervention

Hospitalization to contain disruptive and dangerous behavior. Medical evaluation for presence of medical, neurological, or substance disorders that may be etiologically related. Neuroleptic agents as described above. Psychosocial intervention to complement the use of medication; connecting patient with appropriate aftercare treatment. After acute psychotic episode, goal should be to prevent relapse while adjusting medication to maintenance level. Continued use of neuroleptics reduces relapse rate. Reintegration of patient into community; home environment major treatment milieu. Family treatment shown to reduce relapse in the first year. Day hospital programs for transition may be helpful for patients without support. Social skills training, supportive psychotherapy, and vocational rehabilitation may be indicated.

► Health Maintenance Issues

Designated case manager to coordinate multifaceted treatment plans. Continued monitoring of neuroleptic drug use and side effects. Suicide is common (50% of schizophrenic patients attempt suicide at least once); associated substance abuse; 75% smoke cigarettes, about 30 to 50% may meet diagnostic criteria for alcohol abuse or alcohol dependence; homelessness related to deinstitutionalization of patients (estimates that one-third to two-thirds of homeless people are schizophrenic). Long-term prognosis is variable based on onset; precipitating factors; premorbid social, sexual, and work history; support systems; and presence of positive or negative symptoms. Late and acute onset, obvious precipitating factors, good premorbid history, social support and positive symptoms indicate good prognosis.

F. Other Nonorganic Psychoses

► Scientific Concepts

Various psychoses of nonorganic origin.

► History & Physical

Schizoaffective disorder: Concurrent symptoms of schizophrenia and depression or mania, with at least 2 weeks of psychotic symptoms alone.

Schizophreniform disorder: Same symptoms, history as schizophrenia but duration of < 6 months.

Brief psychotic disorder: Acute-onset psychosis with emotional upset and confusion often following stress. Duration < 1 month. Full return to premorbid functioning. Often seen in young adults.

Shared psychotic disorder: Patient delusional, develops in conjunction with submissive, dependent, isolated relationship with delusional person. Suicide or homicide pacts.

Psychotic disorder not otherwise specified: Psychotic symptoms that do not meet criteria for other disorders. Includes postpartum psychosis (occurs 2 to 3 weeks postpartum, usually primipara, risk of infanticide or suicide), culture-bound syndromes.

► Diagnostic Studies

Lab tests to rule out organic etiology or substance use.

► Diagnosis

Symptoms as specified above.

► Clinical Therapeutics

Schizoaffective disorder: Bipolar type; neuroleptic discontinued or reduced after stabilization; other options include carbamazepine, valproic acid, ECT, lithium for maintenance, clozapine for refractory symptoms. Depressive type; neuroleptic with or without antidepressant, ECT, lithium also used.

Schizophreniform disorder: Neuroleptics for at least 6 months.

Brief psychotic disorder: Neuroleptic or antianxiety agent.

Shared psychotic disorder: Neuroleptics.

► Clinical Intervention

Clinical therapeutics as above with psychotherapy. Hospitalization as needed for patient safety and stabilization.

► Health Maintenance Issues

Follow-up as needed based on diagnosis. Supportive psychotherapy and family support.

II. ANXIETY/MOOD/PERSONALITY DISORDERS

A. Acute Stress Reactions

► Scientific Concepts

Intensity of the trauma (i.e., motor vehicle accident, military combat, rape, etc.) may be strongest predisposing factor. A history of personality disorder, major psychopathology, or low social support may also predict poor psychological adjustment to acute stressor. Expression of dissociation may be culturally influenced.

► History & Physical

Exposure to traumatic event within 4 weeks. Symptoms of anxiety, fear, dissociation (e.g., derealization, numbing detachment, reduced awareness of surroundings, depersonalization), reexperiencing event (images, thoughts, dreams, flashbacks). Avoidance of reminders of event. Impaired ability to perform necessary tasks.

► Diagnostic Studies

None required.

► Diagnosis

Lasts minimum of 2 days; if lasts more than 4 weeks, diagnose posttraumatic stress disorder (PTSD). Symptoms not due to drug effects or other medical condition.

► Clinical Therapeutics

Benzodiazepines or buspirone may be used for short-term treatment.

► Clinical Intervention

Psychotherapy to reduce dissociation, acknowledge trauma.

► Health Maintenance Issues

May have impaired ability to care for self. At risk for PTSD.

B. Adjustment Disorders

► Scientific Concepts

Vulnerability to stress may be related to temperament, constitution, experiences, personality, severity of stressor.

► History & Physical

Identifiable stressor within range of normal experience (acute or chronic illness, employment problems, etc.) within 3 months. Distress in excess of what would be expected. Impaired social or occupational functioning.

► Diagnostic Studies

None required.

► Diagnosis

Emotional disturbance and impaired functioning greater than would be expected from identifiable psychosocial stressor. Stressors include school, divorce, job loss, illness, etc. Onset within 3 months but no longer than 6 months unless stressor is chronic (e.g., chronic illness). If overreaction is part of pattern, diagnose personality disorder. Distress not due to bereavement. Rule out substance abuse. May be classified by predominant symptoms: depressed mood, anxiety, mixed anxiety and depressed mood, disturbance of conduct, mixed disturbance of emotions and conduct, or unspecified. Behavioral symptoms in adolescents; mood, anxiety symptoms in adults. If stressor outside normal range of experiences, diagnose PTSD.

► Clinical Therapeutics

Short-term medication for relief of anxiety, insomnia, and depressive mood.

► Clinical Intervention

Clarify barriers to problem resolution and develop therapeutic plan. Reduce stress (exercise, social support, cognitive restructuring, relaxation techniques, self-care, short-term therapy, group support). Treat substance abuse, underlying psychopathology if present.

C. Anxiety/Panic Disorders

1. Panic Disorder

► Scientific Concepts

Significant evidenc for genetic component; biological basis related to disturbances in norepinephrine and gamma-aminobutyric acid (GABA) neurotransmission. One-year prevalence is 1–2%; onset in third decade of life; more common in women. Often associated with mitral valve prolapse though no causal relationship has been established.

► History & Physical

Recurring, unexpected, sudden "panic attacks" involving intense fear or discomfort to include four or more of the following symptoms: sweating, shortness of breath, trembling/shaking, palpitations, chest pain, choking, dizziness/faintness, nausea/abdominal distress, fear of dying, fear of losing control, chills/hot flashes, paresthesias, derealization/depersonalization. Can be precipitated by stressful event but often occurs unexpectedly without identifiable stressor. Severity and frequency of panic attacks may vary considerably. Persistent concern (> 1 month) regarding occurrence and consequences of recurrent panic attacks; often leads to anticipatory anxiety. May be present with or without agoraphobia (avoidance of leaving the home alone or being in a confined social or physical environment which causes significant anxiety). Primary care provider or cardiologist typically consulted first for somatic complaints. Evaluate for excessive caffeine intake, positive family history, and comorbid depression; childhood anxiety disorder may be a predisposing factor. Physical exam may reveal tachycardia, elevated systolic blood pressure, hyperventilation, sweating, trembling, cold hands. Finding characteristics of mitral valve prolapse may be present.

► Diagnostic Studies

None are diagnostic; carbon dioxide and sodium lactate can precipitate panic.

► Diagnosis

Rule out other anxiety disorders and medical conditions including substance abuse (caffeinism, stimulants, alcohol, or sedative withdrawal) cardiac disorders, hypoglycemia, hyperparathyroidism, hyperthyroidism, hypoxia, pheochromocytoma, seizure disorders, and vestibular disease. Avoid excessive medical workups. Coded as with or without agoraphobia.

► Clinical Therapeutics

Tricyclic antidepressants, SSRIs, and high-potency benzodiazepines are effective.

► Clinical Intervention

Reassurance and relaxation training to manage acute panic attack. Rebreathing into paper bag may be helpful. Prompt referral to psychiatry/psychology for cognitive-behavioral intervention to include relaxation training for panic attacks and systematic desensitization if agoraphobia present. Eliminate caffeine and other stimulants.

2. Generalized Anxiety Disorder

► Scientific Concepts

Familial patterns, possible genetic component.

► History & Physical

Anxiety and worry on most days lasting more than 6 months. Inability to control apprehensive expectations. Anxiety frequency, duration, and intensity is excessive for current life stressors. Associated with three or more of following symptoms: easy to fatigue, sleep disturbance, difficulty concentrating, irritability, restlessness, and muscle tension. Muscle tension, aches, and soreness along with other symptoms of autonomic arousal are common. Significant impairment in occupational, interpersonal, and activities of daily living (ADL) functioning. Often associated with major depression.

► Diagnostic Studies

None required.

► Diagnosis

Not diagnosed if anxiety due to specific anxiety disorders, substance use, or other psychiatric or medical condition.

► Clinical Therapeutics

Although immediately effective, benzodiazepines should be used sparingly and only for up to several months due to potential for abuse. Buspirone is an effective initial treatment, though it does not provide as immediate relief as benzodiazepines. Selective serotonin reuptake inhibitors (SSRIs), tricyclic antidepressants, and monoamine oxidase inhibitors (MAOIs) may be useful in selected patients. May need prolonged or intermittent treatment.

► Clinical Intervention

Cognitive–behavioral therapy. May be at increased risk for panic disorders.

3. Obsessive–Compulsive Disorder

► Scientific Concepts

Affects 2 to 3% of the population. Possible genetic contribution; probable serotonin system abnormality. Often present first to the family care practitioner.

► History & Physical

Persistent and consuming recurrent images, thoughts, and impulses; may be inappropriate and/or intrusive. Perceived as product of own mind (versus delusion or thought insertion). Typical obsessions include a preoccupation with aggression, order, sin, contamination, loss of control, doubt. Obsessions cause significant distress or anxiety that is excessive in respect to current life events. May feel driven to perform ritualistic behaviors (compulsions) to reduce anxiety. Typical compulsions (i.e., repeating words silently, repetitive touching, checking, washing, etc.) are time consuming and interrupt interpersonal, vocational, and ADL functioning. Onset generally by early adulthood; 75% have both obsessions and compulsions. Depressive feelings and major affective disorder very common. May have other anxiety disorders, anorexia nervosa, alcoholism, Tourette's syndrome. Dermatologic complaints may be present secondary to excessive washing.

► Diagnostic Studies
None required.

► Diagnosis
Differentiate excessive pleasure-seeking (i.e., eating, sexual activity, etc.) as opposed to anxiety-reducing (i.e., hand washing, checking, etc.) behaviors. Differentiate from obsessive–compulsive symptoms presenting in depression and schizophrenia that respond to specific treatments.

► Clinical Therapeutics
Fluoxetine (SSRI) and clomipramine (tricyclic antidepressant) effective in 60%; may require higher doses and several weeks to several months. Observe for agitation, sexual dysfunction (fluoxetine), and anticholinergic effects (clomipramine). Most effective when combined with cognitive–behavioral intervention.

► Clinical Intervention
Cognitive–behavioral therapy based on exposure to feared situation, thought stopping, and compulsive behavior blocking. Relapse common.

4. Posttraumatic Stress Disorder

► Scientific Concepts
Disorder is common in individuals exposed to extreme stressors with some prevalence estimates exceeding 50%. Biological basis includes heightened sympathetic nervous system arousal.

► History & Physical
History of exposure to traumatic event threatening or causing serious injury to self or others. Typical events: criminal violence, combat, natural disaster, sexual abuse. Symptoms include intense fear and helplessness; recurrent nightmares, flashbacks, reliving of event; avoidance of event-related stimuli; emotional detachment and loss of interest; emotional distress and/or physiologic arousal on exposure to stimuli resembling or symbolizing traumatic event; persistent hyperarousal (insomnia, hypervigilance, decreased concentration, irritability). Onset usually within 3 months postevent but may be delayed for many months. Often associated with depression and substance abuse; other anxiety disorders may also be present. Lasts 1 month or more and impairs interpersonal, vocational, or ADL functioning.

► Diagnostic Studies
Increased autonomic arousal (i.e., galvanic skin response, electromyogram, heart rate, blood pressure).

► Diagnosis
PTSD symptoms lasting < 1 month represent acute stress disorder; PTSD symptoms following less severe stressor (i.e., divorce, job loss) diagnosed as adjustment disorder.

► Clinical Therapeutics

Benzodiazepines for mild sedation should be used with caution secondary to abuse potential. Antidepressants often useful in those with and without comorbid depression.

► Clinical Intervention

Referral for psychiatric evaluation indicated. Some patients respond to the opportunity to express their feelings (ventilation) and to cognitive–behavioral approaches. Support groups and family education. Treatment for substance abuse and any concurrent disorders. Symptoms often refractory to treatment and accentuated during subsequent stressful periods.

III. ATTENTION DEFICIT HYPERACTIVITY DISORDER

► Scientific Concepts

Familial aggregation; probable genetic contribution in some cases. Probable dysregulation in noradrenergic and dopaminergic neurotransmission. Associated with CNS abnormalities (i.e., Tourette's syndrome, seizure disorders). Greater prevalence in males. Most common mental health diagnosis in children.

► History & Physical

Classic triad involves age-inappropriate impulsivity, hyperactivity, or inattentiveness lasting 6 months or more. Symptom onset must begin before 7 years old. May exhibit careless mistakes, does not follow instructions or appear to listen, easily distracted, forgetful, fidgety, doesn't sit still, talks excessively, accident prone, difficulty awaiting turn during play, often interrupts others. Significant impairment in academic and interpersonal functioning; may be marked by presence of underachievement, substance abuse, suicide attempts, more frequent accidents, low frustration tolerance, and temper outbursts. Physical examination may demonstrate neuromaturational delays, poor psychomotor coordination, or speech and hearing problems including chronic otitis media–associated tic disorder in 10%.

► Diagnostic Studies

Behavioral rating scales are useful in describing classroom and home activities; common scales include the Conner's Parent Rating Scale and the Child Behavior Check List (CBCL), the latter of which assesses for a broader range of psychopathology. Neuropsychological testing may be indicated to detect specific learning disabilities. EEG if seizures are suspected; thyroid function tests if hyperthyroidism is suspected; hematocrit and lead level. Hearing, speech, or vision assessment as indicated by exam.

► Diagnosis

A comprehensive evaluation should be completed before making the diagnosis of ADHD as it may be misdiagnosed if based solely upon limited observation. Classic triad not present in all children; need hyperactivity/impulsivity or inattention/distractibility. Commonly associated with oppositional defiant disorder and conduct disorder, specific learning disorders, anxiety/mood disorders. Rule out schizophrenia, other psychotic disorders, pervasive developmental disorder, or other mental disorders.

▶ Clinical Therapeutics

Stimulants (e.g., methylphenidate, dextroamphetamine, methamphetamine, magnesium pemoline); side effects include insomnia and appetite suppression; long-term therapy may inhibit growth; 25 to 30% do not respond. Antidepressants (imipramine, desipramine, nortriptyline, bupropion) useful for children with associated tics and those experiencing side effects to stimulants; less effective than stimulants. Clonidine for marked aggression or hyperactivity; side effect is sedation, which may assist insomnia associated with stimulants.

▶ Clinical Intervention

Correction of hearing or vision impairments; specific educational interventions for learning disabilities. Family and individual psychotherapy/education. Environmental/behavioral management at home and school. Poorer prognosis associated with coexisting conduct disorder, low IQ, more severe symptoms. Higher risk for child abuse. Symptoms may continue into adulthood.

IV. DEPRESSIVE DISORDERS

A. Major (Unipolar) Depression

▶ Scientific Concepts

Complex psychobiological syndrome involving neurotransmitter dysregulation (primarily decreases in serotonin and norepinephrine) often precipitated by environmental stress, particularly the initial episodes. Probable genetic predisposition. Five to 10% prevalence in primary care settings; greater prevalence in females. Antidepressant medications increase neurotransmitter availability.

▶ History & Physical

Depressed mood (dysphoria) *or* loss of interest or pleasure for ≥ 2 continuous weeks. Four or more of the following: insomnia or hypersomnia, change in appetite, change in weight not due to dieting, psychomotor agitation or retardation, fatigue, feelings of worthlessness or guilt, difficulty concentrating, recurrent thoughts of death or suicide. Often associated with loss of libido, social withdrawal, indecisiveness, obsessive rumination, tearfulness, agitation. Significant impairment in interpersonal, vocational, or ADL functioning. Individuals with "masked depression" may initially present with physical complaints. Children and adolescents may have anxiety, social withdrawal, irritability, behavioral problems, or somatic complaints. Cognitive impairments often prominent in elderly patients. Increased prevalence in those with previous personal episodes or family history. Accentuated in some women during premenstrual period. May demonstrate seasonal pattern. May be precipitated by chronic medical or psychiatric illness. Associated with substance abuse. Increased risk of suicide.

▶ Diagnostic Studies

None diagnostic, though evidence of neuroendocrine dysfunction may be present on dexamethasone suppression test and sleep EEGs. Self-rating instruments (i.e., Beck Depression Inventory, etc.) can be of assistance in assessing depressive symptomatology.

▶ Diagnosis

Rule out bipolar depression and cyclothymia (mania/hypomania), dysthymia (less severe but chronic), self-limited bereavement after personal loss, lifelong pattern of mood instability representing a personality disorder, dementia, or mood disorder caused by medical illness or drugs.

▶ Clinical Therapeutics

As antidepressants tend to be relatively equal in their effectiveness in resolving acute depressive episodes, selection of initial medication often based on a favorable side effect profile. The medication should have few effects hindering patient compliance (i.e., sexual dysfunction), address atypical depression features (i.e., hypersomnia), consider comorbid conditions (i.e., hypertension, cardiac disease), avoid interactions with other drugs (i.e., warfarin), and be consistent with patient preferences and financial resources. SSRIs (fluoxetine, sertraline, paroxetine) as well as nefazodone and venlafaxine are recommended first-line agents. Compared to other antidepressants, SSRIs generally have lower toxicity, fewer side effects, and once-per-day dosing. Side effects include sedation, insomnia, agitation, sexual dysfunction, weight gain, and dry mouth. Non-SSRIs include nefazodone, which is helpful for those with insomnia, and venlafaxine, which is less prone to produce sexual dysfunction. Additional agents include bupropion, which is less frequently associated with sexual dysfunction and fatigue and may facilitate weight loss, and trazodone, which is often coadministered to treat insomnia. Antidepressants should be given for 4 to 6 weeks at a full therapeutic level before assessing response. If necessary, alternative second-line agents include tricyclic antidepressants, which have a higher frequency of side effects (i.e., dry mouth, constipation, sedation, arrhythmia, weight gain, etc.) but cost less. Other medications including MAOIs, which require a tyramine-free diet, and lithium are perhaps best administered under a specialist's care.

▶ Clinical Intervention

Mild depression may be treated with psychotherapy alone; however, moderately to severely depressed patients (as well as those mildly depressed but with significant impairment in daily functioning) should be considered for antidepressant medications as well. Psychotherapy enhances pharmacotherapy effectiveness. Exercise and phototherapy may be of value in those with a seasonal pattern (typical of seasonal affective disorder). Individuals not responsive to initial therapy, having suicidal tendencies, or presenting with comorbid psychiatric or medical conditions may require referral for psychiatric evaluation and treatment. Individuals with significant suicidal risk or major impairment in daily functioning may require hospitalization. ECT is effective for those not responding to antidepressants, who present with psychosis, or who have significant suicidal risk.

► Health Maintenance Issues
Those with a history of recurrent episodes are at increased risk for continued occurrences; hence, long-term maintenance psychotherapy and treatment with antidepressant medication may be needed.

B. Dysthymia

► Scientific Concepts
Complex psychobiological syndrome involving neurotransmitter dysregulation (primarily decreases in serotonin and norepinephrine) often precipitated by environmental stress. Possible genetic predisposition. Greater prevalence in females. Antidepressant medications increase neurotransmitter availability.

► History & Physical
Mood is chronically depressed for a minimum of 2 years (1 year for children/adolescents) with no lapse in symptoms > 2 months' duration. Symptoms must include two of the following: sleep disturbance, appetite disturbance, low self-esteem, fatigue, difficulty concentrating, hopelessness. Symptoms must cause significant impairment in social/occupational functioning or ADL. Onset is insidious and develops in childhood through early adulthood. No history of major depression or manic episode within first 2 years. Greater prevalence in women and in those with a family history of depression. Children with dysthymia often exhibit irritability, poor social skills, and impaired school performance.

► Diagnostic Studies
None required.

► Diagnosis
Rule out chronic psychotic disorder, substance-induced mood disorder, personality disorder (may coexist), or general medical disorder (i.e., hypothyroidism, neurodegenerative or autoimmune conditions, cerebral infarcts, etc.). Major depression can be coexisting condition.

► Clinical Therapeutics
As noted for major (unipolar) depression, SSRIs (fluoxetine, sertraline, paroxetine) as well as non-SSRIs such as venlafaxine are recommended first-line agents.

► Clinical Intervention
Psychotherapy and physical exercise are generally recommended.

► Health Maintenance Issues
Individuals with dysthymia are at significantly increased risk of developing major depression.

C. Bipolar Disorders

► Scientific Concepts
Complex psychobiological syndrome involving neurotransmitter dysregulation. Probable genetic component. Prevalence in females equals males in bipolar I disorder; females greater than males in bipolar II disorder.

► History & Physical
Bipolar I disorder: Essential feature is the presence of one or more manic episodes (distinct period of an abnormally expansive, elated, or irritable mood lasting ≥ 1 week, including three or more of the following: inflated self-esteem, distractibility, talkativeness, decreased need for sleep, flight of ideas, agitation or increased goal-directed activity, or engagement in excessive spending sprees or promiscuity having potentially negative consequences. Onset generally in adolescence or young adulthood. Symptoms lead to impairment in social or occupational functioning or ADL. Manic episode preceded or succeeded by one or more major depressive episodes; may be precipitated by stress. Associated with increased risk of suicide as well as impulsive and violent behavior, which may lead to marital conflict or criminal activity.
Bipolar II disorder: History of one or more hypomanic episodes and one or more depressive periods. Hypomania represents a significant change in functioning involving a milder form of mania both in terms of symptoms and level of impairment. There is no history of mania or a mixed episode of major depression and mania. Associated with a significant risk of suicide, anxiety disorders, substance abuse, and borderline personality disorder.

► Diagnostic Studies
None required.

► Diagnosis
Rule out other mood disorders, including those due to a general medical condition or substance induced, schizoaffective disorder, or another psychotic disorder. Bipolar I and II subtypes are categorized according to more recent episode: manic, hypomanic, depressive, or mixed. An increased cycling rate may be seen as the patient ages.

► Clinical Therapeutics
Approximately 70% respond to lithium after 2 to 3 weeks of therapy for mania, hypomania, and mixed episodes. Lithium has a small therapeutic range; hence, close monitoring of plasma lithium levels is necessary. Significant dose-related toxicity exists at plasma lithium lev-

els > 1.5 mEq/L; symptoms include nausea, vomiting, diarrhea, tremor, and delirium; also closely monitor renal and thyroid function. Other adverse effects include polyuria, hypothyroidism, acne, and weight gain. Teratogenic and cardiac conduction effects require baseline pregnancy test and electrocardiogram (ECG). Anticonvulsants (i.e., valproic acid, carbamazepine) can be used when lithium is difficult to monitor or counterindicated. SSRIs may be initiated to treat depressive symptomatology unresponsive to lithium, though there is some risk of precipitating mania. ECT may also be initiated.

► Clinical Intervention

Psychotherapy, education, and family support may increase medication compliance and overall adaptation. Significant risk of suicide continues. Monitoring for key predictors of relapse and anticipation of high-risk situations; participation in support groups may be helpful. Those with rapid cycling (may increase with age) have poorer prognosis and greater risk of suicide.

► Health Maintenance Issues

Majority of patients will relapse without prophylaxis; lithium generally provided for months or indefinitely in those exhibiting rapid cycling. Women at risk for postpartum episodes.

D. Cyclothymia

► Scientific Concepts

Complex psychobiological syndrome involving neurotransmitter dysregulation. Probable genetic component. Prevalence in females equals males. Often exhibit a family history of affective and substance-related disorders.

► History & Physical

Recurrent, vacillating mood disturbance of at least 2 years' duration (1 year for children/adolescents) with symptoms of depression and hypomania and not pervasive or severe enough to be diagnosed as major depression or bipolar disorder; no lapse in symptoms > 2 months' duration. Symptoms must cause clinically significant impairment in occupation or social functioning or ADL. No history of manic, major depressive, or mixed episode within first 2 years. Disorder onset is generally adolescence, early adulthood. Often associated with a sleep disorder.

► Diagnostic Studies

None required.

► Diagnosis

Rule out schizoaffective disorder, schizophrenia or other psychotic disorder, borderline personality disorder, substance-induced disorder, or disorder due to general medical condition (i.e., hyperthyroidism).

► Clinical Therapeutics

May respond to lithium and anticonvulsant medications as noted under Bipolar Disorders.

► Clinical Intervention
Individual and group psychotherapy may be useful in facilitating adaptation to effects of mood swings on self-esteem and interpersonal functioning.

► Health Maintenance Issues
Substantial risk (15 to 50%) of progression to bipolar I or II disorder.

V. PERSONALITY DISORDERS

► Scientific Concepts
Enduring maladaptive patterns of inner experience (cognition, affectivity) and behavior (impulse control, interpersonal functioning) that substantially deviate from the individual's cultural patterns. Maladaptive pattern is inflexible, pervasive across personal and interpersonal experiences; onset can be traced to adolescence or early adulthood, and causes clinically significant distress or impairment in occupational/interpersonal functioning. Genetic contribution suspected in some (e.g., schizotypal, antisocial, borderline); CNS serotonin dysregulation may be associated with aggressive, impulsive behavior. Symptoms/signs of personality disorders are often precipitated or exacerbated by stress. Most are ego-syntonic in that patients are comfortable with their personality traits even though their behavior may be dysfunctional. Personality disorders are frequently diagnosed in mental health clinics.

► History & Physical
Cluster A Disorders
- *Paranoid:* Pervasive suspiciousness and four of the following characteristics: preoccupied with the trustworthiness of (or reluctance to confide in) others, holds unjustified suspicions regarding sexual partner's fidelity, suspects others of malicious intent, perceives a threatening hidden meaning in benign remarks, or is hypersensitive to criticisms or perceives criticisms where none are apparent.
- *Schizoid:* Significant and pervasive pattern of social isolation and lack of joy in interpersonal/family relationships; demonstrates emotional coldness and poor response to social praise.
- *Schizotypal:* Cognitive distortions, eccentric behaviors, and social deficits, including altered perceptual experiences, magical thinking, ideas of reference, unusual speech patterns (stereotyped, vague, etc.), paranoid ideation, extreme social anxiety, few close friends, constricted or inappropriate affect, unusual behavior. Onset by early adulthood.

Cluster B Disorders
- *Antisocial:* Onset at ≥ 18 years of age, with three or more of the following characteristics since age 15: disregard for social/lawful norms, pervasive lying/conning, physical aggressiveness, impul-

sivity, irresponsibility, disregard for safety of others, lack of re-
morse. Evidence of conduct disorder prior to age 15.

- *Borderline:* Pervasive pattern of impulsivity, unstable relationships, and altered affect with onset in early adulthood. Indicated by potentially self-damaging impulsivity, unstable self-image, marked
mood swings, emptiness, suicidal or self-mutilating behavior, instability in social relationships (vacillates between devaluation
and idealization), perceptions of abandonment, paranoidal
ideation, and difficulty with anger control.

- *Histrionic:* Excessive self-centered orientation characterized by
shallow yet rapidly changing emotions, stylized speech, self-
dramatization, sexually seductive/provocative dress or behavior,
attention seeking, highly susceptible to social influence, exagger-
ates level of interpersonal intimacy.

- *Narcissistic:* Pervasive preoccupation with self as indicated by fan-
tasies of success, perceptions of self-importance or uniqueness,
arrogance, feelings of entitlement, seeks admiration, exploitative,
demanding, lacking in empathy.

Cluster C Disorders

- *Avoidant:* Pervasive social inhibition characterized by preoccupation with social criticism, avoidance of interpersonal situations
that risk embarrassment, fear of being intimate, inhibition in new
social contexts or when unclear of social acceptance.

- *Dependent:* Requires extensive social support as characterized by
inability to perform independent tasks, difficulty making independent decisions, excessive fear of abandonment, attempts to
immediately develop new supportive relationship upon cessation
of old one; passive, submissive, and clingy behavior. May be exacerbated by chronic medical illness.

- *Obsessive–compulsive:* Rigid, perfectionistic, productivity oriented,
preoccupied with rules, reluctance to delegate, excessive hoard-
ing of valuable (i.e., money) as well as invaluable objects, stub-
bornness.

▶ Diagnostic Studies

Standardized testing (e.g., Wechsler Adult Intelligence Scale–
Revised [WAIS-R], Minnesota Multiphasic Personality Inventory
[MMPI], etc.) and projective testing (e.g., Rorschach, etc.) may facili-
tate diagnosis.

▶ Diagnosis

Maladaptive pattern must lead to significant impairment in interpersonal functioning or ADL. Rule out other mental health disorders
(i.e., mood disorders, psychosis [particularly with schizotypal]), substance abuse, adult attention deficit disorder, or medical illness (i.e.,
delirium, CNS trauma or tumor, temporal lobe epilepsy). Mixed personality disorders and atypical presentations are common.

▶ Clinical Therapeutics

In general, medications are of limited value. Patients exhibiting
psychotic decompensation may require major tranquilizers; schizo-

typal and borderline disorders may respond to low-dose neuroleptics; borderline disorders may also respond to SSRIs, MAOIs, or lithium. Those with anxiety may respond to anxiolytic or antidepressant medications.

▶ Clinical Intervention

Treatment of comorbid conditions (i.e., alcohol or other drug abuse, depression); hospitalization if at risk of harm to self and others. Individual and group psychotherapy may be useful for patients and their families.

▶ Health Maintenance Issues

Often resistant to therapy, personality disorders tend to be chronic.

VI. PHYSICAL DISORDERS WITH PSYCHOGENIC ORIGIN

A. Psychological Factor Affecting Medical Condition (Psychosomatic Disorders)

▶ Scientific Concepts

Psychological variables have the potential to influence the development, presentation, and progression of a wide variety of medical illnesses. This diagnostic category is reserved for cases in which psychological/behavioral factors have a clinically significant impact.

▶ History & Physical

Clear evidence (generally including a temporal relationship) between psychological factors (coping styles, emotional state, maladaptive health behavior, psychophysiological stress response) and the development or exacerbation of symptoms of a known medical condition (e.g., asthma, headaches, angina, low back pain, etc.). Psychological factors may also increase risk of medical complications (e.g., continued smoking in the asthmatic patient).

▶ Diagnostic Studies

Temporal linkage between mental stress, excessive psychophysiological arousal, and medical symptoms may be demonstrated (e.g., interpersonal conflict, ambulatory monitoring revealing elevated blood pressure, and angina).

▶ Diagnosis

Establish temporal relationship. Rule out a general medical disorder or substance abuse causing the psychological symptoms, somatoform disorders in which there is no diagnosable medical illness, or the more specific case of pain disorder.

▶ Clinical Therapeutics

Limit addictive analgesics. Antidepressants may be helpful. Pharmacological/surgical therapy for the medical condition should be instituted as appropriate.

► Clinical Intervention

Stress management, including biofeedback, relaxation therapy, hypnosis, breathing exercises. Psychotherapy to facilitate identification and control of psychophysiological responses to stressful situations, enhance and extend range of problem-solving skills.

► Health Maintenance Issues

If limited response to isolated therapies noted above, may respond to intensive, comprehensive interdisciplinary intervention.

B. Factitious Disorder (Munchausen Syndrome)

► Scientific Concepts

Intentional effort to gain benefit from sick role through report of symptoms or behavior suggesting medical disorder. True medical problems may coexist. Onset generally in early adulthood.

► History & Physical

Feigning of symptoms or intentionally inducing signs of disease (e.g., use of medications, thermometer manipulation, self-induced bruises) without obvious external incentives (e.g., avoidance of legal responsibility or work). Often complex or vague medical problems. May present history of repeated hospitalizations and signing out against medical advice. At risk of injury due to attempts to produce signs of medical disease.

► Diagnostic Studies

Studies as appropriate to symptoms to rule out true medical disorder.

► Diagnosis

Rule out true medical or another mental disorder including malingering and somatoform disorders. May have comorbid substance abuse or personality disorder.

► Clinical Therapeutics

None indicated.

► Clinical Intervention

Psychotherapy may be of assistance, particularly in conjunction with confrontation regarding the nature of the disorder.

► Health Maintenance Issues

Often reluctant to accept the diagnosis despite clear evidence, the disorder is generally chronic. Careful monitoring may assist in preventing iatrogenic complications.

C. Malingering

▶ Scientific Concepts
Intentional effort to gain benefit from sick role through report of symptoms or behavior suggesting medical disorder. True medical problems may coexist. Onset associated with external need for medical illness.

▶ History & Physical
Symptoms intentionally produced for obvious reasons (e.g., to avoid occupational, military, legal, or financial responsibilities; obtain drugs; or gain clear secondary social support from sick role). Uncooperative, exaggerated disability claims. May, in some circumstances, represent nonpathologic, adaptive behavior.

▶ Diagnostic Studies
Rule out true medical or another mental disorder including Munchausen syndrome and somatoform disorders. Comorbid antisocial personality disorder is common.

▶ Diagnosis
No objective finding to substantiate symptoms.

▶ Clinical Therapeutics
None indicated.

▶ Clinical Intervention
Eliminate external secondary gain motivating symptoms; confront regarding appropriate diagnosis; supportive psychotherapy.

▶ Health Maintenance Issues
Resolution of conflict with external motivating forces may produce reduction or elimination of symptoms.

VII. SOMATOFORM DISORDERS

A. Somatization Disorder

▶ Scientific Concepts
A broad-ranging pattern of physical complaints causing clinically significant impairment, beginning before 30 years of age and lasting several years. Symptoms inconsistent with medical findings. Onset in adolescence or early adulthood. Some familial association. Occurs primarily in women.

▶ History & Physical
Somatic complaints are not intentionally produced and include at least four pain symptoms, one sexual symptom, two gastrointestinal symptoms, and one pseudoneurological symptom. Symptoms are often vague and presented in a dramatic fashion. Symptoms cannot be

explained by a known medical condition, or if a medical condition is present, the impairment or degree of complaint is clearly excessive. History of treatment by numerous practitioners with potential for extensive evaluations and multiple surgeries. Substance abuse, depression, anxiety, and personality disorders are common comorbid conditions.

▶ **Diagnostic Studies**
Laboratory studies generally do not support symptoms.

▶ **Diagnosis**
Rule out general medical conditions and other mental disorders, particularly pain disorder, schizophrenia, or other somatoform disorder.

▶ **Clinical Therapeutics**
Avoid addictive medications (opiates, benzodiazepines). Antidepressants may be helpful.

▶ **Clinical Intervention**
Psychotherapy particularly for depression, suicidal ideation, or substance abuse. Develop primary care provider rapport with patient and determine appropriate utilization of medical consultative services.

▶ **Health Maintenance Issues**
Therapeutic course is generally chronic over many years; focus on satisfactory management rather than cure.

B. Conversion Disorder

▶ **Scientific Concepts**
Evidence of sensory or voluntary motor dysfunction not well explained by a general medical condition. More common in low socioeconomic status or rural populations; more frequent in women. Thought to represent expression of an unconscious mental conflict or to elicit secondary gain. Onset generally between 10 and 35 years of age.

▶ **History & Physical**
Sensory or voluntary motor function deficits or symptoms suggesting a neurological or other general medical condition. Deficits/symptoms not intentionally induced but may be precipitated or exacerbated by stress. May exhibit lack of concern regarding the symptoms despite clinically significant distress or occupational/interpersonal impairment. Deficits/symptoms include seizures, unconsciousness, paralysis, ataxia, loss of sensation, and blindness; not limited to sexual dysfunction or pain complaints. May have comorbid personality disorder.

▶ **Diagnostic Studies**
Neurological studies show an absence of expected neurological findings given symptoms/signs.

▶ Diagnosis

Symptoms/deficits are not consistent with known neuroanatomy and physiology. Attempt to rule out neurologic or general medical condition recognizing that some patients (~ 25%) may subsequently develop symptoms/signs of a known medical illness. Also rule out drug-induced or culturally sanctioned behavior as cause of symptoms, malingering, major depression, schizophrenia, and other somatoform disorders.

▶ Clinical Therapeutics

Minor tranquilizers may be helpful for anxiety.

▶ Clinical Intervention

Psychoanalysis and cognitive–behavioral therapy helpful for some. Supportive therapy for family; identification and removal of potential for secondary gain. Patients without comorbid psychiatric disorders and who have identifiable stressors precipitating onset of symptoms may have best prognosis.

C. Pain Disorder

▶ Scientific Concepts

Pain is a subjective experience influenced by the patient's cognitive and affective state. The perception of pain and the experience of suffering can occur both with and without recognizable organic pathology. The experience of pain can be reduced through cognitive–behavioral therapy as well as by analgesics and antidepressants intervening in the neurochemical pathways. Onset is generally 30 to 50 years of age; musculoskeletal pain may be more prevalent in women.

▶ History & Physical

Pain causing clinically significant distress and functional impairment is the predominant symptom. No evidence of intent to produce symptoms; but psychological factors appear to precipitate or exacerbate the pain. Physical findings consistent with the development of pain may or may not be present; however, findings are not judged to be sufficient to explain intensity of pain or level of disability. Complaints may be diffuse or vague; excessive analgesic usage and high likelihood of extensive medical care/surgery. Comorbid depression, substance abuse, social isolation, anxiety, and insomnia are common.

▶ Diagnostic Studies

Laboratory studies may identify organic pathology or be negative.

▶ Diagnosis

Psychological factors must have significant influence in precipitating, exacerbating, or maintaining the pain experience. Symptoms must not meet criteria for dyspareunia. Rule out malingering, factitious disorder, or major depression, anxiety, or psychotic disorder as primary diagnosis. Pain disorders classified as associated with psychological factors, or associated with psychological factors and a general medical condition.

► Clinical Therapeutics

Analgesics (in moderation) and antidepressants for pain; non-steroidal anti-inflammatory agents.

► Clinical Intervention

If addicted to analgesics, hospitalization for detoxification may be needed. Pain management training using cognitive–behavioral techniques including physical activity is generally indicated.

► Health Maintenance Issues

Assessment for suicide potential in those with severe depression. Careful review of medical/surgical utilization.

D. Hypochondriasis

► Scientific Concepts

Psychodynamic explanations for this preoccupation with fear of having a serious disease focus on displaced anxiety. Behavioral analyses find that secondary gain may or may not be present. Development and maintenance may depend on misinterpretation of somatic symptoms and signs. Past experience with serious illness, anxiety, and depression are often present. Onset in young adulthood.

► History & Physical

Pervasive fear of having serious disease based on selective attention to, and preoccupation with, somatic signs/symptoms. Fear exists for at least 6 months despite extensive medical evaluation and appropriate reassurance. Anxiety/fear causes clinically significant distress as well as interpersonal or occupational impairment. May or may not recognize that fear is excessive or unreasonable. Reluctant to explore psychiatric basis; excessive utilization of medical resources. Symptoms may exacerbate in response to stress.

► Diagnostic Studies

No evidence of pathophysiology warranting patient's concerns.

► Diagnosis

Rule out body dysmorphic disorder (fears restricted to concern about appearance), delusional disorder, obsessive–compulsive disorder, generalized anxiety disorder, panic disorder, separation anxiety, a major depressive disorder, or another somatoform disorder.

► Clinical Therapeutics

Antidepressant and/or anxiolytic therapy for comorbid depression and anxiety as indicated.

► Clinical Intervention

Psychotherapy may be of some value.

► Health Maintenance Issues

Careful review of medical utilization. Generally chronic course, although remission can occur particularly in those with sudden onset.

E. Body Dysmorphic Disorder

▶ Scientific Concepts

Excessive concern with perceived defect in physical appearance, may be symbolic for perceived personal inadequacies. Onset in adolescence.

▶ History & Physical

Preoccupation with portion of physical appearance, generally the face, which contains an imagined or slight defect. Preoccupation exceeds culturally appropriate expectations, causes clinically significant distress, and/or impairment in occupational or interpersonal functioning (social isolation). Excessive grooming may be present; repeated cosmetic surgery is common. Physical examination does not reveal evidence of anatomical defect warranting severity of patient's concerns.

▶ Diagnostic Studies

None required.

▶ Diagnosis

Rule out normal concerns regarding appearance, anorexia nervosa, major depressive disorder. Comorbid major depressive disorder, social phobia, obsessive–compulsive disorder, and delusional disorder may be present.

▶ Clinical Therapeutics

Antidepressants (SSRIs) may be helpful.

▶ Clinical Intervention

Psychological assessment with particular focus on interpersonal skills proficiency; psychotherapy may be helpful.

▶ Health Maintenance Issues

Severity of preoccupation may wax and wane over time; focus of preoccupation may change. Evaluation for suicidal potential is appropriate, particularly if depression is present.

VIII. EATING DISORDERS

A. Anorexia Nervosa

▶ Scientific Concepts

Occurs in 0.5 to 1% of adolescent girls; 10 to 20 times more often in females. Most frequent in developed countries. Biological, social, and psychological factors implicated. Familiar mood disorders common. Neurochemically diminished norepinephrine and activity suggested. Inverse relationship between 3-methoxy-4-hydroxyphenylglycol (MHPG) and depression; endogenous opioids may contribute to hunger denial.

► History & Physical

Weight loss or lack of weight gain leading to body weight at least 15% below normal expected weight for age and height. Profound body image disturbance, pursuit of thinness often to the point of starvation. Symptoms of bulimia may occur. Postmenarcheal women have absence of at least three consecutive menstrual cycles.

► Diagnostic Studies

As weight loss grows profound, signs include hypothermia, dependent edema, lanugo, and metabolic changes; amenorrhea; impaired water diuresis. ECG changes; endocrinological and medical problems secondary to starvation. Screening lab tests include serum electrolytes with renal function tests; thyroid function tests; glucose amylase and hematological tests; ECG; cholesterol level; dexamethasone suppression test; carotene level. May find decreased thyroid hormone and serum glucose levels. Nonsuppression of cortisol after dexamethasone; hypokalemia, increased blood urea nitrogen; hypercholesterolemia; cardiovascular; hypotension and bradycardia.

► Diagnosis

Symptoms as above. Subtypes:

Restricting type: During current episode has not engaged in binge eating or purging behavior.

Binge eating/purging type: During current episode regularly engages in binge eating or purging behavior.

Complicated by denial of symptoms, secrecy around eating rituals and resistance to treatment; rule out medical illness and various mental disorders, including depressive disorder, somatization disorder, schizophrenia, and bulimia nervosa.

► Clinical Therapeutics

Cyproheptadine, up to 32 mg/d, shows some benefit for nonbulimic patients; cyproheptadine may be helpful due to weight gain side effect; treatment of comorbid depression with antidepressants; serotonergic antidepressants such as fluoxetine, sertraline, and paroxetine may be useful.

► Clinical Intervention

Hospitalization may be necessary due to medical complications and suicidal risk. Treat medical complications; intravenous fluids or nasogastric feedings may be mandated. Evaluate for depression. Supportive, cognitive–behavioral, family therapy with goal of weight maintenance and eating behavior normalization, symptom reduction.

► Health Maintenance Issues

Course varies greatly: spontaneous recovery without treatment, recovery after a variety of treatments, fluctuating and deteriorating course resulting in death caused by complications of starvation; overall mortality rate 5 to 18%; restricting type may be less likely to recover; short-term response to hospital treatment is good; important to monitor medical complications; social relationships often poor, and depression often present.

B. Bulimia Nervosa

► Scientific Concepts

Estimates range from 1 to 3% of young women. More common in women than men, onset often late adolescence. High achievers, decreased serotonin and/or norepinephrine have been implicated; familial depression.

► History & Physical

Recurrent episodes of binge eating; a sense of lack of control over eating. Self-induced vomiting, misuse of laxatives or diuretics, fasting, or excessive exercise to prevent weight gain. Behaviors occur, on average, at least twice a week for 3 months. Self-evaluation unduly influenced by body shape and weight. Does not occur exclusively during episodes of anorexia nervosa. May show dehydration, menstrual disturbance, hypotension, and bradycardia. Check oral cavity for dental enamel erosion and hands for signs of abrasion secondary to self-induced vomiting. Bingeing usually precedes vomiting by about 1 year. Family relationships generally distant and conflictual.

► Diagnostic Studies

Lab studies of electrolytes and metabolism may show abnormalities due to purging and various degrees of starvation (particularly hypokalemia and hypochloremia). May show nonsupression on dexamethasone suppression test. May show dehydration and hypomagnesemia and hyperamylasemia. Complete psychiatric evaluation for comorbid depression, anorexia nervosa, substance abuse, and personality disorders.

► Diagnosis

Symptoms as above; DSM-IV subtypes:

Purging type: Regularly engages in self-induced vomiting or misuse of laxatives, diuretics, or enemas.

Nonpurging type: Uses other inappropriate compensatory behaviors, such as fasting or excessive exercise but not those in purging type.

Seizure disorders; CNS tumors; Kleine–Levin syndrome; Kluver–Bucy syndrome; coexisting borderline personality disorder; anorexia nervosa, binge eating/purging type.

► Clinical Therapeutics

Antidepressant medications including SSRIs such as fluoxetine may be higher than dose typical for treatment of depression (60 to 80 mg/d). Imipramine, desipramine, trazodone, MAOIs helpful at dosages usually given for treatment of depressive disorders.

► Clinical Intervention

Correct medical complications such as electrolyte imbalance. Most treated as outpatients. Individual cognitive–behavioral, group, and family therapy helpful in reducing bingeing. Hospitalization with suicidality, substance abuse, or when extreme purging results in electrolyte and metabolic disturbance. Chronic disorder with waxing and waning course; therapy may be prolonged; after 5 to 10 years, about half recover fully, 20% continue to meet full criteria.

► Health Maintenance Issues

Some patients with mild course may have long spontaneous remissions; often secretive about problem; many have concurrent major depression, anxiety disorder, chemical dependency. Monitor medical complications and long-term medication use. Prognosis dependent on severity of purging sequelae, frequency of vomiting resulting in electrolyte imbalance, esophagitis, salivary gland enlargement, and dental caries.

C. Obesity

► Scientific Concepts

No specific genetic marker; multicausal factors; 80% have family history; metabolic differences, decreased activity, eating behaviors; > 50% of general population, one-third or more of children and adolescents in the United States; six times more common in women of low socioeconomic status than higher status; prevalence increases three-fold between ages 20 and 50.

► History & Physical

Family history; often childhood onset; body weight exceeds by 20% standard weight listed in usual height–weight tables; body mass index (BMI—body weight in kilograms divided by height in square meters) correlates with morbidity and mortality (normal range, 20 to 25).

► Diagnostic Studies

Lab studies for medical complications; correlation with cardiovascular disorders, hypertension, and hypercholesterolemia twice as common; diabetes, gout, hyperlipidemias; proteinuria, nephrosis, and renal vein thrombosis; osteoarthritis; higher-than-normal mortality rate from colon, rectal, and prostate cancer in men; higher-than-normal mortality rate in women from cancer of gallbladder, biliary passages, breast, uterus, and ovaries.

► Diagnosis

Symptoms as above; genetic, developmental, physical activity, brain damage, clinical and psychological factors; close to 50% develop mild anxiety and depression. Night-eating syndrome, in which people eat excessively after evening meal; bulimia; pickwickian syndrome, 100% over desirable weight with associated respiratory and cardiovascular pathology. Associated clinical disorders include Cushing's disease; myxedema; adiposogenital dystrophy; prolonged use of serotonergic agonists may be associated with weight gain.

► Clinical Therapeutics

Amphetamine and congeners, methamphetamine and phentermine work by increasing norepinephrine levels; drugs that prevent absorption of certain macronutrients; perfluoroctyl bromide, orlistat

(Xenical) inhibits fat absorption, must be used in conjunction with a mildly hypocaloric, low-fat diet.

▶ Clinical Intervention

Diet and exercise: Best method, balanced diet of 1,100 to 1,200 calories supplemented with vitamins, particularly iron, folic acid, zinc, and vitamin B_6; total unmodified fasts for short-term weight loss, but have associated morbidity including orthostatic hypotension, sodium diuresis, and impaired nitrogen balance; ketogenic diets, high protein and fat associated with nausea, hypotension, and lethargy; increased physical activity.

Surgery: Gastric bypass, stomach transecting or stapling; gastroplasty, size of stomach stoma is reduced—successful results although vomiting, electrolyte imbalance, and obstruction may occur; lipectomy for cosmetic reasons with no effect on long-term weight loss.

Counseling: Behavior modification somewhat successful; new eating patterns, operant conditioning through rewards; group therapy for support; nutrition education.

Follow-up: Ongoing evaluations of goal achievement negative effects of treatment.

▶ Health Maintenance Issues

Treatment presented within perspective of risk factors; obesity has adverse effects on health, cardiovascular disorders; hypertension and hypercholesterolemia; diabetes, especially type II, can be reduced by weight reduction; may have comorbid depression, anxiety disorder; higher mortality from colon, rectal, prostate, gallbladder, biliary passages, breast, uterine, and ovarian cancer; mortality correlated with degree of obesity; prognosis for weight reduction is poor; of patients who lose significant amounts of weight, 90% regain; particularly poor prognosis for those who had childhood obesity.

IX. SUBSTANCE ABUSE DISORDERS

A. Alcoholism

▶ Scientific Concepts

Type 1: Onset in adulthood; gradually increasing consumption; both males and females; characteristics of perfectionism, dependency, introversion; some family history; amenable to treatment; 75% of all alcoholics.

Type 2: Onset in adolescence and early adulthood; antisocial, risk-taking, impulsive, aggressive characteristics; strong family history; predominantly males; treatment resistant; 25% of all alcoholics.

Some biological features may be inherited: resistance to intoxication, below normal rise in cortisol after drinking, below normal epinephrine release after stress. No typical alcoholic personality identified. Cultural patterns and genetics associated with patterns of drinking and risk of alcohol abuse.

► History & Physical

If not intoxicated, may present with anxiety, tension, insomnia, depression, headache, blackout, nausea/vomiting, or other gastrointestinal symptoms, tachycardia, palpitations, minor injuries due to falls; may attempt to conceal alcohol use. Screen with CAGE (four questions: annoyance with Criticism to drinking; Attempts to cut down; Guilt about drinking; morning Eye-opener); 95% certain diagnosis if three "yes" answers. If intoxicated, may present with alcohol on breath, be lively, emotionally labile, irritable, uncoordinated, have slurred speech and/or ataxia; may be uncooperative, assaultive, dangerous. If in withdrawal, may present with tachycardia, tremulousness, weakness, malaise, nausea/vomiting, diaphoresis, orthostatic hypotension, hyperreflexia, insomnia, hypervigilance, anxiety, irritability, tinnitus, mild illusions and hallucinations, and/or blurred vision worse in the first 12 to 18 hours of the day without drinking. May have convulsions, particularly in the first 2 days of withdrawal. Life-threatening delirium tremens (DTs) in 5% of alcoholics: disorientation, agitation, hallucinations, delusions, sweating, tachycardia, hypertension, tremor, fever, ataxia; increased risk if malnourished or other illness present; 10 to 15% mortality rate, usually due to secondary infection or acute heart failure. Alcohol-induced psychotic disorder presents with intense auditory hallucinations and other symptoms of withdrawal but usually not disoriented; usually self-limited but can become chronic. May have vertebral or rib fractures.

► Diagnostic Studies

Urine drug screen; breath or blood alcohol level. Blood level of 80–110 mg/dL associated with legal intoxication; > 150 mg/dL without intoxication suggests tolerance. May have increased mean corpuscular volume and abnormal liver function tests. Additional studies to consider: folate, vitamin B_{12}, electrolytes (include calcium and magnesium), CBC, EKG, urinalysis, and chest x-ray and CT of head.

► Diagnosis

Presence of impaired social and occupational functioning due to alcohol over 1-year period; inability to stop drinking once started; persistent desire and/or repeated attempts to decrease intake without success; continued drinking despite obviously serious negative consequences (i.e., health, marriage, job, etc.); tolerance to alcohol (increased amounts needed for effect); symptoms of withdrawal and/or compulsive and continuous use. Rule out schizophrenia, bipolar disorder, anxiety, attention deficit disorder, antisocial disorders. If intoxicated, rule out hypoglycemia, CNS infection, other drug toxicities, subdural hematoma.

► Clinical Therapeutics

Disulfiram may be useful as deterrent in cooperative patients.
Intoxicated: May require sedation (e.g., diazepam, 5 to 20 mg).
Withdrawal: Benzodiazepines preferred for sleep, reduce agitation, conserve energy, induce calm; taper off over 4 to 8 days. Barbiturates,

chloral hydrate, carbamazepine may also be used; avoid oversedation. Diazepam and carbamazepine for seizures. Thiamine, 100 mg IM, then 50 mg PO tid × 4 days. Chlordiazepoxide for tremulousness, delirium. Clonidine for sweating, tachycardia, tremor. Antianxiety agents may be useful in 1 to 2 weeks following withdrawal.

▶ Clinical Intervention

Help patient to confront denial; discuss drinking in open, matter-of-fact, nonjudgmental manner. Insist on total abstinence; provide support and encouragement. Expect relapses; encourage patient to continue working and stay socially active. Family therapy/marital therapy may be useful. Group therapy most effective (i.e., 12-step AA).

Intoxicated: Interact in nonthreatening, respectful, patient manner but be ready to use restraints. Consider hospitalization if at risk for withdrawal or becoming comatose; otherwise, consider sending home, jail for observation.

Withdrawal: Hospitalize if severe. Include family/familiar people, lighted room, clear directions and explanations, supportive environment. Use restraints if needed; constant observation. Provide good nutrition, multivitamins, high-carbohydrate diet; correct fluid/electrolyte imbalances. Measure pulse, blood pressure, and temperature every half-hour initially; treat shock with fluids, vasopressors, whole blood. Monitor for hypoglycemia, prolonged prothrombin time, fever. Treat injuries due to falls and/or withdrawal from other substances if present. Possible complications include pneumonia, tuberculosis, urinary tract infection, hypoglycemia, anemia, gastritis with hematemesis, hemorrhagic pancreatitis, cirrhosis, hepatic failure, meningitis. Insomnia, depression, anxiety, irritability may continue for weeks.

▶ Health Maintenance Issues

Counsel patients and follow up for complications including hypertension, gastritis, gastric ulcer, diarrhea, anemia, pancreatitis, cirrhosis, impotence, insomnia, esophageal and rectal varices, Wernicke's encephalopathy. Patients are prone to drug abuse, motor vehicle and other accidents, suicide, poisonings, drownings, assaults, job loss.

B. Caffeine/Tobacco Disorders

▶ Scientific Concepts

Tobacco (nicotine): Conditioned response; some association with other psychiatric, substance use disorders.

▶ History & Physical

Caffeine: Presents with symptoms of agitation, muscle twitching, restlessness, insomnia, diuresis, anxiety, excitement, gastrointestinal disturbance, cardiac arrhythmia. Flushing with intake of two cups of coffee. *Withdrawal symptoms:* headache, fatigue over 4 to 5 days.

Tobacco (nicotine): Assess by number of cigarettes smoked per day, how soon lights up in morning. *Withdrawal symptoms:* irritability, malaise, craving, weight gain, increased appetite, restlessness, anxiety, headache, difficulty concentrating, gastrointestinal distress, bradycardia, cough, insomnia, depression.

▶ Diagnostic Studies
  None.

▶ Diagnosis
  By history.

▶ Clinical Therapeutics
  Tobacco (nicotine): Nicotine patch or gum particularly effective when combined with behavior therapy. Continued smoking with nicotine patch/gum may cause cardiac death. Bupropion (Zyban) may facilitate ability to achieve and maintain smoking cessation. Clonidine may help decrease withdrawal symptoms; side effect: hypotension.

▶ Clinical Intervention
Caffeine: Gradual decrease in consumption may be better tolerated than abrupt cessation.
Tobacco (nicotine): Smoking cessation groups, self-help literature, counseling, behavior modification interventions.

▶ Health Maintenance Issues
  Tobacco (nicotine): Discuss complications of continued use: pulmonary, cardiac, peripheral vascular, neoplastic diseases.

C. Drug Dependence

▶ Scientific Concepts
Stimulants (amphetamines, cocaine, antiobesity drugs, crack, others): May be swallowed, snorted, injected, smoked (crack). Highly addictive. Amphetamines used medically for attention deficit disorder, narcolepsy, depression in elderly. Cocaine used medically in the treatment of nosebleeds and as local anesthetic in ears, nose, throat. Antiobesity drugs usually unsuccessful due to tolerance. No tolerance to tendency to develop psychotic symptoms indistinguishable from schizophrenia although tolerance to other effects develop.
Opioids (heroin, codeine, meperidine, methadone, pentazocine): Street preparation may be tainted with quinine, procaine, lidocaine, lactose, mannitol, and may be contaminated with bacteria, viruses, or fungi. High mortality rate associated with street preparations. Users predominantly in urban areas; more common in males, health care professionals, chronic pain patients, blacks. Can be snorted (heroin), smoked (opium), injected IV or subcutaneously, ingested (pharmaceutic opioids). Associated with depression and antisocial personality disorder.
Sedatives, hypnotics, anxiolytics (benzodiazepines, methaqualone, barbiturates, chloral compounds, others): Effects include euphoria, sedation, psychomotor impairment, amnesia, fatigue, headache, depression, gastrointestinal disturbance. Users often include young drug abusers who combine these with other agents, or patients who become dependent iatrogenically. Short-acting drugs (e.g., amobarbital) more lethal

at lower doses than long-acting compounds (e.g., phenobarbital). Death from overdose of benzodiazepines alone rare.

Hallucinogens (LSD, psilocybin, mescaline, methylenedioxymethamphetamine [MDMA], others): May be taken orally or smoked.

Phencyclidine (PCP, angel dust): Injected intravenously, snorted, smoked, or eaten to produce hallucinogenic effects.

Inhalants (gasoline, volatile glues, solvents, nitrates, cleaners, others): Often used by adolescents to induce euphoria. Possible death by accidental asphyxiation.

Anabolic steroids: Taken orally or intramuscularly, usually in adolescents and/or athletes.

Cannabis (marijuana, hashish, tetrahydrocannabinol [THC]): Most commonly used illicit drug; smoked or eaten.

▶ History & Physical

See Table 13-1.

▶ Diagnostic Studies

See Table 13-1.

▶ Diagnosis

Substance dependence when three or more of the following are present: tolerance (increased amounts required to achieve same effect, or decrease effect with continued use of same amount of substance); withdrawal (substance-specific withdrawal syndrome, or other substance taken to relieve or avoid withdrawal syndrome); increased amounts used or longer time of use than originally intended; inability to decrease use or control substance use; significant amounts of time spent to obtain, use, or recover from substance; discontinuing important social, occupational, or recreational activities due to substance; continuing use despite knowledge/awareness that it is exacerbating or causing physical or mental problems.

▶ Clinical Therapeutics

Amphetamines, cocaine: Intoxication: If symptoms are severe, benzodiazepines for agitation. May need to treat dysrhythmias. *Withdrawal:* Antidepressants for depression after thorough detox. Caution should be exercised with haloperidol and phenothiazines as they may lower the seizure threshold.

Opioids: Intoxication/Overdose: Naloxone administration can be lifesaving in cases of respiratory depression. *Withdrawal:* Be prepared for abstinence syndrome in narcotic-dependent patients. Severe abstinence syndrome may require methadone until symptoms controlled. Clonidine may be useful for anxiety and craving during the detox phase.

Sedatives, hypnotics, anxiolytics: For acute overdose of benzodiazepines, IV flumazenil. Otherwise, long-acting benzodiazepine taper. Phenobarbital with a gradual taper is a second choice. For alcohol, use a long-acting benzodiazepine, multivitamins, thiamine, and magnesium.

Hallucinogens: Intoxication: Benzodiazepines for anxiety; use haloperidol only if additional sedation needed.

► table 13-1

SUBSTANCE ABUSE: DIAGNOSTICS

	Mild–Moderate Intoxication	Severe Intoxication	Withdrawal
Stimulants	Euphoria, increased energy and alertness, talkativeness, sexual arousal, insomnia, increased ability to perform repetitive tasks, decreased appetite, anxiety, irritability, pupillary dilatation, hypertension, increased heart rate, psychomotor agitation, hyperthermia, weight loss, nausea and vomiting. Often associated with sexually transmitted diseases, depression, sexual dysfunction, social isolation. Urinalysis positive for 1–3 days.	*Toxic psychosis:* visual, auditory, tactile hallucinations, delusions, mania, paranoia, aggression, hypervigilance, pupillary dilatation, elevated blood pressure and heart rate, arrhythmias, seizures, exhaustion, coma, intracranial hemorrhage; may progress to delirium or sudden cardiac death.	Dysphoria, hypersomnia or insomnia, increased appetite, fatigue, agitation, anxiety, suicidal ideation, unpleasant dreams; may self-medicate with alcohol or other substances during withdrawal.
Opioids	Euphoria; apathy; analgesia without loss of consciousness; drowsiness; mental clouding; lethargy; dysphoria; hypoactivity; anorexia; constipation; itching; nausea and vomiting; slurred speech; hypotension; bradycardia; constricted pupils; needle tracks; flushed, warm skin (cutaneous vasodilation); dysarthria; impaired attention and memory; illusions. *Dependency:* weight loss, hyposexuality, amenorrhea, criminal involvement, suicide attempts, accidents, other health problems. Urinalysis positive for 1–2 days.	Respiratory depression (may recur up to 24–72 hrs after apparent recovery), depressed reflexes, hypotension, shock, pulmonary edema, pupillary dilation, seizures, coma.	Dysphoria, myalgias, rhinorrhea, fever, nausea and vomiting, diarrhea, dilated pupils, tearing, restlessness, sweating, insomnia, yawning, piloerection, anxiety, craving, hypertension, tachycardia.
Sedatives/ Hypnotics/ Anxiolytics	Slurred speech, mood lability, drowsiness, incoordination, unsteady gait, impaired judgment, impaired attention and memory, nystagmus. Blood and urine tests positive for 1–2 days.	Respiratory depression, depressed reflexes, hypotension, hypoxemia, decreased cardiac output, bullous skin lesions and necrosis of sweat glands, hypothermia, coma, death (usually pneumonia or renal failure).	Insomnia, anxiety, autonomic hyperactivity, psychomotor agitation, anorexia, headache, dizziness, nausea and vomiting, malaise, tremor, transient hallucinations, seizures, death.
Hallucinogens	Depends on substance but, in general, hallucinations, anxiety and panic reactions, dilated pupils, blurred vision, perceptual changes, emotional intensity and lability, increased heart rate and blood pressure, paranoia, sweating, depersonalization, distortion of time sense, inappropriate affect; belief that perceptions, although disturbed, are real; depression. Laboratory evaluation rarely helpful.	Confused, psychotic individuals may be at increased risk for accidents that result in harm to self or others.	No specific withdrawal symptoms; may have flashbacks postcessation.
Phencyclidine	Euphoria, unpredictable violent behavior, paranoia, agitation, nystagmus, dysarthria, hypertension, tachycardia, analgesia, muscle rigidity, hyperreflexia, illogical thinking, ataxia, hyperacusis, hyperthermia, seizures; creatine phosphokinase and serum glutamic oxaloacetic transaminase may be elevated, urinalysis positive for up to several weeks.	Seizures, coma, death.	Agitation, seizures, muscle spasms, flashbacks.

(continued)

► table 13-1 (continued)

SUBSTANCE ABUSE: DIAGNOSTICS

	Mild–Moderate Intoxication	Severe Intoxication	Withdrawal
Inhalants	Euphoria, dizziness, impaired judgment, altered states of consciousness, lethargy, psychomotor retardation, tremor, muscular weakness, blurred vision, perceptual disturbances, delusions, ataxia, disorientation, slurred speech, hyporeflexia, nystagmus. Laboratory analyses for inhalants are not generally available.	Dysarthria, aggression, blurred vision, lethargy, weakness. Can progress to delirium, seizures, coma.	Some sleep disturbance, disorientation, irritability, muscle spasms may be noted.
Anabolic steroids	Enhanced sense of well-being, increased muscle mass, aggressiveness, impulsivity, irritability, mania, psychosis, depression, acne.	Chronic use may lead to hepatic damage, testicular atrophy, hirsutism in females.	Irritability, depression, anxiety.
Cannabis	Euphoria, impaired motor coordination, increased humorousness, distortion of time and space, dry mouth, impaired judgment, increased appetite, pupillary dilation, conjunctival erythema, suspiciousness, dysphoria, anxiety, depersonalization, social withdrawal, tachycardia, impaired memory, decreased libido. Urine positive up to 4 weeks.	*High doses:* psychosis (auditory and visual hallucinations), panic, delirium. *Chronic use:* possible amotivational syndrome.	Irritability and insomnia may be noted.

Phencyclidine: Benzodiazepines for agitation; haloperidol with caution for psychotic symptoms. Dantrolene for hyperthermia, and sodium nitroprusside for severe hypertension.

Cannabis: Oral diazepam sometimes helpful for anxiety.

Inhalants: Anxiolytics may be useful after detox. Propranolol for dysrhythmias. Oxygen by mask may be useful.

► Clinical Intervention

Amphetamines: Supportive therapy, drug-free environment. Treat depression if present following withdrawal; be alert for suicidal ideation. Refer if persistent psychosis.

Opioids: Intoxication: Support vital functions; provide supportive care. *Withdrawal:* Not medical emergency but very uncomfortable.

Sedatives, hypnotics, anxiolytics: Overdose: Emesis if gag reflex is intact and ingestion within 30 minutes; otherwise, gastric lavage. Decrease intestinal absorption with cathartic agent. Close monitoring, maintenance of airway and blood pressure.

Hallucinogens: Intoxication: Reassurance; ensure safe, quiet environment; supervision of behavior. *Flashbacks:* Reassurance if mild; referral if severe or persistent.

Phencyclidine: Ensure safe, quiet, nonstimulating environment. If violent behavior develops, may require physical restraints.

Cannabis: Treatment rarely needed; reassurance in quiet environment; evaluate for polydrug use.

Inhalants: Close supervision, possible restraints may be necessary for acute intoxication. Long-term monitoring to identify relapse and prevent further access to substance.

Anabolic steroids: Evaluate for depression.

▶ Health Maintenance Issues

Inhalants: Important to identify problem early and institute remedial therapy.

X. OTHER BEHAVIORAL/EMOTIONAL DISORDERS

A. Altered Mental Status/Confusional States

▶ Scientific Concepts

Confusion is a disturbance in clarity or coherence of thinking. Often considered a nonspecific sign of organic disorder; but can also occur in schizophrenia and psychotic mood disorders. Several causes of acute confusional state and/or delirium, including metabolic disorders (e.g., hypoglycemia, hyperglycemia, hyponatremia, hypoxia), systemic illness (e.g., anemia, febrile illness, hypertension), CNS disorders (e.g., subdural or epidural hematoma, seizure, stroke, infection, tumor), and drugs and medications (e.g., alcohol, barbiturates, antidepressants). May also indicate dementia; syndrome of the elderly most often caused by Alzheimer's disease.

▶ History & Physical

Cognitive impairment may include reduced attention, disorganized thought with rambling or incoherent speech, shifting levels of consciousness, sensory misinterpretations, illusions, hallucinations, disorientations, memory disturbances. History of delirium is acute with rapid onset of days or weeks in duration. Course and level of consciousness fluctuates, with orientation impaired periodically. Affect is typically anxious, irritable, with disordered thinking; recent memory is markedly impaired. Hallucinations are common; psychomotor skills often retarded, agitated, or mixed. Attention and awareness prominently impaired; symptoms are often reversible. History of dementia is chronic with insidious onset over months or years, progressive. Level of consciousness and psychomotor skills normal. Orientation is intact initially; affect labile but not anxious. Recent and remote memory impaired. Hallucinations less common; attention and awareness less impaired. Majority of symptoms not reversible.

▶ Diagnostic Studies

History, physical, lab studies to diagnose underlying problems. Mental Status Examination (MSE) to screen for wide range of cognitive functions. Workup to include neurological exam, CBC, chemistry profile, thyroid function tests, urinalysis, urine drug screen, blood concentrations of drugs being taken, venereal disease test, ECG, CT, MRI, and EEG as indicated.

► Diagnosis

Important to differentiate acute confusional state from dementia as identified by symptoms in history and physical. Acute loss of orientation to one or more of the parameters of person, place, and time may be related to acute cognitive impairment and/or decrease in level of consciousness. Delirium represents a medical emergency that mandates aggressive medical evaluation and treatment. Dementia is the progressive and chronic development of multiple cognitive deficits manifested in both memory impairment and one (or more) of the following: aphasia, apraxia, agnosia, executive functions. These deficits do not occur exclusively during the course of delirium.

► Clinical Therapeutics

Delirium: Goal is to treat underlying condition. High-potency antipsychotics for psychosis (haloperidol, 2 to 10 mg IM, may be repeated after 1 hour if first dose ineffective). Antipsychotics are less likely than benzodiazepines to worsen cognitive function; however, patients in alcohol or sedative–hypnotic withdrawal are best treated with benzodiazepine.

Dementia: Low dosages of all psychotropic medication in elderly. Antipsychotics such as haloperidol (0.5 to 5 mg/d) for behavior control, but elderly clear drugs more slowly than do young patients due to decreased hepatic and renal function. May have acute side effects including dystonia, parkinsonism, and hypotension. Tacrine (initially 40 mg/d up to a maximum of 160 mg/d in divided doses) for Alzheimer's disease; clinically significant improvement in 20 to 25% of patients who take it. Use with caution in patients with liver dysfunction.

► Clinical Intervention

Delirium: Immediately assess patient's condition; orient and reassure. All cases require hospitalization unless due to rapidly reversible process (e.g., insulin-induced hypoglycemia corrected with glucose infusion). Environmental control of impulsive or unpredictable patient to prevent violence. See Clinical Therapeutics above for acute state. Identify rate of onset of confusion and physical or psychological stressors. Conduct MSE, laboratory tests. Correct any metabolic, nutritional, electrolyte, or fluid abnormalities. Obtain neurological consult. Follow up with treatment when a definitive diagnosis has been made.

Dementia: Discontinue any medications that exacerbate dementia if possible (e.g., the H_2 antagonist cimetidine). Screen for depression and refer to mental health provider. Family support, including development of management plan for long-term care. Some evidence that cholinergic analogs (e.g., tacrine, 80 mg PO qd) may delay the manifestations of Alzheimer's disease.

► Health Maintenance Issues

Delirium: Monitor and follow up for underlying condition.
Dementia: Correct any nutritional and metabolic deficiencies. Preventive measures (changes in diet, exercise, and control of diabetes and hypertension) important in vascular dementia. Continued reassess-

ment of treatment and options for care. Counsel family regarding prognosis, possible need for placement, syndromes that develop in caretakers (burnout, depression, anxiety).

B. Elder/Child Abuse

▶ Scientific Concepts

Elder abuse: Each year, over 1 million cases of elder abuse occur, with as few as 1 in every 14 victimizations reported. Majority of victims are white, widowed women, usually older than 75, living dependently; cognitive impairment and incontinence, nocturnal shouting, wandering, or manifestations of paranoia. Abuser is often a relative in the same household.

Child abuse: There are 500,000 new cases of physical and sexual abuse reported each year, and 2,000 to 4,000 abused children die. An estimated 2 to 4 million children have been abused. Typical child abuser is single, unemployed mother under age 30, although may also be another caretaker such as father, babysitter, or friend. Many victims of physical abuse are also abused sexually. Physical abuse is also called *battered child syndrome.*

▶ History & Physical

Elder abuse: Caregiver often under stress, suffering from alcoholism, marital problems, unemployment, financial difficulties, social isolation, drug abuse. Family history of violence or presence of mental illness or retardation. Key findings:

- *Physical abuse:* Lesions, alopecia and hemorrhaging at nape of scalp, bruises, burns and human bite marks, sexual assault.
- *Neglect:* Pallor, wasting, dehydration, decubitus ulcers, untreated injuries, poor hygiene.
- *Psychological abuse:* Depression, withdrawal, anger, agitation or expression of ambivalent feelings.

Child abuse: Obvious cases present with bruises, fractures, dislocations, burns, lacerations, focal neurological deficits, signs of intracranial bleeding, abdominal injury, malnutrition, or dehydration. Munchausen syndrome by proxy occurs when caretaker brings child with fabricated illness, reporting nonexistent symptoms, altered lab tests, or induced illness. Sexual abuse presents with genital injury or irritation, foreign bodies in the vagina or rectum, excessive masturbation, venereal disease, or pregnancy. May also see PTSD as evidenced by sleep disorder or somatic complaints, regressive behaviors, hypersexuality, generalized low self-esteem, and sense of isolation. Emotional abuse presents as failure to thrive with hypokinesis, apathy, delayed responsiveness, malnutrition, and fearfulness. History of injury may be inconsistent with clinical findings or developmental level; delay in seeking care.

▶ Diagnostic Studies

Elder abuse: Key findings as above. In addition to physical examination and in-depth interview, radiological and metabolic screening, toxicological and drug-level screen, hematological screening, CT.

Child abuse: Key findings as above; in addition to physical examination and in-depth interview, skeletal series, serologies, bleeding screening battery, CBC, creatine kinase as indicated.

▶ Diagnosis

Elder abuse: Seldom reported by its victims. Occurs in three basic categories: domestic, institutional, and self-neglect. Important to rule out normal changes in physical, emotional, and cognitive behaviors due to aging and medical conditions.

Child abuse: Rule out unintentional trauma, bleeding diathesis, dermatologic conditions, vitamin deficiencies, osteogenesis imperfecta, self-inflicted injuries, other medical or metabolic causes for failure to thrive.

▶ Clinical Therapeutics

N/A.

▶ Clinical Intervention

Elder abuse: First priority is to ensure safety while respecting autonomy. Hospitalization; competent patient must first provide consent. Mandatory reporting in most states to Adult Protective Services. Home visit upon discharge by visiting nurse or social worker. Continued mobilization of community, social, and health services.

Child abuse: Interview child alone, expert may be needed to elicit history, separate interview of parents. Treatment of injury or neglect. Hospitalization as needed. Ensure safety of child. Mandatory reporting of suspected abuse; documentation of findings, including pictures. Follow-up. Treatment of child for physical, emotional sequelae. Individual or group psychotherapy indicated. Treatment for abuser ranges from support to mandated therapy, removal of parent abuser or child, legal prosecution.

▶ Health Maintenance Issues

Elder abuse: Education, early intervention with supportive services in high-risk situations. Clear documentation of abuse. Referral and follow-up legal, social, psychiatric, community service including support groups for caregivers.

Child abuse: Follow-up legal, social, psychiatric, and community services. Support group for child and/or parents.

C. Adult Domestic Violence

▶ Scientific Concepts

Battering in 20% of women seeking medical care; 22 to 35% of women presenting to emergency departments; 23% of prenatal patients; 25% of women who attempt suicide; 45 to 58% of mothers of abused children. Risk factors include pregnancy, social isolation, history of child abuse, substance abuse, criminal record.

▶ History & Physical

History may be incompatible with injury. Repeated trauma common. No diagnostic injury pattern, but injuries common in face, head, neck, breast, abdomen.

► **Diagnostic Studies**

Key findings as above. Physical examination and in-depth interview.

► **Diagnosis**

Positive findings on the physical examination and history. Sequelae include PTSD symptoms, low self-esteem, somatic complaints, depression, anxiety, substance abuse, suicide attempts.

► **Clinical Therapeutics**

N/A.

► **Clinical Intervention**

Treatment of injuries; evaluation for suicide risk. Ensure safety of victim and children. Respect victim's judgment regarding safety; increased risk of abuse when abused partner leaves. Assessment of continued risk and resources. Refer for medical, legal, psychiatric, and community services (battered women's shelter). Documentation including photos of injury. Follow-up plan in place.

► **Health Maintenance Issues**

Barriers to leaving abusive relationship should be addressed, including self-blame, feelings of helplessness, financial dependency, fear of retaliation. Continued sensitive questioning on the part of provider to reveal ongoing abuse.

D. Rape/Crisis Adjustment

► **Scientific Concepts**

Rape is the forceful coercion of an unwilling victim to engage in a sexual act. Usually, this act is sexual intercourse; anal intercourse and fellatio also constitute rape. Male rape legally defined in most states as sodomy. Homosexual rape more frequent among men and occurs frequently in closed institutions. Rapist discharges aggression and aggrandizes self. PTSD resulting from aggravated assault, rape, or noncrime trauma affects over 4 million women in the United States. Female victims of aggravated assault are five times more likely to develop PTSD than female victims of noncrime trauma.

► **History & Physical**

Clinicians need high degree of suspicion for unreported rape; 50% are not reported. History and physical should take place in private with patient consent. Rape and sexual abuse victims are often confused after assault. History and physical reveals patient victim of act of violent humiliation, physical trauma. Often occurs in accompaniment to another crime.

► **Diagnostic Studies**

Prior to physical examination and data collection, obtain patient's permission due to possibility of repeated trauma through "medical rape." Physical examination, photographs, specimen collection from vaginal pool for police laboratory. Cervical and rectal cultures for gonorrhea and serology for syphilis, human immunodeficiency virus (HIV) testing.

► Diagnosis

Establishing that a rape has occurred is a legal decision, not a medical diagnosis.

► Clinical Therapeutics

Usually no drug treatment after trauma is indicated. Some patients may experience overwhelming anxiety; short-term treatment with benzodiazepine such as alprazolam (0.5 to 1 mg PO tid), lorazepam (1 to 2 mg PO tid), or oxazepam (10 to 30 mg PO tid) may be needed. Insomnia may also respond to treatment above or with temazepam (15 to 30 mg PO hs) or flurazepam (15 to 30 mg PO hs). To prevent pregnancy, a 5-day course of medroxyprogesterone or diethylstilbestrol may be offered. To protect patient against venereal disease, penicillin should be given.

► Clinical Intervention

Rape: Offer appropriate medical, gynecological, and police services. Immediately treat patient for injuries sustained in the assault. Treat with clinical therapeutics as above.

Crisis adjustment, general: Evaluate victim for possible PTSD, which may not develop immediately; inform patient about possible sequelae. Offer crisis intervention–oriented therapy. Objective is to minimize psychological sequelae of trauma. Refer for ongoing psychotherapy, which should focus on reestablishing sense of control over environment, reducing feelings of helplessness and dependence, and addressing obsessional thoughts and other symptoms of PTSD. Refer to group therapy for trauma victims. Evaluate patient for underlying psychiatric conditions (e.g., substance dependence, schizophrenia) that may cause impaired judgment and place patient in danger of rape or trauma; if present, refer for treatment of underlying psychiatric disorder.

► Health Maintenance Issues

Many trauma victims have symptoms that continue for years, including reliving experience (flashbacks), preoccupation with experience, fear of being alone, nightmares, insomnia, and altered eating patterns. Somatic symptoms include headaches, nausea and vomiting, and malaise. Patient may avoid future sexual relationships or experience sexual symptoms such as vaginismus. Follow-up should include evaluation for PTSD and referral to support groups or mental health provider for symptom resolution.

E. Sudden Infant Death Syndrome (Family)

► Scientific Concepts

Most common cause of death between 7 days and 365 days of age; 5,200 to 5,500 infant deaths per year in the United States; 1.4 sudden infant death syndrome (SIDS) deaths/1,000 live births.

▶ History & Physical

Most deaths between 1 and 3 months of age, peaking at 3 months. Males have higher incidence.

▶ Diagnosis

Diagnosis of exclusion after postmortem examination fails to reveal a cause of death.

▶ Clinical Therapeutics

N/A.

▶ Clinical Intervention

Intense, severe grief reactions common in parents; guilt, anger, somatic symptoms; overactivity, social isolation, psychosis, agitated depression. May lead to health problems, marital difficulties, behavior problems, and fears in siblings. Contact with dead baby, pictures, quick autopsy results; education regarding guilt and blame. Parent support groups; sibling and extended family support; social support; counseling. Look for delayed grief reaction.

▶ Health Maintenance Issues

Association of SIDS with prone sleeping has led to recommendation that all infants be placed in supine position or positioning baby alternating sides and back to help prevent molding.

F. Uncomplicated Bereavement

▶ Scientific Concepts

Not considered a mental disorder; self-limited psychological process; about one-third of bereaved spouses do meet criteria for major depressive disorder.

▶ History & Physical

Intense emotional distress, somatic symptoms, dissociation, preoccupation with deceased, anger, loss of habitual patterns of conduct, mourning; major depressive syndrome with anorexia, crying, loss of concentration, fatigue, anxiety, sleep disturbance; duration up to 1 to 2 years; anniversary reactions common.

▶ Diagnostic Studies

As above.

▶ Diagnosis

As above; rule out major depressive disorder based on symptoms' severity and length, lack of resolution; include preoccupation with worthlessness, hopelessness, suicidal ideation, blame for the death, psychomotor retardation.

▶ Clinical Therapeutics

Medication generally contraindicated unless used to treat an underlying depressive disorder.

► Clinical Intervention

Encourage open grieving, expression of feelings; recognition of variability among family members; anticipatory guidance around anniversary events; referral to support groups, psychotherapy as needed.

► Health Maintenance Issues

Follow-up essential to monitor resolution of grieving process, uncover suicidal ideation, marital and family difficulties; support and reassure around normalcy of uncomplicated grief symptoms and reactions; refer if condition evolves into pathological grieving process or major depressive disorder.

BIBLIOGRAPHY

American Psychiatric Association. *Diagnostic and Statistical Manual of Mental Disorders,* 4th ed. Washington, DC: American Psychiatric Association; 1994.

Berg DD. *Handbook of Primary Care Medicine,* 2nd ed. Philadelphia: Lippincott-Raven; 1998.

Feldman MD, Christensen JF. *Behavioral Medicine in Primary Care: A Practical Guide.* Stamford, CT: Appleton & Lange; 1997.

Goldberg JS. *The Instant Exam Review for the USMLE STEP 3,* 2nd ed. Stamford, CT: Appleton & Lange; 1997.

Kaplan HI, Sadock BJ. *Synopsis of Psychiatry,* 8th ed. Baltimore, MD: Williams & Wilkins; 1997.

Knesper DJ, Riba MB, Schwenk TL. *Primary Care Psychiatry.* Philadelphia: WB Saunders; 1997.

Stoudemire A. *Clinical Psychiatry for Medical Students,* 3rd ed. Philadelphia: Lippincott-Raven; 1998.

Hematology and Oncology | 14

Maura Polansky, MS, PA-C, Kathryn Boyer, MS, PA-C

I. ANEMIAS

► **Scientific Concepts**

Defined by the concentration of plasma to red blood cells; results from decreased production, increased destruction, or both.

► **History & Physical**

Fatigue, weakness, dizziness, shortness of breath, chest pain, pallor; koilonychia (flattened, spooned nail) in chronic states.

► **Diagnostic Studies**

Complete blood count (CBC), mean corpuscular volume (MCV), peripheral smear will determine the presence and severity of anemia and help in distinguishing the type of anemia.

► **Diagnosis**

Normal laboratory values of hemoglobin and hematocrit depend on age and gender. Differential diagnosis of anemia includes pseudo-anemia secondary to increased blood volume (e.g., pregnancy, excess intravascular fluid, hyperproteinemia).

► **Clinical Therapeutics**

Directed at underlying etiology. Except for transfusion when necessary, no therapy should be initiated until the etiology is identified.

► **Clinical Intervention**

No absolute laboratory threshold for transfusion. The decision to transfuse depends on the degree of anemia, rapidity of condition, co-morbidity, and symptomatology.

► **Health Maintenance Issues**

Adequate dietary intake of iron, B_{12}, folate essential. Screening for those at increased risk.

A. Iron Deficiency Anemia

► **Scientific Concepts**

Iron deficiency anemia may be an acute or chronic condition. Causes include frank or occult bleeding; including gastrointestinal (GI) bleeding, trauma, excessive menstrual bleeding. Inadequate dietary intake can occur, but less commonly (e.g., pregnancy).

► **History & Physical**

General symptoms and signs of anemia. With acute blood loss, symptoms and signs of intravascular hypovolemia including orthostatic dizziness and orthostatic hypotension. Since anemia depends on concentration, time after acute blood loss is necessary for fluid shifts to occur and anemia to be present.

► **Diagnostic Studies**

Serum iron, ferritin, total iron-binding capacity (TIBC), transferrin.

▶ Diagnosis

Microcytic, hypochromic anemias; low serum iron, ferritin, and transferrin with high TIBC. Once diagnosed, the etiology must be established.

▶ Clinical Therapeutics

Iron replacement will usually take 2 to 3 months for results. Follow-up is necessary to determine the adequacy of replacement and to ensure no continued blood loss. Discontinue iron once hemoglobin normalizes, as excessive iron use will mask continued or new blood loss.

▶ Clinical Intervention

Treatment of underlying disorder is the most important intervention.

▶ Health Maintenance Issues

Identifying iron deficiency anemia is an important factor in diagnosing serious medical problems such as GI malignancies.

B. Thalassemia

▶ Scientific Concepts

Thalassemia is a diverse group of genetic disorders leading to reduced globin chain production (quantitative abnormality with normal structure) of one or more subunits of hemoglobin, which may include alpha, beta, gamma, or delta. Those at highest risk of inheritance are ethnic groups from malaria-affected regions. However, the disorder can occur sporadically. Alpha- and beta-globin deficiencies are the most common; these are the primary globins present after the first year of life. Manifestation of the disorder ranges from subtle abnormalities to severe disease. Alpha-globin is determined by four genes. Therefore, alpha-thalassemia manifests as a spectrum depending on the number of genes involved from silent carriers with no hematologic abnormalities to Hb Barts with all four genes involved, which is incompatible with life. Beta-globin is determined by only two genes; therefore, beta-thalassemia is divided into thalassemia minor (one gene) and thalassemia major (two genes). Thalassemia minor (thalassemia trait) is usually asymptomatic and often undiagnosed. It may manifest with mild anemia and requires no treatment. Thalassemia major results in severe anemia and usually manifests by 6 months of life.

▶ History & Physical

Symptoms and signs of anemia; splenomegaly may be present.

▶ Diagnostic Studies

CBC, peripheral smear, reticulocyte count, iron studies, hemoglobin (Hb) electrophoresis, alpha/beta-globin chain ratios.

▶ Diagnosis

Microcytic, hypochromic anemia; characteristic target cells, poikilocytosis, elliptocytes, basophilic stippling on Wright stain may be present; elevated reticulocyte count; normal iron studies to differentiate from iron deficiency anemia; Hb electrophoresis is necessary to confirm the diagnosis.

► Clinical Therapeutics

Most require no treatment. Those with severe disease usually present early in life and may become transfusion dependent.

► Clinical Intervention

Bone marrow transplant is the definitive therapy for thalassemia major. Some may benefit from splenectomy.

► Health Maintenance Issues

Genetic counseling is necessary for those at high risk. For those with the disease, folic acid supplementation may be needed due to high bone marrow demand. Iron overload can occur in transfusion-dependent patients and should be tested for and treated. Iron overload may result in organ dysfunction.

C. Lead Poisoning

► Scientific Concepts

Lead acts in two ways: by inhibiting the activity of enzymes in heme synthesis and by injuring red cell membranes. Exposures are common through ingested lead-containing paint and improperly glazed pottery for cooking or eating. Both children and adults are affected.

► History & Physical

Abdominal pain, constipation, vomiting, and muscle weakness are common; neurological and psychological symptoms occur less commonly; lead line (linear blue-black deposit of lead sulfide in gums near teeth), dental caries, motor disturbances.

► Diagnostic Studies

CBC, peripheral smear, reticulocyte count, and lead level.

► Diagnosis

Mild to moderate anemia with mild to moderate hypochromia and microcytosis; basophilic stippling on Wright stain may or may not be present; reticulocyte count elevated, leukocyte count normal or slightly increased. Normal ferritin, marrow iron, and TIBC distinguishes from iron deficiency anemia. Increased transferrin saturation and urinary aminolevulinic acid (ALA) with normal porphobilinogen. Differential diagnosis includes acute intermittent porphyria.

► Clinical Therapeutics

Lead levels guide therapy: Acceptable levels are 15 to 40 µg/dL, treatment needed for > 80 µg/dL. Lead poisoning is treated with ethylenediaminetetraacetic acid (EDTA) to chelate lead. Small amounts should be given as encephalopathy can occur secondary to lead chelate. Lead levels return to normal in a few weeks.

▶ Clinical Intervention
Identify and remove the source of lead.

▶ Health Maintenance Issues
Screening needed for those at high risk (e.g., children).

D. Anemia of Chronic Illness

▶ Scientific Concepts
Secondary to infectious (tuberculosis, pneumonia, chronic fungal disease, osteomyelitis, meningitis), inflammatory (rheumatoid arthritis, systemic lupus erythematosus, myocardial infarction), or malignant disease of more than 1 to 2 months' duration. Mechanisms include:
1. Decreased iron release from storage in macrophages.
2. Shortened erythrocyte survival.
3. Impaired marrow response to shortened red cell life span resulting in no elevation of the erythropoietin level.

▶ History & Physical
Often asymptomatic except for symptoms and signs of underlying disease. It may be symptomatic when associated with certain underlying diseases such as cardiac or pulmonary disease.

▶ Diagnostic Studies
CBC, peripheral smear, reticulocyte count. Iron studies are needed if hypochromic erythrocytes are present.

▶ Diagnosis
Mild to moderate anemia, may be within normal range, but decreased for the individual. Usually normochromic, normocytic, but may be hypochromic; moderate anisocytosis, minimal poikilocytosis; corrected reticulocyte count normal to slightly increased. Serum iron low, with low TIBC (in contrast with iron deficiency with increased TIBC).

▶ Clinical Therapeutics
Erythropoietin may be used.

▶ Clinical Intervention
Directed at underlying illness; transfusion rarely needed.

E. Sickle Cell Anemia

▶ Scientific Concepts
Autosomal dominant disorder resulting in sickling of erythrocytes. Heterozygous (AS) = sickle cell trait; homozygous (SS) = sickle cell anemia. Among those of African-American decent, 8% are AS, 0.1 to 0.2% are SS. Sickling occurs when oxygen decreases at the tissue level. Sickled cells impede blood flow to tissue and organs. Hemolysis is common.

► History & Physical

Pain, fatigue, weakness, pallor; growth and sexual maturation are delayed; cardiomegaly, hepatomegaly with jaundice, splenomegaly. Sickle cell crisis occurs with excessive deoxygenation of red cells often precipitated by infection, dehydration, high altitude. Complications include splenic infarction, renal papillary necrosis, aseptic necrosis, cerebrovascular accident (CVA).

► Diagnostic Studies

CBC, peripheral smear, Hb electrophoresis and sickle cell prep. Prenatal diagnosis by amniotic analysis.

► Diagnosis

Normocytic, normochromic anemia occurring after 6 months of life; sickled cells seen with SS, not AS (trait); anisocytosis, elliptocytes, target cells, ovalocytes, schistocytes; reticulocytosis, leukocytosis, thrombocytosis may all be present; Hb electrophoresis necessary to confirm.

► Clinical Therapeutics

SS crisis—hydration, analgesics, antibiotics for infection. Transfusion may be necessary.

► Clinical Intervention

Bone marrow transplant.

► Health Maintenance Issues

The prevention of crises is important, including the use of vaccines, especially Pneumovax. Crisis precipitated by infection is the primary cause of death. Folate supplementation is usually necessary to maintain adequate erythrocyte production. After CVA, transfusions should continue for years to prevent another stroke.

F. Aplastic Anemia

► Scientific Concepts

Pancytopenia due to severely hypoplastic or aplastic bone marrow. Most serious complications often due to neutropenia and thrombocytopenia. Etiology: congenital, acquired idiopathic, drugs, radiation, infections including hepatitis, miliary tuberculosis, parasites, immune mechanisms.

► History & Physical

Symptoms and signs suggestive of anemia, thrombocytopenia, and neutropenia, such as bacterial infection (not viral) and hemorrhage. Usually normal spleen and no lymphadenopathy.

► Diagnostic Studies

CBC, peripheral blood smear, reticulocyte count, bone marrow aspirate and biopsy.

► Diagnosis

Peripheral blood reveals total white blood cells (WBCs) decreased, normal or mildly decreased lymphocytes; normocytic, normochromic anemia, may be slight macrocytosis of red cells. Red blood cell (RBC) morphology is normal. No immature cells in peripheral blood. Corrected reticulocyte count decreased. Bone marrow aspirate and biopsy reveals hypoplastic or aplastic marrow with increased fat and decreased hematopoietic cells; primarily lymphocytes and plasma cells, megakaryocytes generally absent, patchy areas of cellularity. Differential diagnosis include multiple myeloma, acute leukemia, lymphoma, myelofibrosis, myelodysplastic syndrome.

► Clinical Therapeutics

Blood products, immunosuppressive therapy, and androgens, which stimulate erythropoiesis, granulopoiesis, and thrombopoiesis, may benefit some patients. For patients > 40 years of age, immunosuppressive therapy is recommended over bone marrow transplantation (BMT).

► Clinical Intervention

For patients < 40 years of age, BMT results in higher survival when performed early in the disease, before any blood product transfusions. Occasionally spontaneous remission occurs, especially if cause is a drug that is discontinued.

► Health Maintenance Issues

Can progress to acute leukemia. For BMT recipients, graft-versus-host disease may occur (immune reaction, donor lymphocytes acting against host tissues). BMT requires cyclophosphamide or other intensive chemotherapeutic agent with or without irradiation. Irradiation increases risk of developing a secondary malignancy.

G. Megaloblastic Anemia

► Scientific Concepts

Caused by impaired deoxyribonucleic acid (DNA) synthesis; cell division is slow so cells become large. Causes include cobalamin (B_{12}) deficiency, folic acid (folate) deficiency, drugs, and idiopathic. B_{12} derived from consumption of meat and dairy products; intrinsic factor (IF), produced in stomach, required for intestinal absorption. Dietary deficiency occurs, but is uncommon. Pernicious anemia (i.e., lack of IF) is the most common cause and is a result of atrophy of gastric mucosa. Folate is derived from fruits and vegetables. Folate deficiency can result from dietary deficiency, poor intestinal absorption, or increased demand (e.g., pregnancy). Dietary deficiency is more common, particularly in alcoholics.

► History & Physical

B_{12} deficiency: Pale; mildly icteric; beefy, red, sore tongue; anorexia, weight loss, and diarrhea occur late due to malabsorption; neurologic manifestations (including numbness, paresthesia, weakness, ataxia,

and disturbances in mentation) occur secondary to demyelination ("megaloblastic madness").
Folate deficiency: May appear malnourished, diarrhea, cheilosis, glossitis, no neurologic manifestations.

▶ Diagnostic Studies

CBC, peripheral smear, folate and B_{12} levels. In B_{12} deficiency, Schilling test determines whether pernicious anemia is present.

▶ Diagnosis

Macrocytic anemia (MCV > 100 fL); anisocytosis; decreased levels of B_{12} or folate diagnostic for etiology. Schilling test given when B_{12} deficiency identified to diagnose IF deficiency. Labeled B_{12} is given orally; unlabeled B_{12} is given intramuscularly. B_{12} levels in the urine are then measured. Then test repeated, this time IF also given orally and levels measured in the urine. Differential diagnosis includes liver disease, alcoholism, hypothyroidism.

▶ Clinical Therapeutics

Intramuscular B_{12} replacement given weekly until replaced, then lifelong replacement given monthly is usually required. Folate, given 1 mg PO every day (parenteral rarely needed). *Caution:* Folate can correct megaloblastic anemia even if caused by B_{12} deficiency without correcting or even aggravating neurologic manifestations (which can be permanent). Therefore, the B_{12} level must be checked to rule out B_{12} deficiency before folate is administered.

H. Hemolytic Anemia

▶ Scientific Concepts

Hereditary or acquired disorders with an accelerated rate of erythrocyte destruction. Bone marrow is normal but not capable of keeping up with destruction. Hereditary conditions include glucose-6-phosphate dehydrogenase (G6PD) deficiency, pyruvate kinase deficiency, and hemoglobinopathies. Acquired disorders include infections, hypersplenism, liver and renal disease, and microangiopathic disorders (e.g., disseminated intravascular coagulation). Hemolysis occurs either intravascularly or extravascularly.

▶ History & Physical

Splenomegaly will be present if chronic.

▶ Diagnostic Studies

CBC, peripheral smear, reticulocyte count, Coombs' test, serum chemistries, haptoglobin, urinalysis.

▶ Diagnosis

Normocytic, normochromic, or mildly increased MCV. Elevated reticulocyte count. Microspherocytes and schistocytes on peripheral smear. Elevated lactic dehydrogenase (LDH) and indirect bilirubin.

▶ Clinical Therapeutics

Corticosteroids are often useful.

▶ Clinical Intervention

Treatment of underlying disorder when possible. Splenectomy may be necessary.

▶ Health Maintenance Issues

Avoidance of oxidative states in patients with G6PD deficiency.

II. MALIGNANT NEOPLASMS

A. Leukemias

▶ Scientific Concepts

The leukemias are a group of disorders characterized by the accumulation of abnormal white cells in the bone marrow. These defective cells may cause bone marrow failure, increased WBC, and organ infiltration. Leukemias together comprise 2% of all adult cancers. Leukemias are divided into acute and chronic types, and even further subclassified within these groups. It is essential to accurately diagnose the leukemia because treatment regimens are different and in some types are highly successful. In acute leukemias, the defective cells are unable to differentiate due to a maturation arrest. Rapid proliferation results in over 30% replacement of the normal hematopoietic precursors by the leukemic cells, which are also frequently found in the circulating blood. By definition, acute leukemia is diagnosed when the bone marrow has more than 30% blasts (< 5% is normal); further classification to acute myelocytic leukemia (AML) or acute lymphocytic leukemia (ALL) depends on morphology and which white cell line is most affected. AML is classified further into several subgroups depending on morphology, cytochemistry, immunophenotyping, and cytogenetics. The etiology of this malignant transformation is not known, but viral causes have been postulated. Also, alkylating agents, ionizing radiation, and benzene exposure have all been implicated as causative factors of leukemia, especially of AML and chronic myelocytic leukemia (CML).

1. Acute Myelocytic Leukemia

▶ Scientific Concepts

Acute myelogenous leukemia is a rare malignancy resulting from undifferentiated proliferation of granulocyte precursors, usually the myeloblast, in the bone marrow. This abnormality may disrupt normal production of other cell lines, such as platelets and erythrocytes. AML may be a primary malignancy, or may result as a consequence of prior chemotherapy or radiation exposure. Myelodysplastic syndromes often evolve to AML when the bone marrow blasts reach 30% of the bone marrow. In fact, 25% of adults diagnosed with AML have a history of myelodysplastic syndrome.

▶ History & Physical

Presenting complaints arise from failure of bone marrow to produce red cells, white cells, and platelets. Some patients may actually be asymptomatic, but most have complaints of fatigue, bleeding, persistent infections (including fungal and opportunistic infections), or fevers. Bleeding can be overt hemorrhage or minimal (bruising, petechiae, gingival, epistaxis). On exam, the patient may have pallor, fever, tachycardia, ecchymosis, petechiae, skin lesions (leukemia cutis), lymphadenopathy. Occasionally, splenomegaly is present; rarely one may have hepatomegaly.

▶ Diagnostic Studies

Anemia and thrombocytopenia may be profound; WBC may be elevated (> 100,000) or low, often extremely low. Usually, blasts are present in the periphery, with other immature forms sometimes present. Often, Auer rods (cytoplasmic inclusion bodies) are found in the blasts. The diagnosis is made by a bone marrow aspirate and biopsy; AML has > 30% blasts that are myeloperoxidase positive or esterase positive, terminal deoxynucleotidyl transferase (TdT) negative. Myeloid markers are positive on flow cytometry, and chromosomal abnormalities are often present on cytogenetic analysis.

▶ Clinical Therapeutics

The only treatment for AML is intensive induction combination chemotherapy, regardless of age or initial performance status. The other manifestations of bone marrow infiltration by leukemia (neutropenia, anemia, thrombocytopenia) will not improve unless the disease is treated. Success rates have improved due to a significant improvement in supportive care during chemotherapy. Patients are at risk of dying from complications of anemia, neutropenia, thrombocytopenia (heart failure, infections, bleeding), and occasionally organ infiltration. It is most important to diagnose acute promyelocytic leukemia (APL) because great success can be achieved by early and proper treatment with Idarubicin and a retinoid, all-trans-retinoic acid (ATRA). BMTs should be considered in refractory, resistant, or relapsed cases.

▶ Clinical Intervention

A newly diagnosed AML patient with a WBC > 75,000 is at significant risk of leukostasis with pulmonary infiltration of the blasts, causing respiratory distress and possibly death. This is considered a medical emergency and leukapheresis should immediately be instituted prior to induction chemotherapy, which should be commenced as soon as possible. Other emergencies include tumor lysis syndrome, which can occur when the WBC is high and during induction chemotherapy when the cells are killed. Hyperuricemia, renal failure, hyperkalemia, hypocalcemia, hyperphosphatemia, acidosis, and other metabolic disturbances may occur, leading to multiorgan failure. This syndrome can be prevented with aggressive hydration, alkalinization, and close observation. Disseminated intravascular coagulation (DIC) is another emergency that can be caused by chemotherapy or the disease itself, especially in APL patients. Close observation and supportive care can prevent further complications, and ATRA has prevented this situation by pushing the progranulocytes into maturation prior to chemotherapy. Neutropenic fever in leukemia patients can be fatal, and close surveillance during and after chemotherapy administration is imperative to prevent adverse events. Broad-spectrum intravenous (IV) antibiotics should be started in any leukemia patient who is neutropenic and febrile, whether a source of infection is evident or not. Long-term follow-up is necessary, as late relapses have occurred; however, relapse is less likely after 2 years of remission.

2. Acute Lymphocytic Leukemia

▶ Scientific Concepts

Eighty percent of all childhood leukemias are acute lymphocytic, and 25% of all adult acute leukemias are ALL. The physiology is similar to AML, but the defective cell is the lymphoblast rather than the myeloblast.

▶ History & Physical

Common complaints at presentation include fatigue, bleeding, fevers, lymphadenopathy, bruising, cough and shortness of breath if a mediastinal mass (lymphoblastic T cell) is present. Findings may include pallor, bruising, petechiae, tachycardia, fever, lymphadenopathy, splenomegaly, hepatomegaly. Patients may present with central nervous system (CNS) disease with headaches, neck pain/stiffness, and other signs of increased intracranial pressure. Rarely a testicular mass is present.

▶ Diagnostic Studies

Usually, the WBC is significantly elevated, often > 200,000, with a large percentage of blasts that stain TdT positive. Anemia and thrombocytopenia may be minor or profound; LDH is often elevated. Bone marrow aspiration shows > 30% blasts that are TdT positive, myeloperoxidase negative, lymphoid markers are positive (CALLA, or CD10, and CD19) and may be T cell or B cell. The bone marrow biopsy is hypercellular, and cytogenetic abnormalities may be present. A chest radiograph may show a mediastinal mass (if T cell). A lumbar puncture should be done initially to rule out CNS disease. There are three subclassifications of ALL (L1, L2, L3); however, they are all treated the same.

▶ Clinical Therapeutics

Induction chemotherapy should be started as soon as possible with combination chemotherapy, and supportive care should be similar to that of AML patients, avoiding complications of the anemia, thrombocytopenia, and neutropenia that occurs with treatment. Intrathecal chemotherapy has reduced the CNS relapse rate from > 90% down to < 5%.

▶ Clinical Intervention

Follow-up is important as late relapses have been seen. Bone marrow transplant (BMTs) should be considered in patients with Philadelphia chromosome–positive disease, as this is a very poor prognostic indicator.

3. Chronic Myelocytic Leukemia

▶ Scientific Concepts

Abnormal clonal proliferation of early progenitor stem cells resulting in an excess of cells of myeloid, erythroid, and megakaryocytic lineage. There are three phases (chronic, accelerated, blastic) and, in later phases, maturation arrest is a prominent feature. Associated with the tumor marker Philadelphia chromosome in 85 to 90% of cases, thus can be followed to monitor treatment success. The Philadelphia chromosome is a reciprocal translocation of genetic material between chromosomes 9 and 22 (t(9;22)). Etiology is unknown, but increased incidence in atomic bomb survivors and those who received radiation as treatment for ankylosing spondylitis. CML is usually diagnosed in chronic phase, which is characterized by a high WBC and splenomegaly; usually well controlled with oral chemotherapy or alpha-interferon. Median survival, untreated, is 3.5 years. Accelerated-phase disease is less well defined and more difficult to control; median untreated survival is 6 to 12 months. Blast crisis is similar to an acute leukemia and is treated similarly; median untreated survival averages 3 to 6 months.

▶ History & Physical

Often, CML is diagnosed on a routine CBC. Some patients have complaints of fatigue, early satiety or left-sided abdominal pain (from splenomegaly), shortness of breath, or B symptoms (fever, drenching night sweats, fatigue, weight loss). Usually, the physical exam is normal other than splenomegaly and maybe some minor lymphadenopathy. Hepatomegaly may be present in some cases. In accelerated or blast phase, fever, weight loss, early satiety, and symptoms of worsening anemia and thrombocytopenia, or more commonly thrombocytosis, may be present.

▶ Diagnostic Studies

WBC is elevated, platelets are often elevated, anemia may be mild or absent. LDH is often elevated, and leukocyte alkaline phosphatase is low. Hyperuricemia may be present due to the increased white cell mass. Bone marrow is hypercellular and, in chronic phase, has < 5% blasts; > 30% blasts identifies blast phase. Accelerated phase may contain blasts anywhere from 5 to 29% and may have increased numbers of basophils and megakaryocytes. The Philadelphia chromosome is present on cytogenetic analysis in ~ 90% of patients at diagnosis.

▶ Clinical Therapeutics

Control of WBC and decrease in splenomegaly can be obtained by using hydroxyurea, an oral chemotherapy; however, this treatment does not suppress the Philadelphia chromosome or prevent progression of the disease. Alpha-interferon has been used with success, often eliminates the disease and the Philadelphia chromosome, and prevents progression to more aggressive phases. To date, less success has been found in treating accelerated or blastic disease; however, some chemotherapeutic regimens are promising. A lymphoid blastic transformation can be treated as ALL, with the disease often returning to a second chronic phase.

► Clinical Intervention

Tumor lysis syndrome can occur on rare occasions but is easily prevented with the use of allopurinol and aggressive hydration. Interferon is poorly tolerated in some patients, especially those > age 60, so doses must be adjusted accordingly or other therapeutic regimens must be implemented. Some side effects of interferon are flulike symptoms which rarely last more than the initial 3 weeks of therapy, depression, disturbance in sleep cycle, fatigue, and, after longer periods of use, autoimmune complications. Follow-up is important; cytogenetics should be repeated during treatment and followed for the Philadelphia chromosome.

4. Chronic Lymphocytic Leukemia

► Scientific Concepts

Most common leukemia, usually in older age groups. Characterized by clonal proliferation and accumulation of mature-appearing lymphocytes of B lineage in blood and lymphoid tissues. Etiology is unknown, with no evidence of radiation or chemicals as causative agents.

► History & Physical

Twenty-five percent are asymptomatic at diagnosis; other complaints include B symptoms (fatigue, drenching night sweats, weight loss), frequent and/or persistent infections, lymphadenopathy. Less commonly, skin infections are present at diagnosis, including shingles.

► Diagnostic Studies

Clinical characteristics should be combined with lab results to determine Rai stage at diagnosis Table 14-1. Minimal criteria for diagnosis of chronic lymphocytic leukemia (CLL) are blood lymphocytes $> 10 \times 10^9/L$ and bone marrow lymphocytes $> 30\%$. If anemia and/or thrombocytopenia are present, the Rai stage is higher and more aggressive disease is present. Beta-2-microglobulin should be measured, and prognosis is better if it is < 2.5. Immunophenotyping should be done on both the blood and marrow to determine B- or T-cell lineage. Cytogenetics are often normal, but the most common abnormalities involve chromosome 12. The pattern of infiltration on bone marrow biopsy is yet another prognostic indicator—nodular signifies a lower tumor burden and less aggressive disease than diffuse infiltration.

► Clinical Therapeutics

Usually, observation is recommended with early disease and/or favorable prognostic indicators. Rai stages 0, 1, and 2 are usually observed until signs of disease progression or bulky lymphadenopathy or symptoms of hepatosplenomegaly occur. Chemotherapy (Fludarabine with or without cyclophosphamide) is recommended for more aggressive disease, but not many regimens have shown a survival benefit. Other agents such as cyclosporine A and monoclonal antibodies are being investigated and have shown promising results.

► table 14-1

RAI STAGING SYSTEM

Stage	Clinical/Lab Features	Mean Survival (Months)
0	Lymphocytosis	> 120
1	Lymphadenopathy	95
2	Hepato/splenomegaly	72
3	Anemia (Hb < 11 g/dL)	30
4	Thrombocytopenia	30
Transformed	Richter's transformation (large cell lymphoma)	6

► Clinical Intervention

Herpes zoster infections are more frequent in patients with CLL, so prophylaxis should be considered. CLL patients, for unknown reasons, have a higher incidence than the general population of additional malignancies and therefore should be followed closely, regardless of their CLL status.

5. Hairy Cell Leukemia

► Scientific Concepts

Prior to 1980, this was a universally fatal disease; now curable in almost 100%. B-cell clonal malignancy; cells have characteristic cytoplasmic projections, thus looking "hairy." Patients present with anemia, neutropenia (rarely an elevated WBC), thrombocytopenia, and usually splenomegaly. They usually have an increased incidence of infections that persist longer than in their healthy cohorts.

► Diagnostic Studies

Neutropenia, anemia, thrombocytopenia. Bone marrow with hairy cells present, staining positive on tartrate-resistant acid phosphatase (TRAP) stain. Often a dry tap on bone marrow, thus making diagnosis more difficult.

► Clinical Therapeutics

Treatment formerly was interferon, now preferred treatment is one course of chemotherapy with a single agent, chlorodeoxyadenosine (2-CdA) with excellent results. Pancytopenia should be supported with prophylactic antibiotics/antivirals/antifungals. Transfusion support may be necessary on rare occasions.

B. Lymphomas

1. Hodgkin's Disease

► Scientific Concepts

Etiology of Hodgkin's disease (HD) is unknown, and the cell of origin is not yet completely defined. Current evidence shows that it is from the monocyte–macrophage cell line. Histologically, the cause of

Hodgkin's disease was thought to be infectious, but that remains unproven. EBV may be important in the disease. Hodgkin's comprises 14% of all malignant lymphomas and has a bimodal age distribution, with the first peak in the 20s and the second in the 60s. Histologically, HD is unique in that a small proportion of cells are malignant; most are reactive cells. Reed–Sternberg cells (large polylobulated cells with large nucleoli) are the diagnostic malignant cells found in the background of reactive cells. There are four histologic subtypes; nodular sclerosing and mixed cellularity types make up 90%.

▶ History & Physical

The most common complaint is that of painless lymphadenopathy in young adults, with or without B symptoms, malaise, or pruritus. Usually, the enlarged lymph node is supradiaphragmatic (90%) and is frequently (60 to 80%) in the cervical region. Mediastinal lymphadenopathy may manifest clinically with cough, wheezing, dyspnea, superior vena cava syndrome, and rarely pleural effusions. Affected lymph nodes are firm, mobile, rubbery. Tender nodes usually signify infectious or inflammatory processes. Splenomegaly may be present.

▶ Diagnostic Studies

No specific laboratory findings. On CBC, may find mild neutrophilic leukocytosis, maybe slightly increased platelets, and mild normochromic, normocytic anemia. Liver function tests may be slightly abnormal, and hyperuricemia may be present if there is bulky disease. Serum copper level is often elevated, and the patient is often anergic. Chest radiograph should be done, as well as computed tomographic (CT) scans of chest, abdomen, pelvis. The largest and most central node should be biopsied with the capsule intact and Reed–Sternberg cells must be present in the proper reactive background for the diagnosis to be made.

▶ Clinical Therapeutics

As Table 14-2 illustrates, staging is important for treatment.

HD has become a model of a curable neoplasm—almost 70% are long-term survivors.

▶ Clinical Intervention

Complications of radiotherapy include hypothyroidism, pericarditis, pneumonitis, sterility. Complications of chemotherapy are those

▶ table 14-2

Stage	Clinical Findings	Therapy
I, II	Local disease	Radiation alone
III	Nodal disease both above and below diaphragm	Radiation ± combination chemotherapy
IV	Extranodal disease	Combination chemotherapy

associated with myelosuppression (bleeding, infections, anemia, vomiting, alopecia, paresthesias). Long-term complications include a 17% increased risk of secondary cancers and a 5 to 7% increased risk of acute leukemia.

2. Non-Hodgkin's Lymphomas

▶ Scientific Concepts

Lymphomas are the fifth most common cancer in the United States. Lymphomas are malignant tumors arising from lymphoreticular system and may occur at any site in the body. They are a group of heterogeneous tumors that vary greatly in response to treatment. Progressive increase in incidence with age, but mortality rates are decreasing. Etiology unknown, but several causative relations: increased incidence in immunosuppressed patients and in those with hyperfunctioning immune systems (10% of patients with Sjögren's syndrome develop non-Hodgkin's lymphoma). Some seem to be caused by viruses (EBV, human T-lymphotropic virus-I [HTLV-I]). *Helicobacter pylori* has been implicated in mucosa-associated lyphoid tissue (MALT) lymphomas, but this association is not yet proven. Pathology is very important in classification and treatment. Histological subtypes are determined on the basis of architectural pattern, cellular atypia, and cell type. Progression often disseminates early and widely by hematogenous routes rather than by contiguous nodal extension.

▶ History & Physical

Most common reason for seeking medical attention is unexplained and/or persistent lymphadenopathy. Most patients are asymptomatic, but 20% have constitutional symptoms and waxing/waning lymphadenopathy months prior to diagnosis. Other complaints may be abdominal pain, vomiting, bleeding. Weight loss is common. Most common extranodal site at presentation is GI tract.

▶ Diagnostic Studies

No lab findings are specific for non-Hodgkin's lymphoma. At presentation, CBC is usually normal, but anemia, leukopenia, thrombopenia may occur. Occasionally, lymphoma cells are found in peripheral blood. Bulky disease may cause jaundice, azotemia, bowel obstruction. Studies necessary for staging include biopsy of lymph node, chest radiograph, CT scans of chest, abdomen, pelvis; bilateral bone marrow biopsies; CBC, comprehensive metabolic panel, beta-2-microglobulin, HIV, HTLV serology.

▶ Clinical Therapeutics

Treatment is dependent on specific type of non-Hodgkin's lymphoma and usually involves combination chemotherapy with or without radiation therapy.

3. Polycythemia Vera

▶ Scientific Concepts

Polycythemia vera is one of the myeloproliferative disorders characterized by erythrocytosis (hemoglobin > 17.5 g/dL in men, > 15.5

g/dL in women). It is a clonal disease, and leukocytosis, basophilia, and trilineage hyperplasia of bone marrow with clustering of megakaryocytes occur. The endogenous myeloproliferation of increased red cells decreases the body's erythropoietin levels. Incidence is highest in those 60 to 70 years of age, with an equal male:female ratio.

► History & Physical

Clinically, patients may complain of problems related to hyperviscosity and hypervolemia, such as dyspnea, headaches, blurred vision; night sweats may result from the hypermetabolic state. Pruritus may also be present, probably due to increased levels of histamine or mast cells, and may worsen after a hot bath/shower. On examination, hypertension is found in 30%, splenomegaly in 60%, and the patient may appear plethoric. Peptic ulcers are present in 5 to 10%. Thrombotic and hemorrhagic complications are common as a result of high blood viscosity.

► Diagnostic Studies

Increased Hb, increased hematocrit and red cell count; neutrophils are increased in 50%, some with increased basophils. About half the patients have increased platelets, often three times the normal values. Serum B_{12} and B_{12} binding capacity are increased. Bone marrow is hypercellular with prominent megakaryocytes with or without clonal cytogenetic abnormalities. True red cell volume and erythropoietin levels are necessary for the diagnosis.

► Diagnosis

Primary polycythemia vera should be distinguished from secondary polycythemia, which can be due to hypoxia secondary to chronic obstructive pulmonary disease, cyanotic heart disease, renal causes, tumors, and cigarette smoking. Stress polycythemia is more common than polycythemia vera and may be associated with myocardial infarctions or transient ischemic attacks.

► Clinical Therapeutics

Median survival is 10 to 16 years; in 10 to 15% of patients AML evolves; 15 to 30% of cases evolve into myelofibrosis. If untreated, median survival is approximately 1.5 years. Treatment is therapeutic phlebotomy to keep hematocrit < 44%; that is the point where thromboembolic events increase precipitously. All patients should be given aspirin and maybe dipyridamole. Older patients should also be treated with bone marrow suppressors such as hydroxyurea or busulfan. Platelet count should be maintained < 400,000 to prevent further thrombotic events.

► Clinical Intervention

Thromboembolic events occur frequently in these patients; it is important to therapeutically phlebotomize and keep them on aspirin and other necessary medications long term.

III. OTHER HEMATOLOGIC DISEASES

A. HIV Infection/AIDS

▶ Scientific Concepts

Historically, acquired immune deficiency syndrome (AIDS) was the term given to describe patients who lacked other causes of impaired immunity who developed opportunistic infections or unusual malignancies, and who tested seropositive for the human immunodeficiency virus (HIV). HIV is found in body fluids (blood, semen, saliva, vaginal secretions, breast milk) and is transmitted through direct inoculation of any of these fluids. Manifestations for HIV infection are a consequence of immune defects resulting from dysregulation and destruction of T-helper lymphocytes. Infection causes an increase in the number of T-killer cells (CD8 lymphocytes) and a progressive decline in the number of circulating CD4 cells over several years (mean duration from infection to CD4 count $< 200/mm^3$ is 10 years). AIDS is a global disease, with routes of infection that include sexual, parenteral, and perinatal transmission. High-risk behaviors include rectal receptive intercourse, traumatic intercourse, multiple sex partners, using contaminated drug paraphernalia, prostitution. Heterosexual transmission risk increases in the presence of concomitant genital lesions that disrupt mucosal integrity. The risk of occupational transmission to health care workers is 0.2 to 0.3%. There exists a lack of clinical distinction between HIV infection, AIDS, and ARC (AIDS-related complex). However, four stages have been identified. Progression is not uniform; there is significant overlap among stages.

Stage 1: Asymptomatic infection, initial stage. Still infectious although not necessarily seropositive.

Stage 2: Acute viral syndrome. Mononucleosis-like illness with fever, headache, lymphadenopathy, pharyngitis, macular rash, malaise, aseptic meningitis, hepatosplenomegaly, extreme fatigue, weakness, arthralgias, myalgias; any or all of the above may be present. Usually these symptoms resolve after 2 to 4 weeks, but an AIDS-defining illness may develop. HIV p24 antigens are positive at this stage.

Stage 3: Persistent generalized lymphadenopathy. This stage is defined as lymphadenopathy in at least two extrainguinal sites for > 3 months in absence of any other illness.

Stage 4: Symptomatic infection. Nonspecific complaints (malaise, fever, weight loss, lymphadenopathy, oral thrush, diarrhea) often present in those infected with HIV for > 5 years. Other events during this stage include reactivation of tuberculosis, varicella zoster infection, chronic herpes simplex virus (HSV) lesions, oral leukoplakia, cutaneous fungal infections, *Salmonella* infections.

AIDS-defining illnesses are Kaposi's sarcoma, *Pneumocystis carinii* pneumonia (PCP). The course of HIV infection usually progresses relentlessly.

▶ History & Physical

Because AIDS is a global disease, every patient should be evaluated for risk of HIV. A thorough history should include general health status, immunizations, medication/drug history, sexual history (including gynecologic history), social history, travel, and occupational exposures. Physical examination should include initial height and weight, complete funduscopic, oral, lymphatic, skin, and genital exams. Findings may be completely negative or may be significant, depending on stage and current infection status.

► Diagnostic Studies

Enzyme-linked immunosorbent assay (ELISA) is extremely sensitive and should be used as a screening tool; Immunofluorescent assay (IFA) is more expensive and less sensitive; Western blot is more expensive and is used as a confirmatory test for a positive ELISA. HIV test results should be presented to the patient in person and be accompanied by counseling and referral, if positive. Other lab studies can identify the level of immune dysfunction and determine overall health status. Both the viral load and CD4 lymphocyte count provide important prognostic information and are important in monitoring treatment. Hematologic abnormalities are common; often the WBC is decreased, with absolute lymphopenia. Hepatitis serologies and syphilis titers should be done to diagnose comorbidities. If the patient is febrile, cultures should be sent for acid-fast bacilli (AFB), cytomegalovirus (CMV), Epstein–Barr virus (EBV) titer, and other atypical infectious organisms. In addition, febrile patients often require bone marrow examination with cultures for AFB and other mycobacteria. Lymphomas are diagnosed frequently in AIDS patients.

► Diagnosis

Clinical syndromes for which HIV infection must be considered in the differential include fever, adrenal insufficiency, lymphadenopathy, dysphagia, diarrhea, perirectal pain, acute abdominal pain, cutaneous lesions, dyspnea, headaches, seizures, dementia, blindness, among others. Virtually everything is included in the differential diagnosis. All patients in whom HIV infection cannot be ruled out should be offered HIV testing. A positive ELISA with a positive Western blot is diagnostic of the presence of HIV.

► Clinical Therapeutics

Goals are to improve overall health status and increase survival (and prevent further transmission of the virus). Prompt treatment of infections is important. Antiretroviral therapy initiated early improves morbidity and is now the standard of care. The most recent regimens include double or triple combination therapies consisting of a protease inhibitor, zidovudine, and another reverse transcriptase inhibitor. Prophylaxis for opportunistic infections includes trimethoprimsulfamethoxazole (TMP-SMZ) for PCP; azithromycin or clarithromycin for atypical mycobacterial infections; other prophylactic regimens are under investigation.

► Health Maintenance Issues

The most important issue is preventing the spread of the disease to others. Continuous education is imperative. Identifying life-threatening infections early and treating them successfully is a continuous challenge in this population primarily because of the relentless progression of the disease. Prophylactic measures are also important and should be maintained throughout. Close follow-up with regular checks of viral load and CD4 counts can assist in follow-up and general improvement in overall health status.

B. Infectious Mononucleosis

▶ Scientific Concepts

Infectious mononucleosis is most often found in older children or young adults from higher socioeconomic groups, with the highest incidence in college students and military cadets. Its means of transmission is not well defined, but probably spreads along the respiratory route; intimate contact appears to be necessary for mucosal shedding to infect another. The incubation period is 4 to 7 weeks. The suspected causative agent, EBV, is unique among the herpesviruses in that it replicates in vitro in human B lymphocytes and the EBV genetic material persists indefinitely. Infection occurs from the mucosal shedding to the oropharynx; the resulting inflammatory response produces pharyngeal exudate. The virus is carried via lymphatics to local lymph nodes, then viremia occurs. Viral shedding continues throughout infection and even persists despite clinical recovery. EBV is then permanently established in its latent form in B lymphocytes. EBV is associated with African Burkitt's lymphoma, nasopharyngeal cancer, and non-Hodgkin's lymphomas in transplant recipients.

▶ History & Physical

The hallmark characteristics of mononucleosis are fever, fatigue, cervical lymphadenopathy, sore throat, and the insidious development of increasing malaise, fever, chills, and then within 1 week, pharyngitis. Rarely, it may present as aseptic meningitis or meningoencephalitis with a normal cerebrospinal fluid (CSF), glucose and mononuclear pleocytosis. Neurological manifestations are present in 1% of patients and may include Guillain–Barré syndrome, Bell's or other cranial nerve palsies, or a mononeuritis multiplex. Acute symptoms usually last from 2 to 4 weeks but may last longer, especially if patients exercise. Splenomegaly and lymphadenopathy may persist for several months. In older adults, the presentation resembles a typhoid illness without splenomegaly and lymphadenopathy. A patient inadvertently given ampicillin often rapidly experiences a generalized maculopapular rash, periorbital edema, and palatal petechiae.

▶ Diagnostic Studies

The hallmark lab finding is the presence of heterophil antibodies, which are immunoglobulin M (IgM) antibodies that selectively agglutinate RBCs of other species, especially the horse (Monospot test). This test is positive in > 85% of infected individuals. Atypical lymphocytosis is present on CBC, as well as leukocytosis and absolute lymphocytosis. Liver enzymes (serum glutamic oxaloacetic transaminase [SGOT], serum glutamic pyruvic transaminase [SGPT]) may be mildly elevated. Hematological complications may include a Coombs'-positive hemolytic anemia, profound thrombocytopenia. These complications, in addition to acute splenic congestion and sub-capsular hemorrhages, greatly increase the risk of splenic rupture.

▶ Diagnosis

Tonsillopharyngeal involvement, lymphadenopathy, splenomegaly may be minimal or absent (typhoidal presentation), especially in older patients. Characteristic findings may be overshadowed by complicating features, which include neurological problems, jaundice, thrombocytopenia, bleeding, hemolytic anemia, splenic rupture; however, the disease can usually be confirmed by presence of heterophil antibodies and atypical lymphocytosis. CMV mononucleosis closely mimics EBV mono, but the heterophil test is always negative in CMV mononucleosis. Other diagnoses to include in the differential include toxoplasmosis, hepatitis A, adenovirus infection, herpes infection, pharyngitis, enteroviral infection, Hodgkin's disease, angioim-munoblastic lymphadenopathy, and drug reactions (allopurinol, diphenylhydantoin, para-amino salicylic acid, hydralazine, methyl-dopa).

▶ Clinical Therapeutics

There are currently no known means for prevention. Usually, the illness is benign and self-limiting, and treatment is directed at relief of symptoms and prevention of complications. Acetaminophen is given for headache, fever, pharyngitis; aspirin should be avoided because of the increased risk of splenic rupture/hemorrhage. Corticosteroids may be given for tonsillar hypertrophy to prevent airway obstruction (prednisone, 40 mg PO qd for 5 to 7 days) and parenteral administration may be necessary. Other indications for steroid use include severe hemolytic anemia, thrombocytopenia, or meningitis. Exercise and exertion should be avoided to prevent relapses and expedite resolution of the illness.

C. Thrombotic Thrombocytopenic Purpura

▶ Scientific Concepts

Thrombotic thrombocytopenic purpura (TTP) is a microangio-pathic, hemolytic anemia secondary to platelet aggregates or platelet fibrin thrombi in small blood vessels, intravascular aggregation, and endothelial injury. It is serious, progressive, and rapidly fatal unless intervention is taken. The etiology is unknown, with proposed mechanisms including inappropriate immune response, decrease prosta-glandin formation, stimulation by oral contraceptives. The peak incidence is the third decade of life, with women outnumbering men.

▶ History & Physical

Fever, signs of hemorrhage including pallor and petechiae, neuro-logic signs due to vascular occlusions in brain (e.g., headache, delirium, altered state of consciousness, seizures), and renal dysfunction. However, neurologic symptoms are often remittent.

► Diagnostic Studies

CBC, peripheral smear, serum and urine chemistries, urinalysis, and coagulation profile.

► Diagnosis

Hb is usually < 10 g/dL with diffuse reticulocytosis, polymorphonuclear leukocytosis, schistocytes (characteristic), thrombocytopenia (may be as low as $10 \times 10^{-9}/L$), marked anisocytosis (increased variation in red cell size), elevated bilirubin, hemosiderinuria, hemoglobinuria. Urine studies reveal casts, erythrocytes, and leukocytes. There is increased serum creatinine, blood urea nitrogen (BUN) (secondary to decreased glomerular filtration rate), and LDH. The differential diagnosis includes DIC. In contrast to DIC, there is typically normal fibrinogen, prothrombin time (PT), and partial thromboplastin time (PTT), while the fibrin split products (FSP) may be slightly increased.

► Clinical Therapeutics

High-dose glucocorticoid steroids (prednisone, 60 to 100 mg/d) and platelet inhibitors (aspirin, dextran, sulfinpyrazone, dipyridamole) lead to decrease platelet aggregation. Plasmapheresis, whole-blood exchange transfusion, or plasma infusion is often required. Platelet transfusions should be avoided as they will cause deterioration of the clinical condition. Follow the LDH and platelet count to determine the response to therapy.

► Clinical Intervention

If concurrent DIC present, splenectomy and heparin may be warranted; 60 to 100% show complete response with plasmapheresis.

D. Hemophilia

► Scientific Concepts

The majority of diagnosed congenital bleeding disorders are hemophilia A. Hemophilia A results from a factor VIII: C deficiency. Hemophilia B is a deficiency of Factor IX (i.e., Christmas disease). Both are sex-linked disorders passed on the X-chromosome by women to sons; can occur spontaneously through mutation.

► History & Physical

Patients typically present with spontaneous or excessive bleeding, such as with trauma. Hemophilia B is less severe than hemophilia A.

► Diagnostic Studies

Activated partial thromboplastin time (aPTT), PT, and thrombin time (TT). Assays for factor VIII and IX.

► Diagnosis

Prolonged aPTT, which is corrected by fresh plasma but not by serum, establishes the diagnosis. Disease severity determined by factor level.

► Clinical Intervention

Hemophilia A: Cryoprecipitate is used for bleeding, while mild cases are treated with DDAVP (vasopressin). Antibodies develop against factor VIII: C but may be required in severe cases.

Hemophilia B: Fresh frozen plasma or factor IX in severe cases.

E. Idiopathic Thrombocytopenic Purpura

► Scientific Concepts

Disorder of immune complexes binding to platelets resulting in severe thrombocytopenia. Idiopathic thrombocytopenic purpura (ITP) typically is acute in onset. In children, it is often associated with viral infection. Other associated disorders include lupus, hematologic malignancies, and other infections.

► History & Physical

Symptoms and signs of bleeding predominate the clinical presentation with the presence of easy bruising, epistaxis, and frank bleeding.

► Diagnostic Studies

CBC, peripheral smear, bone marrow.

► Diagnosis

Severe thrombocytopenia is the hallmark finding with the peripheral smear revealing large platelets. The differential diagnoses include aplastic anemia, systemic lupus erythematosus (SLE), and acute leukemias.

► Clinical Therapeutics

Treatment depends on the severity of the illness, with corticosteroids being the standard therapy. Other immunosuppressive drugs such as cyclophosphamide and danazol are used. IV gamma-globulin is only transiently effective.

► Clinical Intervention

Plasmapheresis may be required to reduce the antibody level. Splenectomy sometimes required when medical management fails.

F. Hemolytic Uremic Syndrome

► Scientific Concepts

Acute intravascular hemolysis and renal failure with variable amount of platelet destruction and thrombus formation (primarily affecting kidneys). Causes include mild febrile illnesses, certain immunizations, GI disturbances. Those most frequently affected are infants and children (most < 8 years old), renal transplant patients, pregnant women, and particularly postpartum women.

► History & Physical

Vomiting and diarrhea usually precedes anemia and renal failure, increased blood pressure, pallor, fever, abdominal pain, bleeding from mucous membranes, dark-colored urine, progression to oliguria or anuria. Hepatomegaly, no splenomegaly. Neurological symptoms may be present but less frequent and severe than TTP.

▶ Diagnostic Studies
CBC, peripheral smear, coagulation profile, chemistries, urinalysis.

▶ Diagnosis
Hb may be as low as 4 g/dL, leukocytosis with predominance of neutrophils, thrombocytopenia as severe as anemia, schistocytes, burr cells, coagulation tests usually normal, decreased haptoglobin, increased bilirubin, hemoglobinuria and hemosiderinuria, extreme elevations in BUN and creatinine. Urinalysis—proteinuria, erythrocytes, leukocytes, casts.

▶ Clinical Therapeutics
Conservative management of fluids, electrolytes, blood gases, blood pressure. Dialysis may be required. Mortality rate less than with TTP.

G. Disseminated Intravascular Coagulopathy

▶ Scientific Concepts
Disorder of pathological activation of the clotting cascade with the generation of excess thrombin resulting in concomitant systemic thrombosis and hemorrhage. Precipitators include infection, most common microbes gram-negative organisms (e.g., *Neisseria meningitidis*), intravascular hemolysis, obstetric accidents, burns, malignancies, crush injuries, and closed head injuries.

▶ History & Physical
May manifest with gross bleeding (e.g., bleeding surgical wounds, hematemesis, hemoptysis, hematuria), hematomas, petechiae, and purpura. Thrombosis may manifest with myocardial infarction, CVA, peripheral thrombosis, renal failure, and multisystem organ dysfunction.

▶ Diagnostic Studies
CBC, PT, PTT, DIC profile (fibrin split products [FSP], d-dimer, fibrinogen).

▶ Diagnosis
Known precipitator and evidence of DIC on labs including elevated FSP, d-dimer. Fibrinogen may be elevated early in disease as acute-phase reactant but later becomes consumed; thrombocytopenia (not always in early disease).

▶ Clinical Therapeutics
Supportive care is required until the disease resolves. No specific treatment is available for DIC. Heparin has been used but controversial.

▶ Clinical Intervention

Treatment of precipitator the most important factor in outcome. Transfusion of RBCs and platelets often necessary. Replacement of clotting factors and fibrinogen with fresh frozen plasma and cryoprecipitate is controversial as it may worsen disease.

▶ Health Maintenance Issues

Early detection and treatment of precipitators may prevent or minimize DIC.

H. Splenic Disorders

▶ Scientific Concepts

Splenomegaly occurs in a variety of disease states, including infections (e.g., mononucleosis, malaria, AIDS, viral hepatitis, splenic abscess), immunologic disorders (e.g., rheumatoid arthritis, SLE), congestive heart failure, some anemias (e.g., sickle cell, thalassemia, hemolytic), malignancies (e.g., leukemias, lymphomas, metastatic tumors), and chronic liver disease.

▶ History & Physical

Symptoms and signs associated with the underlying disorder.

▶ Diagnostic Studies

Evaluation should be guided based on history and physical.

▶ Clinical Therapeutics

Treatment of the underlying disorder.

▶ Clinical Intervention

Splenectomy may be required when hypersplenism accompanies splenomegaly.

I. Transfusion Reaction

▶ Scientific Concepts

Hemolytic reactions after a blood transfusion may be immediate or delayed. Life-threatening immediate reactions are associated with intravascular hemolysis and result from incompatible ABO antibodies (complement activating antibodies of IgG or IgM). The severity depends on recipient's titer of antibodies. Extravascular hemolytic transfusion reactions result from a problem with the Rh system, and are less severe, although they may be life threatening. If these are mild, the only sign may be progressive unexplained anemia and/or jaundice.

▶ History & Physical

Clinical features include a hemolytic shock phase and may occur after a few milliliters of blood have been transfused or up to 2 hours after transfusion is completed. The patient may have urticaria, pain in the lumbar region, flushing, headache, precordial pain, shortness of breath, vomiting, rigors, pyrexia, or hypotension. Jaundice and/or DIC may even occur. Moderate leukocytosis is frequent. The oliguric phase is next, and renal tubular necrosis and acute renal failure may ensue. The diuretic phase occurs during recovery from acute renal failure.

▶ Clinical Intervention

The best treatment is prevention of reactions by ensuring compatible transfusions only. If one should occur, management consists of maintaining blood pressure and renal perfusion; administering furosemide, corticosteroids, antihistamines as necessary; and even using epinephrine for severe shock should it occur.

Other transfusion reactions include the following:

Febrile reactions: May occur due to white cell antibodies. Clinical manifestations are rigors, fever, possible pulmonary infiltrates. These can be avoided by transfusing only leukocyte-poor packed RBCs (filtered). Filtered products will also reduce the risk of transfusion-acquired CMV infection.

Nonhemolytic allergic reactions: Occur if there is a hypersensitivity to donor plasma proteins and may result in anaphylactic shock, urticaria, fever, dyspnea, facial edema, rigors. Treatment is the immediate administration of hydrocortisone and antihistamines with or without epinephrine. Transfusing only washed red cells can prevent hypersensitivity reactions.

Post-transfusion circulatory overload: Similar to pulmonary edema; can occur if large amounts of blood products are transfused rapidly, especially in patients with some degree of cardiac decompensation. The first clinical manifestations are usually a dry cough, fullness in head/neck; jugular venous distention may occur. Management is the same as that for congestive heart failure. Slow transfusion with diuretic use can prevent these reactions from occurring.

Post-transfusion hepatitis: Rare with current screening methods, but may still occur.

Transmission of CMV and EBV: Hepatitis C may manifest itself 3 months after transfusion. Other known infectious agents that can be transmitted via transfusion include HIV, mononucleosis, toxoplasmosis, malaria, syphilis.

Post-transfusion iron overload: May develop after repeated transfusions over several years without any blood loss, and may cause damage to the liver, myocardium, and endocrine glands.

IV. ILL-DEFINED PRESENTATIONS

A. Lymphadenitis

▶ Scientific Concepts

Inflammation of the lymph nodes; common in immunocompromised patients.

▶ History & Physical

Enlarged tender regional lymph nodes, may have associated rash, abscess or wound, fever, malaise, anorexia.

► Diagnostic Studies

CBC and cultures with imaging studies as the clinical picture indicates.

► Diagnosis

This is a clinical diagnosis.

► Clinical Therapeutics/Intervention

Heat, elevation, and analgesics are often helpful. Antibiotics, with or without drainage, are necessary for lymphangitis secondary to infection.

B. Fever of Unknown Origin

► Scientific Concepts

Fever is a highly nonspecific sign. Normally, the upper limit of normal is 37.0°C (98.6°F) orally, but normal ranges vary depending on the individual. Normal temperature can increase during the second half of the menstrual cycle, exercise, heavy meals, and normal diurnal variation. Noninfectious causes of fevers include pheochromocytoma, Addison's disease, heat stroke, and anticholinergic drugs. Physiologically, a fever is an endogenous adjustment of the hypothalamic temperature set point to a level greater than normal usually by a disease process distant to the hypothalamus, often caused by endogenous or exogenous pyogens or cytokines. Fever of unknown origin (FUO) is defined by temperature > 38.3°C (101.1°F) persisting > 3 weeks, and a thorough workup is done without a definite diagnosis; all other causes are ruled out. The majority are due to infections, neoplasms, collagen vascular diseases, or granulomatous diseases.

► History & Physical

A detailed history is imperative and should include all major organ systems; careful attention to fever, weight loss, night sweats, rashes, headaches. All previous illnesses should be documented, including dental history, psychiatric illnesses, and surgeries. Other necessary components, in detail, include immunizations, transfusions, family history, work environment, nutrition, travel, drugs, sexual history, recreational habits, animal contacts, tick and mosquito exposure. On examination, fever must be documented. The physical examination should be performed carefully, with special attention given to skin, heart, lungs, lymph nodes, fundi, joints, abdomen. The exam should be repeated daily if patient is in the hospital. Look for rashes, new or changing cardiac murmurs, arthritis, abdominal changes, funduscopic changes, and changes in any lymphadenopathy.

► Diagnostic Studies

At a minimum, should include CBC with differential and peripheral smear, erythrocyte sedimentation rate, serum chemistries, antinuclear antibody, rheumatoid factor, blood cultures, urinalysis and culture, stool culture if GI complaints, sputum culture if pulmonary complaints/findings, CSF analysis/culture (all cultures should be sent for bacteria, mycobacteria, fungus), and serologies (especially HIV,

CMV, EBV, syphilis, toxoplasmosis). Imaging studies initially should include chest radiograph; abdominal ultrasound may be justified. Other studies include purified protein derivative (PPD) with control and electrocardiogram. Additional studies that should be performed, guided by clinical and lab findings, include CT scans of abdomen or chest, endoscopy, echocardiogram, and gallium scan or ventilation-perfusion scan if indicated. Invasive tests should be reserved after all the above are nondiagnostic, and include biopsy of bone marrow, lymph node, liver, or even lap-aroscopy. It may be justified to do a bone marrow aspiration and biopsy on all patients with an FUO. Lumbar punctures should be done if any symptoms of CNS involvement.

▶ Diagnosis

Bacterial causes include abscess, most often intra-abdominal and most often in subphrenic space, liver, retroperitoneal space, or pelvis in women. Tuberculosis must be suspected, and dissemination often occurs, especially in the immunocompromised host. Constitutional symptoms are often present, and chest radiograph may be normal. Cultures require 6 weeks to be considered negative. A focus of mycobacterial/tuberculosis infection may be in the kidney, genitourinary tract, or lymph nodes. Hepatobiliary causes include cholangitis, cholecystitis, gallbladder empyema, bacterial hepatitis caused by alpha-hemolytic streptococcus (an elevated alkaline phosphatase may be the only positive diagnostic finding). Urinary tract infections are rare causes of FUO due to rapid detection on urine analysis. Endocarditis may present with or without a cardiac murmur, and blood cultures may be negative in 10%. Osteomyelitis is another bacterial cause of FUO.

Viral causes are difficult to diagnose and may include the herpesviruses, especially CMV and EBV; they can cause prolonged febrile episodes with constitutional symptoms but no prominent organ manifestations. Fevers of significant duration are common in patients with HIV infection and are caused by opportunistic infections, lymphomas, or HIV itself.

Other causes include fungal (especially in the setting of an immunocompromised patient, broad-spectrum antibiotic use, and intravascular devices), parasites, chlamydia, rickettsia (transmitted from cattle and sheep, hepatic involvement is frequent). Neoplasms, especially lymphomas, leukemias, and solid tumors, can present as FUO. Collagen vascular disorders and autoimmune diseases should be ruled out. Granulomatous diseases, including giant cell arteritis, sarcoidosis, and regional enteritis, are other causes of FUO. Crohn's disease is the most common GI cause of FUO; diagnosis is made on endoscopic biopsy. Less common causes include drug fever (alpha-methyldopa, quinidine, beta-lactam antibiotics, isoniazide, procainamide), pulmonary emboli, and occult thrombophlebitis.

▶ Clinical Therapeutics

Empiric treatment with antibiotics or antituberculosis medicines rarely improves state. Rather than empiric treatment, clinical evaluation should be repeated to find the cause of the fever. Nonsteroidal anti-inflammatory drugs and corticosteroids may be of benefit in treating symptoms but may mask others in the process. Workup should be continued until cause is found and treated.

C. Septic Shock

► Scientific Concepts

Sepsis is the systemic inflammatory response to infection. Septic shock results when sepsis leads to hypotension and/or organ dysfunction due to poor perfusion. It is associated with high morbidity and mortality. Most common microbes are bacterial, but serious infections caused by fungi, mycobacteria, rickettsiae, viruses, protozoans can also result in septic shock. Microbial bloodstream invasion is not required because endotoxin and cytokines (e.g., tissue necrosis factor) and other host response factors can be released systemically. Two-thirds of all cases are hospitalized patients. Predisposers include invasive procedures and devices (e.g., indwelling catheters), drugs causing neutropenia, diabetes mellitus, burns, IV drug injection.

► History & Physical

Hyper- or hypothermia, tachycardia, tachypnea, hypotension, altered mentation, may have signs and symptoms of infection.

► Diagnostic Studies

CBC, lactate, coagulation studies (including DIC profile); pan cultures including blood, urine, and sputum for Gram stain; aerobic, anaerobic microbes and viral and fungal cultures (if indicated); chest radiograph; lumbar puncture; CT scan and other studies may be necessary as history and physical warrants.

► Diagnosis

Confirmed infection plus at least two of the following: hyper- or hypothermia, tachycardia, tachypnea, and hypotension or signs and symptoms of organ dysfunction, including hypoxemia, elevated serum lactate, altered mentation, new coagulopathy, metabolic acidosis, acute renal failure.

► Clinical Therapeutics

Begin antibiotics for suspected sepsis or septic shock as soon as cultures are taken. Consider the likely source of infection, community versus hospital acquired, but empiric therapy should cover both gram-positive and gram-negative organisms and be given IV. Once organism is identified, antibiotic can be streamlined.

► Clinical Intervention

Surgical drainage may be necessary for some infections. Remove source of infection (e.g., remove catheter and culture tip). Provide support including hemodynamic and respiratory.

► Health Maintenance Issues

Prevention and early diagnosis is key. Limit the use of invasive procedures and devices. When invasive devices are necessary, limit the duration of use. Avoid indiscriminate use of antibiotics and glucocorticoid steroids. Consider infection early.

BIBLIOGRAPHY

Berkow R, Fletcher AJ, et al., eds. *The Merck Manual,* 16th ed. Rahway, NJ: Merck Research Laboratories; 1992.

Hoffbrand AV, Pettit JE. *Essential Haematology,* 3rd ed. Oxford: Blackwell Scientific Publications; 1994.

Lotspeich-Steininger CA, Stiene-Martin EA, Koepke JA. *Clinical Hematology.* Philadelphia: JB Lippincott; 1992.

Rosenthal DS, Eyre HJ. Hodgkin's disease and non-Hodgkin's lymphomas. pp. 456–469. In Murphy GP, Lawrence W, Lenhardt RE, eds. *American Cancer Society Textbook of Clinical Oncology,* 2nd ed. Atlanta: American Cancer Society; 1995.

Stein JH et al., eds. *Internal Medicine,* 4th ed. St. Louis: Mosby; 1994.

Waterbury L. *Hematology,* 4th ed. Baltimore: Williams & Wilkins; 1996.

Pediatrics | 15

Ricky E. Kortyna, MMS, PA-C

I. EVALUATION OF THE NEWBORN

► History & Physical

See Table 15-1.

General assessment: High birth weight seen with hyperglycemia, polycythemia; low birth weight with hypoglycemia. TORCH (toxoplasmosis, rubella, cytomegalovirus, herpes simplex) screen if maternal history is positive or congenital infection apparent. Simian crease with trisomy 21 (Down syndrome). Jaundice in 50% by day 4; erythema toxicum common and self-limited; milia in 50% of newborns; lanugo may be present. Check for midline capillary hemangiomas (associated with neural tube defects), other "birthmarks."

Eyes: Pupils constricted for 21 days, then pupillary response; optical blink reflex; bulging or cloudy cornea with glaucoma; red reflex should be visualized.

Ears: Low-set with Down syndrome, renal disease; test hearing, especially if prenatal infection suspected.

Head: Fontanelles sunken with dehydration, bulging with intracranial mass, transillumination with hydrocephalus; caput succedaneum with forceps delivery; limited mobility of the sutures with synostosis.

Mouth/Pharynx/Nose: Check patency of nares with catheter, sucking reflex; cleft lip/palate; thrush; tonsils are not visible; high-pitched cry with increased intracranial pressure (ICP) or drug withdrawal; low-pitched cry with hypothyroidism or hypocalcemic tetany; Turner's syndrome with webbing of the neck.

Chest: Respiratory rate ~ 40 to 60/min, apnea and bradycardia with increased ICP or pulmonary disease; grunting, retraction, or nasal flaring with respiratory distress; plethora with increased hemoglobin, supernumerary nipples; breast discharge for ~ 2 weeks; heart rate > 200 with congestive heart failure (CHF), hypoplastic left heart syndrome; about 60% have murmurs.

Abdomen: If scaphoid, suspect diaphagmatic hernia; marked distention with gastrointestinal/genitourinary (GI/GU) obstruction; umbilical hernia in blacks may suggest hypothyroidism; umbilicus with three vessels should be two arteries and one vein, a solitary artery may

► table 15-1

APGAR CHECKED AT 1 AND 5 MINUTES (BEST SCORE IS 10)

Sign	0	1	2
Color	Blue, pale	Pink body, blue extremities	Completely pink
Heart rate	Absent	< 100	> 100
Reflex irritability	No response	Grimace	Sneeze/cough
Muscle tone	Flaccid	Some flexion of limbs	Good flexion of limbs
Respiratory effort	Absent	Weak/irregular	Good/crying

From: Rudolph AM, Kamei RK. Rudolph's Fundamentals of Pediatrics, *2nd ed. Stamford, CT: Appleton & Lange;*
1998, p. 97.

signify renal disease; check for anal agenesis; passage of meconium—if absent, cystic fibrosis or Hirschsprung's disease, more than just the lower poles may be palpable in congenital polycystic kidney disease.

Genitalia: Check for ambiguity; testes in scrotum in 95% at birth; hypospadias/epispadias; transilluminate hydroceles; labia majora should cover the minora and clitoris; fingertip space between vagina and anus.

Musculoskeletal: Clavicle most frequently broken bone during delivery; brachial palsy after delivery especially with shoulder dystocia; hip dislocation with positive Ortolani/Barlow maneuvers; flat feet normal.

Neurological: If newborn in hyperextension consider meningismus; is newborn hypotonic ("floppy infant") or hypertonic; Babinski upgoing until ~ 4 years of age. Evaluate developmental milestones (Table 15-2) at initial and subsequent visits.

Automatisms: Rooting, sucking, swallowing, plantar and palmar grasp, Moro or startle reflex, placing and stepping responses.

▶ Health Maintenance Issues

Every periodic visit for infants, children, and adolescents should include an age-appropriate history and physical examination, immunizations, evaluation of growth and development, and patient education including anticipatory guidance (see Table 15-3).

II. IMMUNIZATIONS

Note: Because of the dynamic changes occurring in the field of immunization, please contact the Centers for Disease Control or review *Mortality and Morbidity Weekly Report,* both available via the Internet, for the most recent update of the immunization schedule. See: http://www.cdc.gov.

▶ table 15-2

DEVELOPMENTAL MILESTONES DURING THE FIRST YEAR OF LIFE

Age	Gross Motor	Fine Motor	Personal	Language
Newborn	Reflex head turn	—	Regards face	Alerts to bell
1 month	Lifts head when prone	Eyes track horizontally	—	—
2 months	Lifts shoulders when prone	Tracks past midline	Spontaneous smile	Coos; searches for sound
3 months	Lifts up on elbows, head steady	Unfisted > 50%, tracks 180 degrees	—	—
4 months	Lifts up on hands, rolls front to back	Reaches and brings object to mouth	Turns head to voice/noise	—
5 months	Rolls back to front	"Rakes" at bright object	—	—
6 months	Sits alone > 30 sec	Transfers hand to hand	Discriminates social smile	Babbles
7–8 months	Crawls, sits well	Pincer grasp	Stranger anxiety	Mama, Dada
9–10 months	Pulls to stand	Neat pincer grasp	Plays peek-a-boo	Understands "no"
10–11 months	Cruises	—	—	—
12 months	Walks	—	Drinks from cup	3–5-word vocabulary

► table 15-3

ANTICIPATORY GUIDANCE: TOPICS TO DISCUSS WITH PARENTS DURING THE FIRST YEAR OF LIFE

Newborn: Never leave child unattended; use car restraints; feeding topics; crying and sleeping patterns; stooling patterns; hiccups; sneezing and "wet burps"; startle reflexes; care of umbilical cord; circumcision; jaundice; how to take a temperature, when to call the office; fever, vomiting, and diarrhea; postpartum adjustment; sibling reactions

2–4 Weeks: Review above if needed; bath safety and sun exposure; feeding issues, fluoride supplementation; "colic"; bowel and bladder habits; when to call the office; time away from the child; giving time to siblings

2 Months: Review above; car restraints; do not leave unattended on bed/table; caution about hot liquids; do not use walkers; wait to introduce solids at 4–6 months; sleep, crying, and bowel patterns; immunizations; saline nose drops

4 Months: Review above; keep small objects out of reach; introduce solid foods, fruits, and vegetables; night awakening; teething/drooling; talking to baby; responds to vocalizations; immunizations

6 Months: Childproofing the house; syrup of ipecac; Poison Control Center; discourage walkers and encourage stair gates; bathtub safety; electrical outlets; introducing finger foods; discourage milk or juice as pacifier substitute; resistance to sleep; teething; shoes; separation and stranger anxiety; immunizations

9 Months: Toddler car restraint; ingestants such as peanuts, grapes; finger foods, self-feeding; weaning from bottle and introducing cup; sleep awakening; favorite toy; dental care; separation and stranger anxiety; imitation; social games; discipline, limit setting; distraction; child care support

12 Months: Reinforce above; kitchen, stairs, water, and car safety; fences, gates, and latches; table foods, decreased food intake; speech development; autonomy; limit setting, discipline

Adapted from Rudolph A, Kamei R. "Anticipatory Guidance—Suggested Topics at Each Visit." Rudolph's Fundamentals of Pediatrics, 2nd ed. Stamford, CT: Appleton & Lange; 1998, p. 22, Table 1–16.

A. Diphtheria and Tetanus Toxoids and Pertussis (DTP)

Given intramuscularly (IM) in anterolateral thigh or deltoid; contraindications include acute febrile illness, seizures, an evolving or suspected neurological disease, and/or severe reaction to prior dose of DTP; DTP may be delayed for the above reasons; contraindicated if patient has seizures after dose; reactions include local swelling and tenderness, fever, and irritability; acetaminophen given beforehand may decrease the symptoms; if the schedule for DTP is interrupted, it is resumed, not restarted.

B. Polio

Oral polio vaccine (OPV) is live attenuated, IPV is inactivated; OPV not given if someone in household has decreased immunity such as acquired immune deficiency syndrome (AIDS); IPV given to adults not previously immunized and to immunocompromised children; adverse reactions may include a rare case of polio caused by the vaccine; IPV form contains small amounts of neomycin, streptomycin, and polymyxin B, and should not be given to persons with sensitivity to these drugs.

C. Measles, Mumps, Rubella (MMR)

Contraindications include pregnancy, as vaccine may cross placenta and cause spontaneous abortion; immunodeficiency; therapeutic immunosuppression or acute febrile illness. Measles and mumps component is grown in chick embryo cultures and should not be given to those with anaphylactic reaction to egg products, although other egg-allergic reactions do not lead to contraindication; adverse reactions include fever, rash, transient arthralgia, and paresthetic pains; encephalopathy rare with measles: vaccine contains small amounts of neomycin and is contraindicated in those allergic to it.

D. *Haemophilus influenzae* Type B (Hib)

Indications that carry an increased risk include sickle cell disease, asplenia, and chemotherapy-treated malignancies; no known contraindications.

E. Hepatitis B Virus

At high risk are children born to infected mothers; rarely Guillain–Barré may occur; no known contraindications.

III. NUTRITION

A. Growth Patterns

The average baby weighs 3.5 kg, is 50 cm long, and has a head circumference of 35 cm. Newborns lose 5 to 10% of body weight during the first few days of life and then gain it back by day 10; newborns gain about 30 g/d for the first 3 months of life; then 10 to 20 g/d for the remainder of the first year; infants double their birth weight by 6 months and triple it at 1 year; average child weighs 10 kg at age 1, 20 kg at age 5, and 30 kg at age 10.

B. Breast Feeding

Newborn nurses 8 to 12 times every 24 hours, with each feed around one-half hour; at around 4 months, most infants temporarily lose interest in breast feeding; breast-fed infants urinate about 8 to 10 times per day with colorless urine, stools seedy, yellow; postnatal bilirubin rises more in a breast-fed infant then formula-fed—if it continues to rise, halt breast feeding; human milk can be stored for 24 hours in refrigerator, 30 days in freezer; most medications and illicit drugs can be transmitted via breast milk; mother should suspend feeding if she has group B streptococcal disease, herpes simplex or syphilitic lesions around the breast, pertussis, chickenpox, human immunodeficiency virus (HIV), and non-B hepatitis; infants with galactosemia are not to receive galactose from any source. Colostrum, the first milk produced, contains proteins, immunoglobulins, and secretory immunoglobulin A (IgA); mature milk occurs at 7 to 10 days.

C. Breast Milk Versus Formula

Both have 20 kcal/oz.; casein:whey ratio in human milk is 40:60, 80:20 in most formulas; polyunsaturated fat in human milk, saturated in cow milk; greater amount of lactose in human milk; breast-fed infants may need supplements of vitamins K and D and iron and fluoride (newborns should receive prophylactic dose of vitamin K); iron in breast milk is in smaller amounts but is more bioavailable; infections are less frequent in breast-fed infants.

Most formulas are interchangeable; they attempt to reproduce human milk; formula-fed infants do not require supplements. Bottle should not be propped as this causes pooling of feeds and secondary caries. Formulas do not have to be warmed and should never be microwaved. Infants should be burped every several ounces; stomach capacity at birth is 1 to 3 ounces; therefore, a newborn cannot take a 4-ounce feeding. Formula intolerance includes diarrhea, vomiting, abdominal pain, failure to thrive, asthma, eczema, and shock.

D. Addition of Other Foods

Risk of increasing food allergies may stem from too early introduction of solids as may childhood obesity; solid food added around 3 to 6 months; single-grain cereals first, then fruits, vegetables, and later meats; add only one new food/week in case of allergies. "Baby food" is given as per the label, and child should not eat out of the jar as saliva may cause the food to liquefy. Open jars may be kept for 2 to 3 days; finger foods introduced at 9 months when child has pincer grasp; 1 year old should be able to eat same food as adults; avoid raw carrots, nuts, and hard candies as these may be aspirated. Cow's milk, peanuts, egg whites, and citrus before age 1 year may be associated with allergies later on.

Honey is not recommended during the first year of life as it may contain *Clostridium botulinum* and cause botulism; breast feeding should not be stopped if mother on antibiotics except for metronidazole and tetracycline; mothers with silicone breast implants who breast feed risk giving child esophageal scleroderma. Infant milk need not be sterilized. Infants who drink cow's milk at risk for hypocalcemia; signs of vitamin E deficiency in the neonate are hemolytic anemia, peripheral edema, and thrombocytosis.

IV. BEHAVIOR PROBLEMS

A. Toilet Training

Age varies from 2 to 4 years; takes 2 weeks to 2 months to learn; frustration of parents with this is a leading cause of child abuse; occasional accidents months after training are not uncommon.

B. Breath Holding

Not uncommon during first year of life; child may pass out or have seizure; cyanotic child with emotional provocation, pallid child with physical provocation. Differential includes seizures, syncope, arrhythmias, vertigo, cataplexy, central or obstructive apnea. Treat with atropine sulfate for pallid episodes.

C. Temper Tantrums

Occurs from 12 months to 5 years; ~ 20% of children have one daily; > 5/d is abnormal; treatment is behavior modification.

D. Crying

At 2 weeks, the average crying time is 2 hr/d; at 6 weeks 3 hr/d, and at 12 weeks 1 hr/d; If > these times, consider colic and infections, flatus, trauma, behavioral problems, drug reactions, child abuse, sickle cell crisis, CHF.

E. Thumb Sucking

Occurs in 50 to 90% of all children; nonnutritive sucking occurs longer on the average than nutritive sucking during a typical day; do not try to stop until child is at least 4 years old; if > 4, then possible upper incisor protrusion may occur; the risk for dental problems is lower with pacifiers.

F. Enuresis

▶ Scientific Concepts

Ten to 20% of first-grade boys and 8 to 17% of first-grade girls; epidemiology—poverty, large family size, low birth weight, low intelligence quotient (IQ), poor speech and coordination, encopresis; family stresses such as a divorce may play a role; 97% nonpathological. Pathological causes include ectopic ureter, urinary tract infection (UTI), neurogenic bladder, bladder calculi, obstructive sleep apnea.

▶ Diagnostic Studies

Renal ultrasound, vesicourethrogram (VCUG), urinalysis, blood urea nitrogen (BUN), complete blood count (CBC), lytes.

▶ Clinical Therapeutics

Desmopressin acetate and imipramine; normal bladder capacity of child in ounces is child's age + 2.

G. Encopresis

▶ Scientific Concepts

Occurs in 2% of 8-year-old boys and 0.7% of 8-year-old girls. May lead to megacolon.

▶ History & Physical

Distended loops of bowel, tight sphincter tone, fistulas, pus and mucus on undergarments.

▶ Diagnosis

Differential includes Hirschsprung's, disorders of intestinal motility, disorders of anal tone and anatomy, spina bifida.

▶ Clinical Therapeutics

Dietary manipulation, laxatives, and enemas.

V. ANEMIA, BLEEDING DISORDERS, LYMPHADENOPATHY

A. Physiologic Anemia

▶ Scientific Concepts

Newborn has high hemoglobin and hematocrit; progressive decline from week 1 to 8 secondary to cessation of erythropoiesis with onset of respiration and expansion of blood volume.

▶ Diagnostic Studies

Hemoglobin and hematocrit, ferritin.

▶ Diagnosis

Vitamin E and folic acid deficiencies, failure to thrive.

▶ Clinical Therapeutics

Transfusion, but large transfusion may inhibit erythropoiesis.

B. Iron Deficiency Anemia

▶ Scientific Concepts

Most common hematologic disease of infancy; most common cause is dietary deficiency. Need to have daily intake to counterbalance losses. Most common in ages 9 to 24 months.

▶ History & Physical

Pallor, then irritability, anorexia, tachycardia, cardiac dilation, systolic murmurs, splenomegaly, pica.

▶ Diagnostic Studies

Ferritin < 10 mg/mL; serum iron < 30 g/dL; reticulocyte count > 600,000; hypochromic microcytic anemia with anisocytosis and poikilocytosis (basophilic stippling with lead poisoning).

▶ Diagnosis

Peptic ulcer, Meckel's diverticulum, polyps, hemangiomas, chronic intestinal blood loss by ingestion of cow's milk.

▶ Clinical Therapeutics

Supplementation with 4 to 6 mg/kg of elemental iron in three divided doses for at least 4 to 6 weeks; adequate response is increase of hemoglobin > 1 g/dL in 10 days.

▶ Health Maintenance Issues

Children at increased risk for lead poisoning secondary to pica. Prophylactic iron supplementation for all but exclusively breast-fed infants.

C. Megaloblastic Anemias

▶ Scientific Concepts

Uncommon, peaks at 4 to 7 months, secondary to deficient intake of folic acid in diets of goat's milk or to B_{12} deficiency.

▶ History & Physical

Pallor, irritability, failure to thrive, chronic diarrhea.

▶ Diagnostic Studies

Smear with macrocytic red blood cells (RBCs), increased indices, low reticulocyte count, and low serum folate levels.

▶ Diagnosis

Associated with thrombocytopenia, neutropenia, hypersegmentation; confused with aplastic anemias or leukemia.

▶ Clinical Therapeutics

Change formula.

▶ Health Maintenance Issues

B_{12} deficiency may lead to neurological abnormalities.

D. Folic Acid Deficiency Anemia

▶ Scientific Concepts

Infants require 10 times more folate/body weight than adults; folic acid absorbed through small intestine. Etiologies include celiac disease, chronic infectious enteritis, and enteroenteric fistulas; other etiology is phenytoin or trimethoprim.

▶ Diagnostic Studies

Smear with macrocytic RBCs, increased indices, low serum folate levels of < 140 ng/mL.

▶ Clinical Therapeutics

Folate 0.5 to 1.0 mg/d to start then 0.05 to 0.10 mg/d.

E. Sickle Cell Anemia

▶ Scientific Concepts

Countries associated—all of Africa, Italy, Greece, Middle East, and India; those with homozygosity for the sickle gene have disease and those heterozygous have the trait.

▶ History & Physical

Symptoms do not appear before 6 months; painful or vaso-occlusive crises with painful swelling of the hands and feet secondary to infarctions of the small bones, severe abdominal pain, cerebrovascular accidents (CVAs), pulmonary consolidation, splenomegaly, aplastic crisis; pain precipitated by cold, dehydration, infection, stress but mostly indeterminate; about one-third develop pneumococcal sepsis in first 5 years.

► Diagnostic Studies

Hemoglobin electrophoresis conclusive study.

► Clinical Therapeutics

Consider patient as a compromised host; no antisickling drugs, narcotics for pain, correct dehydration and infections; prophylactic penicillin to prevent sepsis, bone marrow transplants.

F. Coagulation Disorders

► Scientific Concepts

Platelet disorders, clotting factor abnormalities.

► History & Physical

Questions—bleeding with circumcisions; immunizations; tooth eruption; after minor trauma; frequent epistaxis; drug intake such as aspirin, anticonvulsants, antibiotics, ingestion of warfarin containing rat poison; purpura, mucosal bleeding with platelet disorders, soft-tissue bleeding, hemarthrosis with plasma clotting factors, hepatomegaly, splenomegaly, angiomatous skin and mucous membrane lesions in child with GI bleeding with hereditary hemorrhagic telangiectasia.

► Diagnosis

Consider thrombocytosis, von Willebrand's, disseminated intravascular coagulation (DIC), vitamin K deficiency.

► Clinical Therapeutics

Treat underlying abnormality.

G. Lymphadenopathy

► Scientific Concepts

May be pathologic or nonpathologic; *Staphylococcus aureus* and *Streptococcus pyogenes* most common infectious; noninfectious collagen vascular disease, Kawasaki's, thyroglossal duct cyst, cystic hygroma, neoplasms.

► History & Physical

Prior illness, exposure to cats (cat scratch fever and toxoplasmosis), travel with histoplasmosis in southeastern United States, coccidioidomycosis in California. Measure size of nodes at widest diameter; note redness, tenderness, warmth, mobility, hepatomegaly, splenomegaly; lymph drainage in anatomical pattern, tender nodes with infection and fixed hard nodes with malignancy.

► Diagnostic Studies

Aspirate for culture and sensitivity, CBC, erythrocyte sedimentation rate (ESR), liver function test (LFT), purified protein derivative (PPD), throat cultures, viral studies, antinuclear antibody (ANA), rheumatoid factor (RF), biopsy to rule out lymphoma.

► Clinical Therapeutics
Antibiotics, PPD, surgical removal/biopsy if present > 3 months.

► Health Maintenance Issues
Awareness of travel, presence of cats.

H. Hodgkin's Versus Non-Hodgkin's Lymphoma

► Scientific Concepts
Hodgkin's peaks in adolescence, similar human lymphocyte antigen (HLA) typing in families; more common in higher socioeconomic groups. Non-Hodgkin's lymphoma (NHL) is 1.5 times as common as Hodgkin's; peak age is 7 to 11 years; seen with varied inherited disorders, chronic immunosuppressive therapy, long-term phenytoin usage.

► History & Physical
Hodgkin's with painless lymphadenopathy of cervical, supraclavicular, axillary, or inguinal nodes noted incidentally; night sweats, fever; weight loss; affected nodes rubbery, nontender, and may be matted; NHL: 30% with GI involvement with right lower quadrant pain, nausea, vomiting, and abdominal distention; 25% with mediastinal involvement including the superior vena cava syndrome (plethora/edema of face, neck, and upper chest with dilated veins in these areas); tonsils and nasopharynx may be affected.

► Diagnostic Studies
Hodgkin's: Must obtain lymph node for pathology; CBC, ESR to follow success of treatment, chest x-ray (CXR) to ascertain mediastinal adenopathy, computed tomographic (CT) scan.
NHL: Must obtain lymph node or remove mass; the following as needed—CBC, bone marrow aspirate, lumbar puncture, LFTs, BUN/creatinine, uric acid, phosphorus, calcium, gallium or technetium bone scan, CT of chest, pelvis, abdomen.

► Diagnosis
Staging of Hodgkin's and non-Hodgkin's similiar but not the same.

► Clinical Therapeutics
Hodgkin's: Radiation preferred treatment, varied chemotherapeutic agents, combination therapy beneficial.
NHL: Chemotherapy, surgery for resection of lesions, radiation for head/neck involvement, bone marrow transplantation.

VI. CARDIOVASCULAR DISEASES

► Epidemiology and Prevalence of Congenital
  Heart Disease
Eight per 1,000 live-born infants have a heart malformation; 25% of beds in pediatric intensive care unit secondary to heart disease.

Frequency of common defects: ventricular septal defect (VSD), 30%; patent ductus, 8.6%; pulmonary stenosis, 7.4%; atrial septal defect (ASD), 6.7%; aortic coarctation, 5.7%; tetralogy of Fallot, 5.1%.

A. Transposition of the Great Vessels

▶ Scientific Concepts

Aorta originates from right ventricle, pulmonary artery from left ventricle; therefore, principal problem is severe hypoxia.

▶ History & Physical

Cyanosis with or without murmur, loud single second heart sound and a prominent right ventricular impulse.

▶ Diagnostic Studies

Electrocardiogram (ECG) with right axis deviation (RAD) and right ventricular hypertrophy (RVH) (normal in newborn), echocardiogram (ECHO) important for diagnosis.

▶ Clinical Intervention

Surgical with arterial switch repair, including transplantation of both coronary arteries into the reconnected aorta.

▶ Health Maintenance Issues

Prognosis unknown for the latest techniques, atrial arrhythmias for techniques of the 1960s and 1970s.

B. Tetralogy of Fallot

▶ Scientific Concepts

Spectrum of abnormalities that have in common a large unrestrictive VSD, dextroposition of the right aorta, subpulmonary stenosis, and RVH.

▶ History & Physical

Asymptomatic to severely hypoxic; systolic murmur heard best over left sternal border; may be associated with cleft lip and palate, hypospadias, skeletal malformations, Klippel–Feil syndrome (congenital cervical vertebral body anomalies); cyanosis secondary to increase in left-to-right shunting; exertional dyspnea, decreased exercise intolerance, squatting is position of comfort; episodes of paroxysmal hypoxemia occur, are self-limited, last < 30 minutes, occur mostly in morning, precipitated by fright, characterized by increasing cyanosis and increased rate and depth of respiration; clubbing if severe pulmonary stenosis.

▶ Diagnostic Studies

CXR with "boot-shaped" heart, enlargement of right ventricle with concavity of the upper left heart border secondary to absence of the main pulmonary artery segment; ECHO with increased blood flow in main pulmonary artery.

► Clinical Intervention

Subpulmonary stenosis worsens with age; medical management for secondary polythycemia, etc.; definitive treatment surgical with modified Blalock–Taussig shunt.

C. Hypoplastic Left Heart Syndrome

► Scientific Concepts

Term describes a spectrum of disease, usually with underdeveloped left ventricle and ascending aorta, mitral stenosis, mitral hypoplasia, or mitral atresia; male preponderance.

► History & Physical

Normal at birth, symptoms develop by day 2 to 3 with cyanosis, tachypnea, tachycardia, absent peripheral pulses, occasional rales, soft grade I/VI systolic murmur at left sternal border.

► Diagnostic Studies

ECG with right axis deviation (RAD) and RVH; CXR with increased vascular markings; ECHO definitive.

► Clinical Intervention

Surgical reconstruction or transplantation.

D. Atrial Septal Defects

► Scientific Concepts

Third most common congenital heart defect; hole in septum between right and left ventricle; small defects of no hemodynamic significance, larger defects with shunting of blood.

► History & Physical

Symptoms range from asymptomatic to exercise intolerance; CHF; atrial arrhythmias, often with decreased height and weight; cyanosis; hypoplastic thumb; heart sounds: first sound split, pulmonary systolic murmur that peaks in early systole; crescendo–decrescendo murmurs, fixed wide splitting of the second heart sound; diastolic murmurs are middiastolic.

► Diagnostic Studies

ECG sinus rhythm usually, atrial arrhythmias after second decade, CXR with cardiac enlargement and increased pulmonary vascularity, ECHO diagnostic.

► Clinical Intervention

Large defect surgically closed.

E. Ventricular Septal Defects

► Scientific Concepts

Most common cardiac abnormality in children; hole in septum between right and left ventricle that may occur in either the membraneous or solid part of the septum.

► History & Physical

Harsh, high-pitched, holosystolic murmur heard best at left sternal border; first and second heart sounds normal; large defects may cause CHF without murmur.

► Diagnostic Studies

ECG with left ventricular hypertrophy (LVH) if large defect, ECHO diagnostic.

► Clinical Therapeutics

Medical management of CHF.

► Clinical Intervention

Surgical repair if medical treatment fails—small defects close spontaneously.

F. Patent Ductus Arteriosus

► Scientific Concepts

Persistence of a normal fetal blood vessel that connects the main pulmonary artery with the descending aorta; second most common heart defect.

► History & Physical

Hypoxia from high altitude, pulmonary disease, and rubella during first trimester may predispose to patent ductus, incidental murmur to florid heart failure, propensity to pulmonary infections, continuous murmur, maximum at the first and second left intercostal spaces at the left midclavicular line, bounding pulses.

► Diagnostic Studies

ECG with LVH and atrial enlargement, CXR with cardiomegaly, prominent main artery segment, large ascending aorta and arch and increased pulmonary vasculature markings, ECHO diagnostic.

► Clinical Intervention

Generally closes by itself within several weeks of birth. If severe at birth, pharmacological closure with indomethacin. Surgical intervention by age 2 to 3 years if above not effective.

G. Coarctation of the Aorta

► Scientific Concepts

A constrictive ring of tissue distal to the left subclavian artery. Increased in males and Turner's syndrome.

► History & Physical

Need blood pressures in all four extremities—elevated in upper and decreased in lower; no true cardiac symptoms; discrepancy in pulses when taking brachial and femoral in regard to timing and pulse volume; left-sided infraclavicular murmur, right upper sternal border thrill.

► Diagnostic Studies

ECG normal at birth, later with LVH; CXR with normal heart size, reverse 3 sign (dilatation of the aorta, coarctation, postcoarctation dilatation), rib notching secondary to enlargement of the intercostal collaterals.

► Clinical Intervention

Anticongestive measures, surgical.

H. Rheumatic Fever

► Scientific Concepts

Sequela to upper respiratory infection (URI) with group A beta-hemolytic strep, diffuse inflammatory disease that involves the heart, blood vessels, joints, central nervous system (CNS), and subcutaneous tissues; occurs most commonly in the winter and spring as does pharyngitis.

► History & Physical

Antecedent streptococcal pharyngitis 1 to 5 weeks prior to symptoms; Jones criteria major: polyarthritis of large joints, carditis with apical systolic murmur, ECG with prolongation of PR and QT intervals, second-degree or complete block; chorea, subcutaneous nodules on extensor surfaces and bony prominences of the arms and legs, erythema marginatum over trunk and proximal parts of the limbs. Jones criteria minor: pallor, epistaxis, fever, tachycardia, anorexia, weight loss.

► Diagnostic Studies

Increased ESR, C-reactive protein, and antistreptolysin-O (ASO). May see anemia and leukocytosis.

► Diagnosis

Use Jones criteria.

► Clinical Therapeutics

Treat streptococcal pharyngitis, antibiotics, aspirin, steroids.

► Health Maintenance Issues

Must treat and follow up group A beta-hemolytic streptococcal pharyngitis.

VII. GASTROINTESTINAL DISORDERS

A. Vomiting

► Scientific Concepts

Vomiting is forceful expulsion of food, regurgitation is effortless, rumination is voluntary induction of regurgitation; 50% of infants have spitting up or vomiting as isolated complaint; occurs secondary to various stimuli.

► History & Physical

A.M. vomiting without nausea may be secondary to increased ICP; check ears for otitis; abdominal masses; peristaltic waves with pyloric stenosis.

► Diagnosis

Infants: Structural abnormalities—the higher the lesion, the earlier the symptoms; esophageal atresia; overfeeding in bottle-fed infants (not really vomiting but parents call it that); food allergies especially cow's milk; gastroesophageal reflux; rarely metabolic disorders, associated with otitis and URIs; pyloric stenosis.

Children: Usually gastroenteritis; URI; otitis; delayed gastric emptying secondary to diabetes mellitus; CNS problems; Reye's syndrome; medications, especially theophylline, erythromycin, and digitalis; appendicitis and other surgical lesions.

Adolescents: Ingestion of illicit drugs/alcohol, pregnancy, eating disorders, migraine.

► Diagnostic Studies

Stool for leukocytes, occult blood, and possibly viral cultures; CBC/differential, electrolytes, urinalysis, metabolic workup last; ultrasound or contrast-enhanced CT to rule out obstructive lesions.

► Clinical Therapeutics

Hydrate, PO better than IV, clear liquids, discourage antiemetics; further management dependent on diagnosis.

B. Diarrhea

► Scientific Concepts

Characterized by an increased volume of stool of looser consistency and increased frequency; average child with one episode yearly (more if in day care center) that may be associated with fever, vomiting, bloating, abdominal pain, dehydration, and weight loss; infants excrete 5 to 10 g/kg of stool daily. *Osmotic diarrhea*—stooling stops with cessation of diet; *secretory diarrhea*—bowel secretes water and electrolytes. Steatorrhea is fat in stools—occurs with giardiasis, liver, cystic fibrosis, pancreatic disease, and acute gastroenteritis; chronic diarrhea is defined as lasting > 2 weeks.

► History & Physical

Look for dehydration, growth retardation.

► Diagnosis

Most common cause is viral gastroenteritis, usually rotavirus, preceded by URI, followed by fever, vomiting, hypernatremia, and 10% with otitis. Bacterial causes include *Shigella, Salmonella, Campylobacter; Shigella/Campylobacter* with blood/mucus in stools, febrile, seizure prone; *Giardia, Entamoeba,* and *Cryptosporidium* need to be cultured separately; *Escherichia coli* with epidemic outbreaks and large explosive watery green stools without blood. Necrotizing enterocolitis with blood and watery stools in infants; consider food intolerance/allergies, overfeeding of fruit juices/sorbitol-containing products, cow milk intolerance with associated steatorrhea, growth retardation, anemia, hypoproteinemia, edema, eczema, eosinophilia, elevated IgE; inflammatory bowel disease, Crohn's, irritable bowel disease; antibiotics and heavy metals; cystic fibrosis with large, bulky, foul-smelling stools and failure to thrive. Celiac disease related to allergy to wheat proteins/gluten.

► Diagnostic Studies

Evaluate gross appearance; undigested food secondary to poor chewing; chemical and microscopic analysis for unabsorbed nutrients such as carbohydrates/fats; blood and leukocytes. Carmine red for fat; methylene blue for white blood cells (WBCs); ova/parasites; sodium, potassium, and osmolality; endoscopy last.

► Clinical Therapeutics

Hydrate and correct electrolyte imbalances, dietary manipulation with BRAT diet (bananas, rice, applesauce, toast). Antibiotics for pathogens such as *Shigella, Campylobacter,* and *Giardia.* DO NOT use antidiarrheal agents as this retains the toxins. Usually self-limited; may lead to malnutrition.

C. Constipation

► Scientific Concepts

Stools are hard, dry, and difficult to pass; about 3% of outpatient visits.

► History & Physical

Hard, dry stools; infrequent stooling; abdominal pain, hematochezia; painful defecation; anorexia; fecal soiling. Examination usually normal but may be able to palpate feces. Relaxed anal tone with spinal cord disease, tight sphincter with loose stools after exam with Hirschsprung's disease.

► Diagnostic Studies

Flat plate, barium enema, thyroid function tests, stool for botulism, rectal biopsy to rule out Hirschsprung's disease.

► Diagnosis

Hirschsprung's disease if meconium delayed > 24 hours, may not be diagnosed until age 5 to 6 years. Hypothyroidism—if secondary to hypopituitarism, not diagnosed through newborn screening process because of normal thyroid-stimulating hormone (TSH). Imperforate anus may not be recognized early. Botulism—constipation between the ages of 6 weeks and 6 months, history of exposure to honey, corn syrup, homegrown herbal teas; often febrile, hypotonic, lethargic with flattened facies, inability to gaze away from light shone directly in eye. Gentamicin administration may potentiate neuromuscular blockade and precipitate respiratory arrest; other considerations include medications such as aspirin, codeine, vincristine, anticholinergics, iron, bismuth (Pepto-Bismol), dehydration, neurologic disorders.

► Clinical Therapeutics

Dietary manipulation, discontinue iron, add fruit and vegetables, Maltsupex, *no* corn syrup. In older children, mineral oil, Milk of Magnesia, lactulose, cleanout enemas.

► Clinical Intervention

Surgical intervention for Hirschsprung's and imperforate anus.

D. Congenital Diaphragmatic Hernia

► Scientific Concepts

Varied presentations, 80% left-sided.

► History & Physical

Respiratory distress, scaphoid abdomen, absent breath sounds on affected side, displacement of the apical impulse.

► Diagnostic Studies

CXR positive.

► Clinical Therapeutics

Nitric oxide for pulmonary hypertension.

► Clinical Intervention

Surgical repair.

► Health Maintenance Issues

Lung on affected side hypoplastic, mediastinal shift, pulmonary infections, associated cardiac and GI abnormalities.

E. Hirschsprung's Disease

► Scientific Concepts

Absence of ganglion cells in the mucosal and muscular layers of the colon; rectum and rectosigmoid usually affected; increased in males and Down syndrome.

► History & Physical

Failure to pass meconium, then vomiting, abdominal distention, anorexia, bouts of enterocolitis; older children present with constipation with foul-smelling, ribbon-like stools. Examination with enlarged abdomen, prominent veins, peristaltic pattern visible, rectal exam without solid feces in anal canal, usually with gush of liquid stool as finger is withdrawn.

► Diagnostic Studies

Biopsy of bowel to detect ganglion cells; x-ray of abdomen with dilated proximal colon/absence of gas in pelvic colon; barium enema with narrowed segment distal to dilated portion.

► Clinical Intervention

Surgical with colostomy and resection of a ganglionic segment at 6 months of age.

► Health Maintenance Issues

Chronic constipation, fecal incontinence, strictures.

F. Acute Appendicitis

► Scientific Concepts

Most common childhood emergency surgery, obstruction of the appendix by fecaliths.

► History & Physical

Low-grade fever, periumbilical pain that localizes to right lower quadrant, peritonitis, anorexia, vomiting, constipation, diarrhea; localized mass, tenderness on rectal exam, positive psoas/obturator signs on some.

► Diagnostic Studies

Mild leukocytosis, negative urinalysis; ultrasound with noncompressible, thickened organ with localized fluid collection; human chorionic gonadotropin (HCG) in females at childbearing age, radiopaque fecalith on two-thirds of flat plates.

► Diagnosis

Pneumonia, URI, ectopic pregnancy, mechanical obstructions, and inflammatory diseases.

► Clinical Intervention

Appendectomy.

► Health Maintenance Issues

Appropriate postoperative antibiotics.

G. Intussusception

► Scientific Concepts

Most frequent obstruction in first 2 years of life; increased in males; associated with celiac disease, cystic fibrosis.

► History & Physical

Paroxysmal abdominal pain with drawing up of knees; vomiting, diarrhea afterward, then bloody bowel movement or "currant jelly stools"; fever, tender, distended abdomen with palpable sausage-shaped mass in the upper midabdomen. May last several days and be recurrent.

► Clinical Therapeutics

Conservative with diagnostic and therapeutic barium enema.

► Clinical Intervention

If barium enema not effective, surgical correction.

H. Hypertrophic Pyloric Stenosis

► Scientific Concepts
Hypertrophy of circular muscle of pylorus, increased in males and full-term; possible defect in innervation.

► History & Physical
Nonbilious vomiting during the first few weeks after birth with increasing intensity of vomiting to projectile; infants take feedings; dehydration; abdominal exam may yield palpation of "olive," hypochloremic hypokalemic metabolic alkalosis.

► Diagnostic Studies
Flat plate with absence of air distal to pylorus, barium with "string sign," ultrasound with thickened and elongated pylorus.

► Clinical Therapeutics
Correction of dehydration/electrolyte imbalance.

► Clinical Intervention
Pylorotomy.

I. Neonatal Jaundice

► Scientific Concepts
Breakdown of heme; metabolism of heme is not complete in the newborn; defective bilirubin conjugation.

► History & Physical
Irritability, vomiting, poor feeding with metabolic disorders; check jaundice in skin/sclera, unusual facies, hepatomegaly, other masses.

► Diagnosis
Physiologic jaundice peaks at 3 to 5 days postpartum, breast milk jaundice at 2 to 3 weeks; hemolytic disease; erythrocyte defects, glucose-6-phosphate dehydrogenase (G6PD); polycythemia; vitamin K; varied syndromes; antibiotics. Intestinal obstruction for unconjugated hyperbilirubinemia; for conjugated hyperbilirubinemia intrahepatic disorders, alpha-1-antitrypsin deficiency, cystic fibrosis, hepatitis.

► Diagnostic Studies
Need to differentiate unconjugated from conjugated hyperbilirubinemia; peripheral blood smear to rule out hemolysis, blood and urine cultures, viral titers, thyroid function tests, sweat chloride, alpha-1-antitrypsin phenotype, urine Clinitest to rule out galactosemia, scintigraphy to rule out hepatitis, ultrasound for choledochal cyst/cholelithiasis, biopsy.

► Clinical Therapeutics
Photochemical reduction for unconjugated hyperbilirubinemia.

► Health Maintenance Issues
Kernicterus with subsequent neurologic problems.

VIII. RESPIRATORY DISORDERS

A. Sinusitis

▶ Scientific Concepts

One to 5% of URIs complicated by sinusitis; predominant organisms are *Streptococcus pneumoniae, Moraxella,* and *H. influenzae;* adenoviruses, parainfluenza, and rhinoviruses may be present.

▶ History & Physical

Nasal discharge, cough at night, malodorous breath, periorbital swelling, rarely facial pain, mucopurulent discharge in nose or posterior pharynx, nasal mucosa erythematous, throat with moderate injection, no lymphadenopathy, possible tenderness over the sinuses; transillumination rarely helpful.

▶ Diagnostic Studies

X-ray with air–fluid levels or opacification of sinus cavities (air–fluid level rare in children < 5 years); CT is best way to diagnose. Aspiration gives precise diagnosis; nasal, throat, or nasopharyngeal cultures do not reflect bacteria in sinuses.

▶ Clinical Therapeutics

Antimicrobials such as amoxicillin, erythromycin, trimethoprim-sulfamethoxazole (TMP-SMZ), cefaclor.

▶ Clinical Intervention

Enlargement of natural meatus.

▶ Health Maintenance Issues

Complications include orbital abscess/cellulitis, optic neuritis, frontal osteomyelitis, epidural abscess, subdural empyema, sagittal sinus thrombosis, meningitis, brain abscess.

B. Pharyngitis

▶ Scientific Concepts

Etiologic agents are more often viruses, with adenovirus most common, then influenza, parainfluenza; bacterial etiologies are group A beta-hemolytic strep, *Mycoplasma pneumoniae, Chlamydia,* and *Neisseria gonorrhoeae* (in sexually active teens).

▶ History & Physical

Fever, conjunctivitis, exudates; may be associated with headache, nausea, vomiting, and occasionally abdominal pain. Examination with pharyngeal erythema, tonsillar enlargement, cervical adenitis; follicular, ulcerative, and petechial lesions. Cannot make diagnosis by visualization only.

▶ Diagnostic Studies

Rapid cultures specific but may lack sensitivity; streptococcal infections must be diagnosed because of sequelae.

► Clinical Therapeutics

Supportive, specific treatment pending cultures.

► Health Maintenance Issues

Untreated may lead to rheumatic fever, glomerulonephritis. Keep child out of school until cultures return.

C. Otitis Externa

► Scientific Concepts

Etiologies include trauma, swimming, excessive cleaning, high temperature and humidity; *S. aureus, Pseudomonas,* group A strep, often polymicrobial.

► History & Physical

Ear pain, itching, and fullness; purulent discharge with red/swollen walls; ipsilateral cervical lymph node enlargement; pain on pulling the pinna or movement of the tragus.

► Clinical Therapeutics

Remove moist cerumen, keep canal dry. Topical antibiotic and steroid drops (e.g., Cortisporin otic suspension) are usually sufficient for most infections.

D. Otitis Media

► Scientific Concepts

One-third of all pediatric visits, increased in boys, most common from 6 to 36 months. Predisposing factors include cleft palate, poverty, bottle feeding in horizontal position, secondhand smoke, day care attendance, winter months. Organisms are *Streptococcus pneumoniae, H. influenzae, Moraxella.*

► History & Physical

Fever, otalgia, hearing loss, irritability, anorexia, loose stools, scratching at ears. Examination reveals hyperemic opaque tympanic membrane (TM) with distorted or absent light reflex, pneumatic otoscopy with decreased or no movement of TM; redness alone may be secondary to crying.

► Clinical Therapeutics

Acetaminophen, local heat, antibiotics acutely such as amoxicillin, TMP-SMZ, erythromycin, cefuroxime, axetil, cefixime, amoxicillin/clavulanate or prophylactic prescription with amoxicillin or sulfisoxazole if > three episodes in the past 6 months.

► Clinical Intervention

Pneumococcal vaccine, myringotomy tubes.

► Health Maintenance Issues

Complications include purulent labyrinthitis, mastoiditis, osteomyelitis of temporal bone, facial nerve paralysis, epidural and subdural abscesses, meningitis, lateral sinus thrombosis, brain abscesses.

E. Epiglottitis

▶ Scientific Concepts

This is an emergency situation. Ninety percent by *H. influenzae, S. aureus, S. pyogenes,* and *S. pneumoniae;* viral causes are parainfluenza and herpes; usually 2 to 7 years of age; year-round.

▶ History & Physical

Abrupt onset of sore throat and dysphagia, high temperatures; shortly thereafter, child becomes toxic, has respiratory distress, prefers to sit up, drools when leans forward; cough, hoarseness, stridor late if at all; onset of symptoms to arrival in emergency room about 12 hours.

▶ Diagnosis

Laryngotracheobronchitis with secondary bacterial infection, uvulitis, diphtheria.

▶ Diagnostic Studies

Lateral neck x-ray with "thumb sign"; diagnosis confirmed in operating room under direct visualization.

▶ Clinical Therapeutics

Secure the airway, IV antibiotics.

▶ Health Maintenance Issues

Rifampin prophylaxis to those in close contact and susceptible to *H. influenzae* type b disease; complications include death, pulmonary edema.

F. Croup

▶ Scientific Concepts

Most common between 1 and 3 years; boys > girls; etiologies include parainfluenza, respiratory syncytial virus (RSV), adenoviruses.

▶ History & Physical

Starts as cold with nasal congestion, sore throat, cough and fever, slow development; disturbing the child increases the likelihood of crying and further laryngeal swelling. As laryngeal inflammation increases, respiratory distress develops.

▶ Clinical Therapeutics

Cool mist, racemic epinephrine, corticosteroids may be helpful, oxygen, IV hydration.

G. Sudden Infant Death Syndrome

▶ Scientific Concepts

A leading cause of death in infancy, unexplained, peaks at 2 months, occurs mostly at night, increase during peak respiratory virus season, male predominance; history of low birth weight, maternal drug addiction, and smoking; family history; association with prone position, history of hypoxia, apnea.

H. Foreign Body Aspiration

► Scientific Concepts

Peaks at 6 months to 4 years; principally small objects such as peanuts, hard candy, toys.

► History & Physical

Upper: Respiratory distress, laryngospasm, stridor, sudden onset; if partial, child may be able to vocalize and cough; if complete, aphonia and cyanosis.
Lower: Large airway obstruction with respiratory distress; in lower respiratory tract, cough and wheeze may resolve only to recur; asymmetric breath sounds.

► Diagnostic Studies

Inspiratory and expiratory CXRs, with former showing hyperinflation of a segment and possibly the object itself.

► Clinical Intervention

Upper: Allow child to cough, if < 1 year, deliver five measured back blows with heel of hand with child face down, then five rapid chest compressions as per basic life support; do not probe blindly, possible emergency intubation, tracheostomy, needle cricothyrotomy.
Lower: Bronchoscopy followed by beta-adrenergic nebulizer treatment. If upper not treated, progressive cyanosis, loss of consciousness, seizures, bradycardia and cardiac arrest, with lower bronchiectasis and lung abscess.

► Health Maintenance Issues

Monitoring small objects, toys, and food.

I. Bronchiolitis

► Scientific Concepts

Common in winter in children < 2 years; RSV most common, then parainfluenza, influenza, adenovirus, *Mycoplasma, Chlamydia, Ureaplasma, Pneumocystis.*

► History & Physical

With RSV, 1 to 2 days of fever, rhinorrhea, cough then wheezing, tachypnea, respiratory distress, shallow breathing, nasal flaring, cyanosis, retractions, rales/rhonchi.

► Diagnostic Studies

Mild lymphocytosis, CXR with hyperinflation, mild interstitial infiltrates.

► Clinical Therapeutics

Oxygen, oximeter, hydration, intake and output, beta-adrenergics and corticosteroids, rapid diagnostic testing for RSV, ribavirin for hospitalized patients, RSV immune globulin (RespiGam) for infants at risk.

J. Cystic Fibrosis

► Scientific Concepts

Most common lethal genetic disease in the United States; median survival ~ 28 years.

► History & Physical

Fifteen percent with meconium ileus at birth, 50% with failure to thrive, respiratory compromise, frequent respiratory infections with *Staphylococcus aureus* and later *Pseudomonas aeruginosa*, productive cough, rales, clubbing, decreased exercise tolerance. Other system involvement includes GI with abdominal distention; bulky, greasy stools; flatulence; hypoalbuminemia; edema; hepatomegaly; inspissated stools; rarely portal hypertension; > 95% of males and 50% of females infertile.

► Diagnostic Studies

Elevated immunoreactive trypsinogen, sweat chloride > 60 mmol/L; pulmonary function studies with decreased flow rates.

► Clinical Therapeutics

Pancreatic enzyme supplementations for GI, no dietary restrictions. For respiratory, chest physical therapy, antibiotics, bronchodilators, anti-inflammatory agents (NSAIDs).

► Health Maintenance Issues

Side effects from steroids, questionable effectiveness of lung transplants and gene therapy.

K. Pneumonias

► Scientific Concepts

Viral: RSV, parainfluenza, and influenza for > 75% of infections.
Myocoplasmal: Two- to 3-week incubation; onset of symptoms is slow.
Hypersensitivity: Exposure to birds/bird droppings or organic dusts such as moldy hay, compost, tree bark, aerosols.
Bacterial: S. pneumoniae, H. influenzae, S. aureus.

► History & Physical

Viral: Preceded by URI, wheezing, stridor, cough, retractions, grunting, nasal flaring, rales, decreased breath sounds.
Mycoplasmal: Fever, cough, headache, malaise, sputum production later, associated sore throat, otitis media, rales, decreased breath sounds, dullness to percussion. Complications include hemolytic anemia, coagulation defects, thrombocytopenia, cerebral infarction, Guillain–Barré syndrome, cranial nerve involvement, psychosis, erythema multiforme, Steven–Johnson syndrome.
Hypersensitivity: Episodic cough/fever, chronic exposure with weight loss, fatigue, dyspnea, cyanosis, death.

S. pneumoniae: Abrupt onset of fever, restlessness, and respiratory distress with diminished breath sounds, crackles, and dullness on the affected side.
H. influenzae: No unique findings.
S. aureus: Rapid progression of respiratory distress in a toxic-appearing child, formation of pneumatoceles and empyema.

► Diagnostic Studies

Viral: Mild leukocytosis, rapid viral diagnostic tests, CXR with perihilar streaking, increased interstitial markings, patchy bronchopneumonia, lobar consolidation, hyperinflation, pneumatoceles with adenovirus.
Mycoplasmal: CBC and differential normal, cold hemagglutinin titer > 1:64 supports diagnosis; CXR with interstitial or bronchopneumonic infiltrates in middle or lower lobes.
Hypersensitivity: Eosinophilia, obstruction on pulmonary function test acutely, restrictive chronically.
S. pneumoniae: Leukocytosis, positive blood cultures, and CXR with lobar consolidation.
H. influenzae: CXR with lobar consolidation, positive tracheal, blood, urine, or pleural fluid cultures.
S. aureus: CXR with pneumatoceles, empyema, and pyopneumothorax; positive blood, pleural fluid, or bronchial washings.

► Diagnosis

Viral: Asthma, airway obstruction, viral/bacterial tracheitis.
Hypersensitivity: Asthma, collagen-vascular, immunologic, interstitial disease.

► Clinical Therapeutics

Viral: Supportive care, rimantadine or amantadine hydrochloride for high-risk infants, respiratory isolation.
Mycoplasmal: Dehydration, antipyretics, erythromycin × 7 to 10 days.
Hypersensitivity: Elimination of precipitant, steroids.
S. pneumoniae: Penicillin or erythromycin.
H. influenzae: IV cefuroxime or cefotaxime.
S. aureus: Nafcillin and cloxacillin; cefazolin and cefuroxime also considered.

► Health Maintenance Issues

Viral: Most recover, but death possible in those with underlying cardiorespiratory disease or superimposed bacterial pneumonia.
Mycoplasmal: Excellent recovery if no extrapulmonary complications.

L. Asthma

► Scientific Concepts

Reversible, 5 to 10% of the population, increased in boys. Triggers include URI, allergic reactivity, foods, cigarette smoke, air pollution, cold air, exercise, rapid change in temperature, aspirin; "atopic triad" is exzema, seasonal rhinitis, and asthma.

► History & Physical

Wheezing, dyspnea, excessive secretions, "noisy" breathing, cough, intercostal and suprasternal retractions; may occur in the absence of wheezing. Examination with prolongation of expiration; wheezes; rhonchi; higher-pitched wheezing with increasing obstruction; silence with poor air exchange; restlessness; apprehension; cyanosis of lips, gums, and nail beds; pulsus paradoxus.

► Diagnostic Studies

Eosinophil accumulations in sputum, leukocytosis, elevated hematocrit, respiratory acidosis; CXR with hyperinflation, patchy atelectasis, flattening of diaphragm, decreased flow rates on pulmonary function test.

► Diagnosis

Croup, bronchiolitis, bronchopneumonia, pertussis, gastroesophageal reflux disease, cystic fibrosis.

► Clinical Therapeutics

Cromolyn sodium, nedocromil sodium, and inhaled steroids to control disease; if not controlled then methylxanthines, long-acting inhaled beta-2 agonists. If admitted to hospital—hydration, moisturized oxygen, arterial blood gases, atrovent with albuterol, corticosteroids, aminophylline, antibiotics if indicated, intubation.

► Health Maintenance Issues

Avoid allergins and aggravating factors; education; peak flow meters at home; spacer devices; exercise encouraged; close follow-up.

IX. MUSCULOSKELETAL AND RHEUMATOLOGIC DISORDERS

A. Osgood–Schlatter Disease

► Scientific Concepts

Related to growth and/or repetitive trauma (usually sports related).

► History & Physical

Swelling and pain over apophysis of proximal tibia at insertion of patellar ligament, activity worsens symptoms, often bilateral; more common in boys; may avulse patellar tendon from tibial tuberosity.

► Diagnostic Studies

Fragmentation of tibial tubercle, soft-tissue swelling.

► Diagnosis

Other fractures.

► Clinical Therapeutics
Rest, restrict activity, NSAIDs.

► Health Maintenance Issues
Symptoms resolve at termination of growth.

B. Scoliosis

► Scientific Concepts
Defined as > 10° coronal curve, but this is a finding, not a diagnosis; therefore, workup is needed.

► History & Physical
Usually discovered on routine exam; idiopathic is painless. If painful, consider other causes, question bowel/bladder function. If resolves in sitting position, may be leg length inequality; having patient bend over to touch toes shows asymmetry. Look for neurocutaneous markers secondary to spina bifida. If change in reflexes, consider neuromuscular etiology.

► Diagnostic Studies
Anterior posterior (AP) x-ray measuring curve with Cobb method (geometric measurement of the severity of a curve).

► Diagnosis
Idiopathic occurs during growth spurt, more common in females; curve may progress if onset before menses. Congenital associated cardiac and renal anomalies. Paralytic secondary to neuromuscular problems.

► Clinical Intervention
Idiopathic with > 25° curve gets bracing, surgical correction if > 50°. Congenital not braceable; if progressive, needs surgery. Paralytic is progressive and not braceable; surgery may be indicated.

► Health Maintenance Issues
Screening to detect early curves that may be corrected with bracing.

C. Legg–Calvé–Perthes Disease

► Scientific Concepts
Idiopathic with capital femoral epiphysis becomes avascular and is resorbed, then later revascularized. More common in short boys ages 4 to 10 years.

► History & Physical
Slowly progressive limp with groin and knee pain, decreased abduction, and inward rotation of hip.

► Diagnostic Studies
Plain x-ray sufficient to show abnormality.

► Clinical Intervention
Abduction bracing or surgery.

► Health Maintenance Issues
Eighteen to 36 months for healing after surgery.

D. Slipped Capital Femoral Epiphysis

► Scientific Concepts
Etiology not known; capital femoral epiphysis slips off metaphysis through the growth plate.

► History & Physical
Obese boys; insidious limp that becomes worse after vigorous activity; pain in knee, thigh, or groin; examination with outward rotation with hip flexion and reproduction of pain.

► Diagnostic Studies
AP and frog lateral views of hip show widening of physis with gross deformity as disease progresses.

► Clinical Intervention
Surgical emergency.

E. In-Toeing and Out-Toeing

► Scientific Concepts
Arises from foot, tibia, or femur; may be from intrauterine positioning except for femoral origin.

► History & Physical
With foot, curved lateral border of foot, may be flexible or rigid. With tibia inward, foot/thigh angle; with femur, increased inward hip rotation.

► Clinical Intervention
For foot, serial casting sometimes works; for others, none.

F. Developmental Dysplasia of Hip

► Scientific Concepts
Spectrum of problems; mechanical, genetic, hormonal factors as etiology.

► History & Physical
Positive Galiazzi (compares level of knees when patient flat on bed with legs flexed); Ortolani (hip clunk) and Barlow tests (the examiner attempts to dislocate the femur).

► Diagnostic Studies
X-ray and/or ultrasound confirm diagnosis.

► Clinical Intervention

Pavlik harness; closed or open reduction with spica cast.

G. Foot Abnormalities

Clubfoot: May be from intrauterine positioning, dysplasia, associated with birth defects; depending on etiology treatment ranges from stretching, serial casting to surgery.

Calcaneovalgus foot: Due to uterine positioning; dorsum of foot lies on tibia; resolves with stretching.

Vertical talus: Rare, usually of neurologic etiology, "rockerbottom" deformity, serial castings and surgery to treat.

Pes planus (flat feet): Flexible flat foot is usually benign; rigid may be associated with neurological disease, trauma, infection, tumors; orthotics appropriate but other treatments controversial.

H. Kawasaki Disease

► Scientific Concepts

Affects children < 5 years, boys > girls; has well-established criteria.

► History & Physical

Fever > 40°C × 5 days unresponsive to antibiotics <u>and</u> four of the following: extremity changes—palmar/plantar erythema, indurative edema, desquamation of hands/feet, Beau lines; polymorphous exanthem—changes often in perineum, urticaria, morbilliform papules, scarlatiniform erythroderma; lymphadenopathy—unilateral cervical, > 1.5 cm, firm, nonfluctuant; mucosal changes—erythema, dry fissured lips, strawberry tongue, erythema of propharyngeal mucosa; conjunctival injection—bilateral bulbar, limbal sparing, nonexudative, painless. Other symptoms include arthralgias, arthritis, abdominal pain, diarrhea, vomiting, hepatic dysfunction, irritability, urethritis.

► Diagnostic Studies

Elevation of cytokines.

► Diagnosis

Scarlatina, measles, Rocky Mountain spotted fever, erythema multiforme.

► Clinical Therapeutics

IV immunoglobulin, 2 gm/kg, and high-dose salicylates.

► Health Maintenance Issues

Coronary artery dilatation and aneurysms may occur.

I. Juvenile Rheumatoid Arthritis

► Scientific Concepts

Varied presentation secondary to immunogenetic factors.

► History & Physical

Three major patterns: acute febrile with salmon pink macular rash, arthritis, hepatosplenomegaly, leukocytosis, polyserositis, remission within a year; polyarticular chronic pain and swelling of joints in symmetric fashion, low-grade fever, fatigue, rheumatoid nodules, anemia possible; arthritis waxes and wanes, occasionally iridocyclitis; pauciarticular with chronic arthritis in few joints, asymptomatic iridocyclitis.

► Diagnostic Studies

RF-positive in ~ 15%; ANA with pauciarticular, ESR not specific; joint aspirate with 5,000 to 60,000 WBCs, mostly neutrophils, x-ray with soft-tissue swelling, regional osteoporosis, magnetic resonance imaging (MRI) with early joint damage.

► Diagnosis

Orthopedic problems, reactive arthritis, infections, collagen-vascular disease, neoplastic, psychological.

► Clinical Therapeutics

NSAIDs, aspirin, physical therapy, methotrexate, injectable gold salts, steroid injections, joint replacement; iridocyclitis should be treated by ophthalmologist.

► Health Maintenance Issues

If articular, may resolve; worse prognosis with those with hip involvement, RF-positive, synovitis.

J. Fracture Facts

► Scientific Concepts

Physeal (growth plate) and metaphyseal (ends of long bones) fractures are most common in children. Most frequent sites are clavicle, distal radius, distal ulna. Growth plate fractures classified by Salter–Harris method. Pathologic fractures often secondary to bone cysts. Distal fifth metacarpal fracture after teenager punches object in anger. Colles' fracture from fall on outstretched arms. Visibility of the posterior fat pad on an elbow x-ray is indicative of bleeding, inflammation, or fracture. In adolescent with wrist trauma, the scaphoid is commonly fractured leading to "snuffbox" tenderness with high risk for nonunion or avascular necrosis.

X. GENITOURINARY DISORDERS

A. Hematuria

► Scientific Concepts

Common, gross—red/brown urine versus microscopic which is 3 or more positive dipsticks and 6 or more RBCs per high-power field.

► History & Physical

Patients with microscopic present with dysuria; question trauma, recent skin infection, pharyngitis, dysuria, abdominal or flank pain. Examine for rashes/petechiae; palpate for renal masses; check for arthritis, funduscopic, peripheral edema; check genitalia; check blood pressure.

► Diagnostic Studies

First morning urine to differentiate upper/lower; if RBC casts, then ASO titer, ANA, C3 complement, CBC and differential, BUN/creatinine, albumin; if no casts, urinalysis for culture and sensitivity, platelets, prothrombin time and partial thromboplastin time (PT/PTT), sickle cell tests, renal ultrasound or CT, CXR.

► Diagnosis

Urinary tract infection (UTI), perineal irritation, meatal stenosis, trauma, coagulopathy, stones, nephritis, cystitis, tumors, vaginitis, prostatitis, renal artery or vein thrombosis, insertion of foreign objects into urethra, after vigorous exercise, hypercalciuria with secondary stones, hemolytic anemias, drug-induced hemolysis, mismatched blood transfusions, myoglobinuria secondary to rhabdomyolysis, varied drugs/dyes/pigments.

► Clinical Intervention

Treat underlying disease.

B. Proteinuria

► Scientific Concepts

Small amount normally present; levels may increase with exercise, fever, trauma, CHF, or surgery; dipstick detects albumin but not reliable in alkaline urine.

► History & Physical

Periorbital morning edema, check height/weight for gain/loss, blood pressure, impetigo to rule out strep infections, joints for swelling, ascites, organomegaly.

► Diagnostic Studies

If detected in asymptomatic patient, should be repeated. Best determined by timed collection (24-hour), orthostatic proteinuria with A.M./P.M. dipstick (A.M. neg/P.M. pos), urine protein/creatinine ratio, lytes, BUN, creatinine, serum protein and albumin, ANA, C3, ASO titer, hepatitis B surface antigen.

► Diagnosis

Glomerulonephritis, orthostatic.

► Health Maintenance Issues

If abnormal 24-hour collection, refer to nephrologist. If physiologic/orthostatic, evaluate annually/no restrictions on physical activity.

C. Posterior Urethral Valves

▶ Scientific Concepts

Rare, congenital, prostatic urethra, male only.

▶ History & Physical

Detected prenatally with ultrasound; at birth with distended bladder, palpable kidneys, UTI, renal insufficiency, poor stream; later with failure to thrive, vomiting, hematuria, enuresis, hesitancy.

▶ Diagnostic Studies

Ultrasound, voiding cystourethrogram best.

▶ Clinical Intervention

Transurethral catheter, correction of underlying medical problems, transurethral ablation of valves, temporary vesicostomy.

▶ Health Maintenance Issues

Best predictor is drop in serum creatinine after treatment, renal failure and dialysis in those whose creatinine stays > 1.0, vesicoureteral reflux, voiding problems.

D. Hypospadias

▶ Scientific Concepts

Maldevelopment of distal or anterior urethra, most common penile abnormality. Consider virilization disorder, familial tendency.

▶ History & Physical

Located anywhere along the shaft, midline scrotum, perineum; ventral foreskin absent.

▶ Clinical Intervention

Surgical at 6 to 18 months.

▶ Health Maintenance Issues

Repeat surgeries not uncommon; delay circumcision.

E. Vesicoureteral Reflux

▶ Scientific Concepts

Retrograde movement of urine into kidney.

▶ Diagnostic Studies

Voiding cystogram.

▶ Clinical Intervention

Low-dose prophylactic antibiotics, ureteral reimplantation.

▶ Health Maintenance Issues

Lower grades of reflux spontaneously resolve; increased incidence in siblings.

F. Cryptorchidism

▶ Scientific Concepts

Undescended testicles, 3 to 4% of full-term infants.

▶ History & Physical

Examination in warm environment, multiple positions, palpable/nonpalpable.

▶ Diagnosis

Retractile testes secondary to hyperactive cremasteric.

▶ Clinical Therapeutics

Intramuscular hCG controversial.

▶ Clinical Intervention

Surgical at 6 to 18 months.

▶ Health Maintenance Issues

Malignant degeneration, infertility.

G. Urinary Tract Infections

▶ Scientific Concepts

Second to URI; increased in males in neonatal period only, higher in uncircumcised.

▶ History & Physical

Dysuria, hematuria, incontinence, flank tenderness, lethargy, fever; in neonates, weight loss, irritability, fever, cyanosis, CNS disorders; vomiting, high fever, flank pain, lethargy with upper tract infections.

▶ Diagnostic Studies

Bladder tap; catherized specimen; clean catch, bagged, voiding cystourethrogram; after diagnosis ultrasound, intravenous pyelogram, nuclear scan to determine anatomy.

▶ Clinical Therapeutics

Seven- to 10-day course of antibiotics with follow-up culture, prophylactic antibiotics if needed.

H. Acute Poststreptococcal Glomerulonephritis

▶ Scientific Concepts

Most common postinfectious nephritis, possible genetic susceptibility, always preceded by group A streptococcal throat or skin infection with clinical glomerulonephritis 10 to 14 days later.

▶ History & Physical

Asymptomatic to renal failure, periorbital or peripheral edema, oliguria, CHF, hypertension, encephalopathy. Common presenting symptoms are hematuria, proteinuria, lethargy, anorexia, vomiting, fever, abdominal pain, headache.

▶ Diagnostic Studies

Urinalysis with RBC casts, serum ASO, antihyaluronidase (AHT) and anti-Ndase B (antideoxyribonuclease-B titer) titers, throat and skin cultures, depressed serum C3, BUN elevated disproportionately to creatinine.

▶ Diagnosis

Benign hematuria, IgA nephropathy, hereditary nephritis, idiopathic hypercalciuria.

▶ Clinical Therapeutics

Supportive, treat hypertension, restrict fluids versus diuretics, antistreptococcal antibiotics for throat/skin infections.

▶ Health Maintenance Issues

Full recovery in > 95%, some with chronic renal failure, hematuria/proteinuria for up to 3 months—if longer, question diagnosis, C3 raises after 8 weeks or diagnosis is membranoproliferative glomerulonephritis.

I. Ambiguous Genitalia

▶ Scientific Concepts

Intersex abnormality, pseudohermaphroditism, hermaphroditism, 1/4,000 live births.

▶ History & Physical

Varied, enlarged phallus, labioscrotal fusion, hyperpigmented labia, labial rugae, perineal hypospadias, inguinal hernia; look for nongenital dysmorphic features, palpate testes; hypospadias and cryptorchidism together associated with intersex disorder 50% of time.

▶ Diagnostic Studies

Serum 17-hydroxyprogesterone, urine 17-ketosteroids and pregnanetriol, karyotype, sex steroids, electrolytes, pelvic ultrasound/CT for müllerian structures.

▶ Diagnosis

Congenital adrenal hyperplasia, adrenogenital syndrome, maternal androgen ingestion, biochemical defects, chromosomal mosaicism.

▶ Clinical Therapeutics

Hormonal supplementation, cortisol for adrenogenital syndrome, surgical procedures after medical treatment.

▶ Health Maintenance Issues

Excellent prognosis; females with amenorrhea/sterility.

XI. PSYCHOLOGICAL AND DEVELOPMENTAL PROBLEMS

A. Mental Retardation

▶ Scientific Concepts

Describes symptom, not etiology. IQ < 70 on Wechsler; increased incidence in males; etiologies include inborn errors of metabolism, chromosomal, intrauterine infections, pre- or postmaturity, endocrinopathies, infections, poisoning, abuse, low family intelligence.

▶ History & Physical

Syndromic appearance, developmental delay, speech/swallowing problems, incoordination, seizures, behavioral, difficulty adapting.

▶ Diagnostic Studies

Metabolic screen, further workup if syndromic.

▶ Diagnosis

Autism.

▶ Health Maintenance Issues

Treat associated problems, impact on families, education, rehabilitation, protection.

B. Attention Deficit Hyperactivity Disorder

▶ Scientific Concepts

Increased in males; possible genetic link.

▶ History & Physical

Distractibility; short attention span; hyperactivity; impulsivity; previously evident, especially at school; > 6 months without associated psychosis, onset prior to age 7 years, neurological exam may be normal.

▶ Diagnostic Studies

ADD-H: Comprehensive Teachers Rating Scale (ACTeRS) profile.

▶ Diagnosis

Parents or teachers who are inexperienced or overly critical may provide attention deficit hyperactivity disorder history for child. Other disorders that may mimic include specific developmental disorders, anxiety, adjustment disorder, hyperthyroidism or drugs.

▶ Clinical Therapeutics

Behavior modification or psychiatric therapy prior to or concurrent with stimulants—methylphenidate (Ritalin), dextroamphetamine (Dexedrine).

► Health Maintenance Issues
Prognosis better with higher intellect.

C. Autism

► Scientific Concepts
Rare, increased in males, two-thirds with mental retardation, possible genetic association.

► History & Physical
Qualitative impairment in social interaction and communication and repetitive stereotypical patterns of behavior; infants fail to make eye contact; impaired imitation; self-injurious behavior.

► Diagnosis
Mental retardation.

► Health Maintenance Issues
Incurable, behavior modification, limited success with medication.

D. Child Abuse

► Scientific Concepts
Nonaccidental physical/psychological harm; wide spectrum from obvious trauma to failure to thrive.

► History & Physical
Family stress, unknown injury, injury not consistent with story, previous inadequate medical care, physical findings must match history; check genitalia and other orifices; retinal hemorrhages and full fontanelle with "shaken baby."

► Diagnostic Studies
Funduscopic, x-rays—extremities, skull and ribs, spiral fractures, chip fractures, skeletal survey shows multiple fractures in different stages of healing.

► Diagnosis
Platelet disorders, leukemia with bruising, rickets, osteogenesis imperfecta with fractures.

► Clinical Intervention
Protection of child is priority. Mandatory reporting in many states.

XII. NEUROLOGICAL PROBLEMS

A. Febrile Seizures

► Scientific Concepts
Fever may cause a solitary seizure in a patient without a seizure disorder or may provoke a seizure in a patient with a seizure disorder.

► **History & Physical**
Rapid onset of fever, normal neurological exam.

► **Diagnostic Studies**
Electroencephalogram (EEG) not indicated; consider lumbar puncture (LP).

► **Clinical Therapeutics**
Antipyretics, anticonvulsants not given for solitary febrile seizure.

► **Health Maintenance Issues**
Treating febrile seizures does not decrease the risk of afebrile seizures.

B. Weakness

► **Scientific Concepts**
Static versus evolving weakness, central versus peripheral, upper versus lower motor neuron.

► **History & Physical**
In older children, upper motor neuron lesions with spasticity, hyperreflexia, Babinski, lower with hypotonia, hyporeflexia, but in infancy may have overlap of symptoms; also cortical thumb, persistent primitive reflexes; Gower's maneuver.

► **Diagnosis**
Cerebral palsy, myelitis, spina bifida, polio, spinal muscle atrophy, inflammatory, hereditary polyneuropathies, myasthenia, botulism, muscular dystrophy.

► **Diagnostic Studies**
Electromyography/nerve conduction velocity (EMG/NCV), biopsy.

► **Clinical Therapeutics**
Treat underlying cause.

C. Abnormal Head Size

► **Scientific Concepts**
Brain growth drives skull growth, serial measurements with tape measure over the eyebrows anteriorly and occipital protuberance posteriorly, compare to growth charts; bulging anterior fontanelles seen with hydrocephalus, intracranial tumors, or arachnoid cysts.

► **History & Physical**
Head size is two or more standard deviations from normal; transillumination for macrocephaly.

► **Diagnosis**
Chromosomal syndromes, craniosynostosis, TORCH, radiation,

toxemia, familial, perinatal, hypoxia, metabolic, Tay–Sachs for microcephaly. Hydrocephalus, subdural hematomas, tumors, congenital, familial, achondroplasia for macrocephaly.

▶ Diagnostic Studies
TORCH screen, IgM, serum and urine amino acids for microcephaly, ultrasound/CT/MRI for macrocephaly.

▶ Clinical Intervention
Surgical for some macrocephaly, supportive for microcephaly.

D. Bacterial Meningitis

▶ Scientific Concepts
E. coli, group B streptococci, *Listeria monocytogenes*, *H. influenzae*, coagulase-negative staphylococci for 0 to 2 months; *S. pneumoniae*, *N. meningitidis*, *H. influenzae* for 2 months to 6 years; *S. pneumoniae*, *N. meningitidis* for 6 to 18 years.

▶ History & Physical
Headache, stiff neck, fever or hypothermia, hyperirritability, seizures, focal sensory/motor changes, Kernig's and Brudzinski's signs; bulging fontanelle and increased head size in newborns; papilledema and cranial nerve palsies in older children.

▶ Diagnostic Studies
CBC and differential, chemistry panel, obtain cerebrospinal fluid (CSF) (after intracranial mass is ruled out), expect increased polymorphonuclear leukocytes, elevated protein, decreased glucose (with viral, expect no or mild leukocytosis, elevated protein, and normal glucose), CT/MRI to rule out intracranial masses and show meningeal inflammation; EEG nonspecific.

▶ Clinical Therapeutics
Hydrate at two-thirds maintenance, correct electrolytes, acidosis, NPO. Empiric broad-spectrum antibiotics until Gram stain/culture returned: cefotaxime/ampicillin if < 3 months; ceftriaxone, cefo­taxime, or ampicillin/chloramphenicol for > 3 months, add vancomycin/rifampin if *S. pneumoniae* not ruled out.

▶ Health Maintenance Issues
Seizures, subdural effusions, cerebral edema; long-term effects include blindness, hearing loss, seizures, hydrocephalus, cranial nerve deficits, mental retardation, behavioral problems. Prevention with good hand washing and patient isolation.

E. Cerebral Palsy

▶ Scientific Concepts
Generic term, nonprogressive, varied, increased in small infants; intrauterine hypoxia/bleeding, infections, toxins, congenital malformations/infections, genetic.

► History & Physical

Impaired function of voluntary muscles—75% spastic, 15% ataxic, 5% dyskinetic, rarely hypotonic, any combination of limbs affected. Associated with seizures, mental retardation, speech/sensory deficits. Examination with claspknife rigidity, possible contractures, hyperactive reflexes, clonus, extensor plantar responses, decreased fine motor voluntary responses, "floppy infant," 25% microcephalic, smaller hand/foot.

► Diagnostic Studies

No routine studies, hip films to rule out dislocation, EEG, urine screening for amino and organic acidurias.

► Diagnosis

Progressive neurological change is *not* cerebral palsy; consider other neurological disorders/metabolic.

► Clinical Intervention

Physical and/or occupational therapy, special education, diazepam/baclofen for spasicity, family support, rhizotomy.

► Health Maintenance Issues

Ranges from resolution for mild to death for severe.

F. Amblyopia and Strabismus

► Scientific Concepts

Amblyopia is reduction in central visual acuity. Strabismus is misalignment of the visual axes of the two eyes.

► History & Physical

Amblyopia may occur in strabismic patient, with untreated refractive errors, with cataracts, media opacities, or complete ptosis. Strabismus with esotropia (excessively convergent) or exotropia (excessively divergent).

► Clinical Intervention

Amblyopia: Correct refractive errors, cataracts, opacities, visual rehabilitation, patching good eye.
Strabismus: Surgical correction, patching, glasses.

XIII. COMMON CHILDHOOD DISEASES

A. Respiratory Syncytial Virus

► Scientific Concepts

Accounts for most hospitalizations for pulmonary reasons of children < 2 years, midwinter and spring outbreaks, transmitted by nasal secretions.

► History & Physical

Four- to 7-day incubation, rhinorrhea, fever, irritability, poor feeding, progressive cough, wheezing and shortness of breath; younger infants may have lethargy, apnea; also with otitis media, pharyngeal hyperemia, conjunctivitis.

► Diagnostic Studies

WBC count variable, CXR with overaerated lungs, flat diaphragm, horizontal ribs, diminished heart size, nasal secretions positive via enzyme-linked immunosorbent assay (ELISA)/direct fluorescent antibody.

► Clinical Therapeutics

Oxygen, supportive, ribavirin, adrenergic bronchodilators, *no* steroids.

► Health Maintenance Issues

One percent morbidity, respiratory isolation, good handwashing techniques, gamma globulin with anti-RSV antibody for high-risk preterms. RSV immune globulin (RespiGam) for infants at high risk.

B. Infectious Mononucleosis

► Scientific Concepts

Epstein–Barr virus (EBV) is the etiologic agent.

► History & Physical

Fever, malaise, nontender cervical lymphadenitis, tonsillopharyngitis, hepatosplenomegaly, rhinitis, rash, abdominal pain, eyelid edema, failure to thrive, otitis media, possible rash with ampicillin administration.

► Diagnostic Studies

Atypical lymphocytes, relative neutropenia, mildly elevated serum transaminase levels; heterophil antibodies, EBV-specific serologic testing.

► Diagnosis

Bacterial/viral tonsillopharyngitis, phenytoin/isoniazid hypersensitivity reactions.

► Clinical Therapeutics

Bedrest, avoid ampicillin, artificial airway if respiratory compromise, steroids for swollen pharyngeal lymphoid tissue with secondary respiratory compromise.

► Health Maintenance Issues

Pneumonia, seizures, meningitis, thrombocytopenia, bacteremia, jaundice, glomerulonephritis; no contact sports for 6 to 8 weeks if patient has splenomegaly.

C. Roseola

► Scientific Concepts

Incidence 6 months to 3 years.

► History & Physical

Abrupt onset of fever to 40°C for 3 days, normal appetite/behavior. Examination shows eyelid edema, suboccipital lymphadenopathy, pharyngeal erythema, bulging fontanelle, pale pink macular rash of neck/trunk after fever breaks for 1 to 2 days.

► Diagnostic Studies

Mild WBC elevation with neutrophilia, also with relative lymphocytosis.

► Clinical Therapeutics

Acetaminophen.

► Health Maintenance Issues

Febrile seizures.

D. Varicella-Zoster (Chickenpox)

► Scientific Concepts

Lifelong immunity; virus lies in dorsal root ganglion and may reappear as "shingles"; infectious 1 to 4 days prior to rash; transmitted via sneezing; most cases in spring.

► History & Physical

Macule to papule to vesicle to crusted visicle, trunk and extremities; prodrome with malaise and low-grade fever, progresses in stages.

► Diagnostic Studies

Rarely need antigen detection studies.

► Clinical Therapeutics

Acetaminophen, Calamine lotion, diphenhydramine HCl. If immunosuppressed, varicella-zoster immune globulin, acyclovir early, vaccination.

► Health Maintenance Issues

Secondary bacterial infection of lesions, pneumonitis, hepatitis, arthritis, pericarditis, glomerulonephritis, meningitis, myelitis. Prevention with vaccination.

E. Rubella (German Measles)

► History & Physical

Prodrome in older children with low-grade fever, coryza, conjunctivitis, cough and lymphadenopathy, soft palate erythematous pinpoint Forschheimer spots; rash that descends and is erythematous, discrete, maculopapular, noncoalescing, rarely encephalitis.

▶ Diagnosis

Viral isolates from nasopharyngeal secretions, enzyme immunoassay, latex agglutinations, indirect immunofluorescence.

▶ Clinical Therapeutics

Supportive, acetaminophen, aspirin for rubella arthritis only.

▶ Health Maintenance Issues

Prevention with vaccination.

F. Rubeola (Measles)

▶ Scientific Concepts

Highly contagious, transmitted via respiratory secretions, winter/spring disease.

▶ History & Physical

Incubation ~ 10 days, 3- to 5-day prodrome of fever, coryza, cough, conjunctivitis, Koplik's spots (white papules on reddened base on the buccal mucosa) then descending confluent erythematous maculopapular rash ~ 14 days after exposure that lasts ~ 7 days, pharyngitis, splenomegaly, diarrhea, vomiting, abdominal pain.

▶ Diagnostic Studies

ELISA that peaks 2 to 6 weeks after rash; two specimens 3 weeks apart simultaneously measured.

▶ Diagnosis

Infectious mononucleosis, rubella, enteroviruses.

▶ Clinical Therapeutics

Acetaminophen, humidified air, increased fluids, consider ribavirin.

▶ Health Maintenance Issues

Complications include pneumonia, laryngitis, bronchiolitis, otitis media, myocarditis, pericarditis, appendicitis, corneal ulcerations, encephalitis, seizures, prevention with vaccination.

G. Mumps

▶ Scientific Concepts

Contagious, transmitted by direct contact/infected droplets.

▶ History & Physical

Parotitis, fever, headache, malaise, anorexia, abdominal pain, orchitis, meningocephalitis.

► **Diagnostic Studies**

Viral cultures from Stensen's duct, urine, or CSF; serologic with paired sera 2 to 4 weeks apart.

► **Diagnosis**

Other viral parotitis, adenitis, Stensen's duct calculus, parotid gland tumors.

► **Clinical Therapeutics**

Supportive, acetaminophen, respiratory isolation if hospitalized, vaccine.

► **Health Maintenance Issues**

Auditory nerve neuritis with deafness, facial nerve neuritis, arthritis, myocarditis; prevention with vaccination.

H. Rotavirus

► **Scientific Concepts**

"Winter gastroenteritis," 6 months to 2 years; nosocomial in pediatric wards, transmitted by contact with infected feces, respiratory, or waterborne (swimming pools).

► **History & Physical**

Fever; URI; vomiting, then profuse watery diarrhea for 3 to 5 days.

► **Diagnostic Studies**

Rotavirus in feces seen with electron microscopy, ELISA, latex agglutination.

► **Health Maintenance Issues**

Hydrate, correct electrolytes; antibiotics/antidiarrheals not indicated; good handwashing techniques to prevent spread.

XIV. ENDOCRINE DISORDERS

A. Juvenile Diabetes Mellitus

► **Scientific Concepts**

Most common type in < 40 year old, ketosis-prone; immunologic damage to beta cells; strongly genetic.

► **History & Physical**

Polyuria, polydypsia, polyphagia, glucosuria on routine urinalysis.

► **Diagnostic Studies**

Fasting glucose > 200 mg/dL or random > 300; glycosylated hemoglobin every 3 months, cholesterol yearly, TSH yearly, 24-hour urine for albumin if patient diabetic > 5 years.

► Clinical Therapeutics

Insulin, dietary, exercise, stress management; frequent glucose monitoring, close clinical follow-up.

► Health Maintenance Issues

Hypoglycemia, ketonuria/ketoacidosis, microvascular, ophthalmology yearly for retinal photographs.

B. Short Stature

► Scientific Concepts

Defined as height that is ≥ 2.5 standard deviations below the mean for age. Nonendocrine etiologies include chronic renal failure, inflammatory bowel disease, liver disease, CHF, asthma, cystic fibrosis, hemoglobinopathies, rickets, radiation treatment, malnutrition, Turner's syndrome, Down syndrome. Endocrine etiology centers around primary or secondary growth hormone deficiency.

► History & Physical

Perinatal events, growth patterns, height, weight, head circumference, height velocity for all. If growth hormone deficiency, then normal size at birth but growth failure after 6 months, excessive adiposity, hypoglycemia in 20%, and normal head circumference.

► Diagnostic Studies

Thyroid function tests, BUN/creatinine, LFTs, calcium, growth hormone levels (random and with clonidine challenge), bone age.

► Clinical Therapeutics

Directed toward the cause of growth failure.

► Health Maintenance Issues

The long-term effects of growth hormone treatment are not yet known.

C. Abnormalities of Puberty

► Scientific Concepts

Pubertal delay defined as lack of increase of testicular size above prepubertal size by age 14 in boys and lack of initiation of breast development by age 13 in girls. Etiologies include trauma, infection, autoimmune, chemotherapy, radiation, hypopituitarism, chronic diseases, Prader–Willi syndrome, Turner's syndrome, Kleinfelter's syndrome. Precocious puberty is defined as the development of secondary sexual characteristics before age of 8 years in girls, or 9 years in boys.

► History & Physical

Pubertal delay: No signs of puberty as listed above.
Precocious puberty: When and rate of change; palpate thyroid; check for abdominal mass; measure size of penis and testes; examine clitoris, labia, and vagina.

► Diagnostic Studies

Pubertal delay: Follicle-stimulating hormone (FSH) and luteinizing hormone (LH) response to gonadotropin-releasing hormone, karyotope.

Precocious puberty: Bone age, FSH, LH, estradiol, gonadotropin-releasing hormone, ultrasound or CT of abdomen to rule out ovarian masses, cranial MRI, dehydroepiandrosterone (DHEA), adrenocorticotropic hormone (ACTH) stimulation test.

► Clinical Therapeutics

Pubertal delay: Replacement of sex steroids.

Precocious puberty: Gonadotropin-releasing hormone analogs, thyroid replacement if indicated.

► Health Maintenance Issues

Long-term studies not available.

XV. POISONINGS

A. Acetaminophen

► Scientific Concepts

Acetaminophen (Tylenol) is a frequently used antipyretic/analgesic metabolized in the liver. Whereas 150 mg/kg is considered a toxic overdose in an adult, the same dose may have little effect on a child under 10 years. Chronic overdose leads to hepatic damage. With acute overdose, there is initially GI disturbances, then an asymptomatic period from 12 to 48 hours followed by signs of liver damage after 48 hours.

► History & Physical

History does not correlate with examination; hepatic failure with encephalopathy, then coma and death. Children unlikely to have toxic levels if there was spontaneous vomiting after ingestion; many remain asymptomatic; diaphoresis 6 to 12 hours after ingestion. Asymptomatic period from 12 to 48 hours, after which the hepatic enzymes rise, and by 48 hours there is evidence of hepatic injury clinically and via lab.

► Diagnostic Studies

Acetaminophen level, liver panel, and glucose.

► Diagnosis

Acute gastroenteritis, encephalopathy, and chemical hepatitis.

► Clinical Therapeutics

Stabilize patient, emesis/lavage; do *not* give ipecac if patient vomited; charcoal; acetylcysteine 20% (Mucomyst) diluted fourfold to a 5% solution in water, cola, or grapefruit juice within the first 8 hours of ingestion if acetaminophen level within toxic range. If levels not available, may start then withdraw treatment. Dose is 140 mg/kg/dose followed by 70 mg/kg/dose × 17 doses orally, or IV 10 mg/kg/dose q4h.

▶ Health Maintenance Issues
All patients requiring Mucomyst should be admitted to the hospital.

B. Anticholinergics

▶ Scientific Concepts
Multiple drugs including antihistamines, atropine, scopolamine, chlorpromazine, prochlorperazine, haloperidol, thiothixene, amitriptyline, imipramine, doxepin, dicyclomine, propantheline bromide, tropicamide, Excedrin PM, Midol, Sominex, Cogentin, and Artane. Varied plants such as jimson weed, nutmeg, potato, and wild sage.

▶ Diagnostic Studies
Tachycardia; hyperpyrexia; hypertension; dry, flushed skin and mucous membranes; dilated pupils; urinary retention; decreased bowel sounds; dysrhythmias; delirium with disorientation; uncontrollable agitation; hallucinations; movement disorders such as myoclonus and choreoathetosis and picking and grasping movements; seizures; coma; respiratory failure and cardiovascular collapse.

▶ Diagnostic Studies
Must notify lab; glucose, ECG, arterial blood gases; flat plate may show nondissolved tablets of phenothiazines.

▶ Clinical Therapeutics
Supportive care: IV dextrose and naloxone at 0.1 mg/kg up to 2 mg IV. Physostigmine for supraventricular dysrhythmias, hallucinations, agitation, and coma. Dose is 0.02 mg/kg/dose up to 0.5 mg/dose IV. Side effects: Seizures, bradycardia, asystole, hypersalivation. Contraindications: asthma, gangrene, GI/GU obstruction. This is *not* a first-resort drug. Phenytoin may be used to treat seizures/dysrhythmias.

▶ Health Maintenance Issues
Hospitalize/monitor.

C. Carbon Monoxide

▶ Scientific Concepts
Odorless/colorless. Seen after fires and with methylene chloride (paint strippers) which is metabolized to carbon monoxide. Binds to hemoglobin 212 times more avidly than oxygen.

► **History & Physical**

Dysrhythmias, myocardial ischemia, pulmonary edema, renal failure, encephalopathy with agitation, seizures, coma, and possible long-term neuropsychiatric changes and memory loss.

► **Diagnostic Studies**

Hemoglobin carbon monoxide levels elevated. Pulse oximetry *not* reliable. Arterial blood gas with measured, not calculated, oxygen saturation. CXR normal in first 24 hours and may show pulmonary edema after 1 to 4 days.

► **Clinical Therapeutics**

Hyperbaric oxygen if possible. Otherwise 100% oxygen. Half-life of hemoglobin carbon monoxide is ~ 4 hours.

► **Health Maintenance Issues**

Admit those with hemoglobin carbon monoxide > 20%, abnormal neurological exams or ECGs, pregnant patients.

D. Cocaine

► **Scientific Concepts**

May be teratogenic.

► **History & Physical**

Dilated pupils, tachycardia, dysphoria, agitation, respiratory stimulation. Complications include dysrhythmias, intestinal ischemia, pneumomediastinum, intraventricular hemorrhage, rhabdomyolysis, seizures, and cardiovascular collapse.

► **Clinical Therapeutics**

Stabilize, treat seizures, treat dysrhythmias with phenytoin, activated charcoal, clean nose with petrolatum-tipped cotton swab.

► **Health Maintenance Issues**

Hospitalize.

E. Iron

► **Scientific Concepts**

Ingestion of > 60 mg/kg is dangerous.

► **History & Physical**

Pattern of progression.

Stage I: Vomiting, hematemesis, diarrhea, hematochezia, and abdominal pain.

Stage II: 2 to 12 hours. Patient improves.

Stage III: 4 to 2 hours. Systemic toxicity with shock, metabolic acidosis, fever, hyperglycemia, bleeding, death.

Stage IV: 48 to 96 hours. Hepatic failure with seizures, coma.

Stage V: 2 to 5 weeks. Pyloric stenosis.

► Diagnostic Studies

Serum iron > 350 µg/dL should worry the practitioner, > 500 is toxic. Diarrhea, vomiting, leukocytosis, hyperglycemia, and positive x-ray suggest level > 300. Obtain CBC, electrolytes, glucose, LFT.

► Diagnosis

Acute gastroenteritis, GI bleed, shock.

► Clinical Therapeutics

Fluid and acid–base corrections. Emesis or lavage. Deferoxamine; 100 mg can chelate 8.5 mg of elemental iron. This drug may cause hypotension, facial flushing, rash, urticaria, tachycardia, shock. Transfusion.

► Health Maintenance Issues
If level > 350, admit.

F. Theophylline

► Scientific Concepts
Becoming less common.

► History & Physical

Irritability, seizures, tachycardia, dysrhythmias, hypertension, nausea, vomiting, diarrhea, abdominal pain. Mean theophylline level of patient with seizures is 45 µg/dL.

► Diagnostic Studies
Blood level.

► Clinical Therapeutics

Emesis or lavage, serial doses of charcoal and/or whole bowel irrigation. Diazepam for seizures.

► Health Maintenance Issues
Admit if level > 30 mg/dL.

G. Aspirin

► Scientific Concepts

In over-the-counter medications such as Alka-Seltzer. Single dose of 250 mg/kg may produce toxicity.

► History & Physical

Tachypnea with deep, labored breathing; hyperthermia; tinnitus; vomiting; lethargy or excitability; seizures; coma; slurred speech; hallucinations; vertigo; pulmonary edema; cardiovascular collapse. Complications include hypoglycemia, metabolic acidosis, respiratory alkalosis, potassium deficit, hyponatremia, pulmonary edema, seizures secondary to lab abnormalities, coma, bleeding secondary to hypothrombinemia and platelet dysfunction, chemical hepatitis, allergic manifestations.

▶ Diagnostic Studies

To 5 mL of urine, add a few drops of 5% ferric chloride—urine will turn purple if salicylates present. Salicylate level, lytes, glucose, arterial blood gas, coagulation studies, ECG.

▶ Diagnosis

Uremia, diabetes mellitus, starvation, meningitis, other ingestants, Reye's syndrome.

▶ Clinical Therapeutics

Stabilize; emesis with ipecac or lavage and charcoal; IVs to correct electrolytes and metabolic abnormalities; cooling blanket for hyperpyrexia, diazepam for seizures, vitamin K for bleeding problems. Patients who need dialysis: renal failure, CNS deterioration, nonfalling salicylate level, unresolving metabolic acidosis, pulmonary edema.

▶ Health Maintenance Issues

Admit.

BIBLIOGRAPHY

Bates B. *A Guide to Physical Examination and History Taking*, 6th ed. Phildelphia: JB Lippincott; 1995.

Berkowitz C. *Pediatrics: A Primary Care Approach*. Philadelphia: WB Saunders; 1996.

Hay W, Groothuis J, Hayward A, Levin M, eds. *Current Pediatric Diagnosis and Treatment*, 13th ed. Stamford, CT: Appleton & Lange; 1997.

Johnson K, Oski F. *Oski's Essential Pediatrics*. Philadelphia: Lippincott-Raven; 1997.

Polin R, Ditmar M. *Pediatric Secrets*, 2nd ed. Philadelphia: Hanley and Belfus; 1997.

Rudolph A, Kamei R. *Rudolph's Fundamentals of Pediatrics*, 2nd ed. Stamford, CT: Appleton & Lange; 1998.

Seidel H, Ball J, Dains J, Benedict G, eds. *Emergency Pediatrics*, 2nd ed. St. Louis: Mosby-Year Book; 1991.

Index